ADVANCED NUTRITION:
Macronutrients

MODERN NUTRITION
Edited by Ira Wolinsky and James F. Hickson, Jr.

Published Titles
Manganese in Health and Disease, Dorothy Klimis-Tavantzis
Nutrition and AIDS: Effects and Treatment, Ronald R. Watson

Forthcoming Titles
Calcium and Phosphorus in Health and Disease, John B. Anderson and
    Sanford Garner
*Nutrition Care for HIV-Positive Persons: A Manual for Individuals and
    Their Caregivers*, Saroj M. Bahl and James F. Hickson, Jr.
Nutrition and Health: An International Perspective, Saroj M. Bahl
Zinc in Health and Disease, Mary E. Mohs

Edited by Ira Wolinsky

Published Titles
Practical Handbook of Nutrition in Clinical Practice, Donald F. Kirby and
    Stanley J. Dudrick
Childhood Nutrition, Fima Lifshitz

Forthcoming Titles
Laboratory Tests for the Assessment of Nutritional Status, 2nd Edition,
    H. E. Sauberlich
Nutrition and Cancer Prevention, Ronald R. Watson and Siraj I. Mufti
Nutrition and Health: Topics and Controversies, Felix Bronner
Nutrition and Hypertension, Michael B. Zemel
Nutrition: Chemistry and Biology, 2nd Edition, Julian E. Spallholz and
    L. Mallory Boylan
Nutritional Concerns of Women, Ira Wolinsky and Dorothy Klimis-Tavantzis

ADVANCED NUTRITION:
Macronutrients

Carolyn D. Berdanier
Professor, Foods and Nutrition
University of Georgia
Athens, Georgia

Illustrations by: Toni Kathryn Adkins

CRC Press
Boca Raton   Ann Arbor   London   Tokyo

Library of Congress Cataloging-in-Publication Data

Berdanier, Carolyn D.
    Advanced nutrition / Carolyn D. Berdanier : Illustrations by Toni
Kathryn Adkins.
        p.   cm. -- (Modern nutrition)
    Includes bibliographical references and index.
    Contents: v. 1. Macronutrients
    ISBN 0-8493-8500-8 (v. 1)
    1. Nutrition. 2. Metabolism. 3. Energy metabolism. I. Title.
II. Series: Modern nutrition (Boca Raton, Fla.)
QP141.B52 1994
612.3′9—dc20
                                        94-11519
                                          CIP

SERIES PREFACE FOR MODERN NUTRITION

The CRC Series in Modern Nutrition is dedicated to providing the widest possible coverage to topics in nutrition. Nutrition is an interdisciplinary, interprofessional field par excellence. It is noted by its broad range and diversity. We trust that the titles and authorship in this series will reflect that range and diversity.

Published for a scholarly audience, the volumes of the CRC Series in Modern Nutrition are designed to explain, review, and explore present knowledge and recent trends, developments, and advances in nutrition. As such, they will also appeal to the educated layman. The format for the series will vary with the needs of the author and the topic, including, but not limited to, edited volumes, monographs, handbooks, and texts.

Contributors from any bona fide area of nutrition, including the controversial, are welcome.

Ira Wolinsky, Ph.D.
Series Editor

PREFACE

At the turn of the century and for a few decades after, nutrition research was conducted by biochemists seeking to unlock the secrets of metabolism. The vitamins were discovered one by one and the mysteries of such endemic diseases as pellagra, beriberi, goiter, and rickets were no more. We learned that ingestion of the "vital amines" could be accomplished by including foods rich in these substances in our diets. The needs for certain of the fatty acids, the amino acids, and many minerals were likewise discovered during this golden age of nutrition.

Now we have another period of great discovery upon us. Today's discoveries are no less exciting for they are showing how the genetics of the consumer affect his/her use of the food that is consumed and, in turn, how the components of the consumed food can affect the expression of the genetic heritage of the consumer. The science of nutrition and its study as an advanced topic has evolved from one in which the student learned the names of the macro- and micronutrients and their chemistry, their requirements, and their deficiency symptoms. Today, the student must have a strong science background with emphasis in biochemistry, genetics, and physiology to be able to integrate this knowledge with an understanding of each of the nutrients and how the body uses them. The student needs to be able to look forward to new discoveries by understanding where our gaps in knowledge exist. The basic sciences have been incorporated into the text and clinical examples have been used to illustrate the importance of particular steps in the metabolic pathways. While the animal of primary interest is the human, this text is useful for the study of other species as well. The basic science of nutrition is all-inclusive and we can learn a lot through interspecies comparisons.

This volume contains text relating only to the needs for and use of the macronutrients. It will serve as the basis for an upcoming volume, which will address the micronutrients. The two volumes can be integrated so that the student will gain a comprehensive view of this composite science called nutrition.

Carolyn D. Berdanier

ACKNOWLEDGMENTS

This book would not have been possible without the encouragement and support of the faculty and graduate students in the University of Georgia Nutrition Science graduate program. Particular appreciation is extended to those who read and criticized the initial draft: Richard Lewis, Anne Dattilo, James Hargrove, Martin Hulsey, Brenda Marques, Martin Kullen, John Parente, Krystyna Kras, Shelly Nickols-Richardson, and the members of my Advanced Nutrition class who provided constructive criticism of the content and who found innumerable errors in punctuation, spelling, grammar, and so forth. The book would not have been possible without the manuscript preparation skills of Lula Fields, Betty Brown, and Kathy Adkins. I am especially grateful for the encouragement and support of my editor, Harvey Kane.

AUTHOR

Carolyn D. Berdanier, Ph.D., is a Professor of Nutrition at The University of Georgia in Athens, Georgia. She received a B.S. degree from The Pennsylvania State University and M.S. and Ph.D. degrees from Rutgers University in Nutrition in 1966. After a post-doctoral fellowship year with Dr. Paul Griminger at Rutgers, she served as a Research Nutritionist with the Human Nutrition Institute which is part of ARS, a unit of the U.S. Department of Agriculture. In 1975 she moved to the University of Nebraska College of Medicine where she continued her research in nutrient gene interactions. In 1977 she moved to the University of Georgia where she served as Head of the Department of Foods and Nutrition. She stepped down from this post ten years later and devoted her full time efforts to research and teaching in her research area. Her research on the diet and genetic components of diabetes and vascular disease has been supported by NIH, USDA, U.S. Department of Commerce, The National Livestock and Meat Board, and the Egg Board. She is a member of the American Institute of Nutrition, the American Society for Clinical Nutrition, The Society for Experimental Biology and Medicine, and several honorary societies in science. She has served on the Editorial Boards of the *FASEB Journal, The Journal of Nutrition,* and *Nutrition Research and Biochemistry Archives.* She is also a Contributing Editor for *Nutrition Reviews* and Editor of the AIN News Notes. Current research interests include studies on aging, the role of diet in damage to mitochondrial DNA, and the role of specific dietary ingredients in the secondary complications of diabetes.

TABLE OF CONTENTS

Unit 1

HUMAN HEALTH, FOOD, AND NUTRITION

TABLE OF CONTENTS

I. OVERVIEW

For centuries people have sought the fountain of youth. The early conquistadors explored the New World hoping to find the secret to long life. What they found were new foods and, probably, new diseases. In the 1500s, the expected life span was half that of today in the advanced nations of the world. Yet, today, there are populations that are no better off with respect to life span than those early explorers. Today, we are still discovering new foods and new diseases. Our discoveries are no less exciting nor less promising than those of yesteryear, but today's discoveries are not merely additive to those already in hand. New knowledge seems to be exponential. Each discovery leads to a multitude of related discoveries and each discovery makes possible the integration of prior knowledge. While new nutrient needs are still being discovered, most of the new knowledge allows the nutrition scientist to better understand why different animals (including humans) need certain nutrients in certain amounts to ensure a healthy, productive life span. To the scientist, it seems obvious that individuals would or could ensure a long life by consuming the appropriate amounts and kinds of foods that contain the needed nutrients, however, this is not so obvious to everyone. There are a number of barriers that interfere with the appropriate exercise of the obvious. Among these are our incomplete knowledge of the need for and tolerance of specific nutrients, the social and economic status of the population, the availability of sanitary facilities and safe water, the availability and acceptance of modern medical care, the education of the consumer with respect to food choices, and the availability of a wide selection of safe food. All of these factors impinge upon the simple premise that a healthy, long life can be achieved simply by consuming the "right" amounts of the "right" foods.

How do we know what the "right" amounts of the "right" foods are? What does health mean? What is long life? These are not simple questions. If they were, we would already know the answers and further study of the relationships of food choice to health and well-being would be unnecessary.

One of the challenges in today's world is understanding how nutrition, or more properly, food, can affect the health and well-being of humans and animals. We must understand how the body works, its anatomy, its physiology and biochemistry, as well as how the individual interacts with members of his/her cultural/social group. Nutritionists are also concerned with the economic and educational status of the consumer because these will affect how much and what kind of foods are purchased, prepared, and consumed. While nutrition researchers specialize in single aspects of these concerns, they are aware of the larger arena in which the community of nutrition scholars perform.

Early in the history of nutrition science, a healthy diet was defined as one which contained a sufficient variety of raw and cooked foods that, all together, provided sufficient nutrients to prevent such diseases as beriberi, pellagra, rickets, xerophthalmia, goiter, and scurvy. The prevention of such deficiency diseases was the key element in nutrient intake recommendations. While this is still true today, we have learned that one's genetic heritage may dictate both the need for and tolerance of the nutrient. We have begun to unravel the mystery of the role of inheritance in dictating nutrient need. In the future, nutrient intake recommendations based on genotype will be made so as to potentiate the expression of traits for health while suppressing traits for disease.

Throughout this text, genetic errors in macronutrient metabolism will be described. Where possible, nutrient-gene interactions will also be indicated. Before the use of the macronutrients can be addressed, the reader should be aware of those aspects of the study of nutrition that justify the detailed examination of the biochemistry and physiology of these nutrients at the organismic and cellular levels.

II. POPULATION STUDIES

Epidemiology is the study of disease incidence and distribution or prevalence in a defined population. The population may be defined by gender and/or age and/or geography and/or sociocultural status and/or economic status and/or other descriptors. Such population studies have been responsible in large part for the discovery and description of nutrition-related diseases. Among the first of these were reports of scurvy in British sailors on long voyages and the reports of beriberi in Japanese sailors also on long sea duty. Both reports provided data on the incidence, severity, and mortality of these seafaring men and both noted the fact that their diets consisted of a limited variety of foods. Only those foods that could be stored for long periods of time were found on these ships — hardtack (a sort of very stale, often maggot infested, bread) and a meat preserved in brine were the staples of the British sailors' diet. In the Japanese navy, rice replaced the hardtack, and this rice was frequently polished and milled white rice. The officers supplemented these items with fresh fruit, meat, and vegetables when these items were available and the officers had the money to buy them. The officers were thus less likely to develop deficiency diseases.

The physician-scientists who studied these sailors noted the difference in disease patterns between the officers and seamen, and likewise noted the difference in diet. Although at that time no one knew that vitamins existed or were essential nutrients, there was a recognition of a possible relationship between disease and food intake. This tradition continues today as we seek to understand the diet and disease connection. Population studies may be very detailed, with specific assessments of the foods consumed together with clinical and biochemical assessments of health status, or they may be very general. The design of the study and its methodology is dictated by the question the scientists wish to answer. If the question relates to the incidence and severity of heart disease in 40-year-old white professional males in Chicago, the methods used will be very different from a study designed to answer questions about rickets in preschool children in rural Mississippi or about the growth of children in the state of Hawaii. In each instance, the investigators have designated a specific population and a specific health concern. In each instance, the information about food intake can be either very specific or very general. The amount of detailed information collected depends on many factors. These include the population size, the amount of money available for the study, and the detail needed to answer the question asked. Population studies can be labor intensive if they involve the study of representative groups within the population. However, there are ways to study disease patterns and food intake using large computer-based data sets. There are several sources for these data.

III. MORTALITY STATISTICS

Until there was a universal recognition of the causes of infectious diseases and the development of appropriate therapeutic and preventative strategies for these diseases, they were the leading causes of death. Death from cholera, bubonic plague, typhoid disease, smallpox, whooping cough, pneumonia, appendicitis, childbirth, typhus, and scarlet fever were common prior to improved sanitation, clean water, the development of antibiotics and immunization programs, and the development of aseptic techniques and anesthesia that made simple surgeries possible and effective. Infectious disease is still a leading cause of death in third-world nations where education and economics combine to effectively limit the adoption of health care practices that educated citizens of more wealthy nations take for granted. Shown in Figure 1 is a comparison of the leading causes of death in India and the U.S. Other country comparisons might show slightly different causes of death, depending on the nations in question. For example, a nation enduring a devastating food production failure might have death due to starvation in the list of ten top causes. A nation at war or a nation at the epicenter of a communicable disease such as AIDS likewise might have a different list from that given for the U.S. The reader should be aware of these country differences and recognize that mortality statistics can be misleading if one selects only one or two diseases and tries to relate the incidence of these diseases to the food choices of the populations in these different nations. One must always remember that the causes of death must be taken all together — the percentages of the different causes of death must add up to 100%. If one nation or population has 35% of its population dying from heart disease and another nation has only 5% dying from this cause, one cannot ignore the reasons for death of the other 65 or 95% of the respective populations. Perhaps the latter population has a greater problem with infectious disease or a greater infant mortality. Perhaps this population has an average life span of only 35 years. In other words, in the final analysis, all the deaths have a cause and all causes add up to 100%. Whether these causes are nutrition related cannot be assumed merely by examining these death statistics. Chronic diseases now rank high in the ten leading causes of death in the U.S. These are shown in Table 1.

Years of potential life lost (YPLL) is a public health term that reflects the impact of deaths occurring in years preceding a conventional cut-off of age, usually 65 years. This number, YPLL, is calculated using final mortality data from the U.S. Department of Public Health Center for Disease Control. The CDC, as it is commonly called, tracks the incidence and prevalence of all diseases and keeps records of causes of death. The CDC also conducts a health and nutrition survey and monitors the public health not only in the U.S. but throughout the world. The National Health and Nutrition Survey is discussed in Section V of this unit.

The YPLL is based on the population estimate provided by the U.S. Census Bureau. While the YPLL is updated yearly based on the reports of deaths made to the CDC, the census of the U.S. population is taken only every ten years. Thus, the YPLL is only an estimate which becomes less reliable as the years from the last census increase. Nonetheless, YPLL is very useful in providing estimates of the social and economic impact of death from leading causes.

During 1990, YPLL from all causes totaled 12,237,379 for the U.S. (Table 2). Accidents or unintentional injuries leading to death accounted for 17.5% of this total. This was followed by deaths from cancer (15.1%), homicide and suicide (12.2%), cardiovascular disease (11.2%), and congenital diseases (birth defects) (5.4%). Although AIDS does not claim as many lives

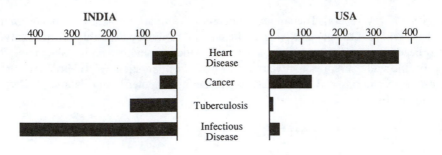

FIGURE 1.   Comparison of death rates per 100,000 population from selected causes in India and the United States.

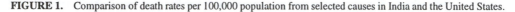

TABLE 1
Leading Causes of Death in the U.S.
in 1990

Rank	Cause of death	% of Total
1	Heart diseases	33.5
2	Cancers	23.4
3	Strokes	6.7
4	Accidents	4.3
5	Lung diseases	4.1
6	Pneumonia and flu	3.6
7	Diabetes mellitus	2.3
8	Suicide	1.4
9	Homicide	1.2
10	Liver diseases	1.2
11	AIDS	1.1
12	All other causes	<u>17.2</u>
		100.0

Taken from: Vol. 39, Month Vital Statistics Report of
the National Center for Health Statistics, 1991.

as any of the above, because its victims are often young adults, its associated YPLL is a significant percentage of the total, 5.4%. Cardiovascular disease, while accounting for more than half of all deaths, strikes much older persons so the years of potential life lost is a much smaller number than one would expect. In addition, therapies have been developed that attenuate the progress of cardiovascular disease such that the affected individual has his/her life span extended frequently beyond the cut-off age of 65 used for the calculation of YPLL. Table 2, published by the CDC in April of 1993 in its weekly report (Volume 42, *MMWR*), also indicates that some gains have been made to forestall death. Note in Column 4 the figures on percentage change from 1989 to 1990. Accident prevention programs, more effective treatments for heart disease, improved prenatal and postnatal care, plus better treatments for alcoholism and lung diseases are indicated by the negative figures in this column. The number of years lost has decreased from the previous year and hopefully this means that the public health efforts are worthwhile.

As noted, the calculation of YPLL is based on age 65. This age is used because it has been considered to be the age at which retirement from full-time employment is considered. Years lost from this age are considered to have a more significant social and economic impact on the population than years lost from the total expected life span. In the U.S. at this age, retirement income from Social Security can be received without penalty. Retirement benefits from Social Security are reduced if one retires prior to age 65. The Social Security Act of 1935 was designed to ensure income for retirees. Its cost was based on the actuarial tables in use

TABLE 2
Years of Potential Life Lost Before Age 65[a] (YPLL-65), by Cause of Death—United States, 1989 and 1990 (Final), and 1991 (Provisional)

Causes of death	YPLL-65 for persons dying in 1989	YPLL-65 for persons dying in 1990	% Change from 1989 to 1990	VPLL-65 for persons dying in 1991[c]
All causes (total)	12,339,045	12,237,379	−0.8	12,276,349
Unintentional injuries	2,235,335	2,143,002	−4.1	2,102,923
Malignant neoplasms	1,832,039	1,846,719	0.8	1,867,263
Suicide/homicide	1,402,524	1,493,672	6.5	1,563,507
Diseases of the heart	1,411,399	1,375,923	−2.5	1,382,789
Congenital anomalies	660,346	666,684	1.0	607,980
Human immunodeficiency virus (HIV) infection	585,992	660,261	12.7	776,240
Prematurity	487,749	442,664	−9.2	438,600
Sudden infant death syndrome	363,393	349,397	−3.9	333,465
Cerebrovascular disease	237,898	240,942	1.3	225,374
Chronic liver disease and cirrhosis	233,472	224,355	−3.9	206,127
Pneumonia/Influenza	184,382	176,618	−4.2	168,148
Diabetes mellitus	145,501	145,895	0.3	149,322
Chronic obstructive pulmonary disease	135,507	132,743	-2.0	129,655

[a]   YPLL-65 is calculated as 65 minus the middle age for each age group, times the number of deaths from a specific cause within that age group, added for all age groups to 65.
[b]   International Classification of Diseases, Ninth Revision.
[c]   Death rates are from a 10% sample of all deaths and are adjusted for reporting lags. HIV infection including acquired immunodeficiency syndrome. These codes are from addenda to the ICD-9 (3).
[d]   Category derived from disorders relating to short gestation, unspecified low birthweight, and respiratory distress syndrome.
Taken from: *Morbidity Mortality Weekly Report (MMWR)*, 42: 251–53, 1993.

at that time, but since then both life span (the total years of life) and life expectancy (the years of life one can expect to live) have changed significantly. This has had a dramatic effect on the cost of this program. Since 1900, life expectancy at birth has increased 66% for males and 71% for females. In some countries, life expectancy for males has doubled. Shown in Figure 2 are some of the changes in life expectancy observed in a few selected countries. The U.S. Census Bureau maintains an international data base that tracks the births and deaths in a number of countries in the world. As can be seen in Figure 2, the largest gain in life expectancy occurred between 1900 and 1950. Recall that it was during this period that antibiotics were discovered and many public health measures were put in place. The importance of many of the micronutrients in the diet was likewise uncovered. All together, these discoveries and practices resulted in an improvement in the general health of the population and, as a consequence, the life span increased. Today, as health-related research continues, health and expected life span can be expected to steadily increase, but not at the same dramatic rate as occurred between 1900 and 1950. Nonetheless, a child born today in the U.S. can expect to live 72.1 years if he is a male and 79 years if she is female. In some parts of the country, even longer life expectancies have been observed.

During this century, gender differences in life expectancy have developed and broadened. Prior to this century, many females died in childbirth. If they survived the child-bearing years, they lived as long or longer than their male counterparts. After the implementation of more sanitary procedures for childbirth, the development of medical practices which could success-fully manage and care for pregnant women, and the development of safe and effective birth control measures, female mortality associated with childbirth decreased. Thus, early in the 20th century as more females survived childbirth, a gender gap in life expectancy began to

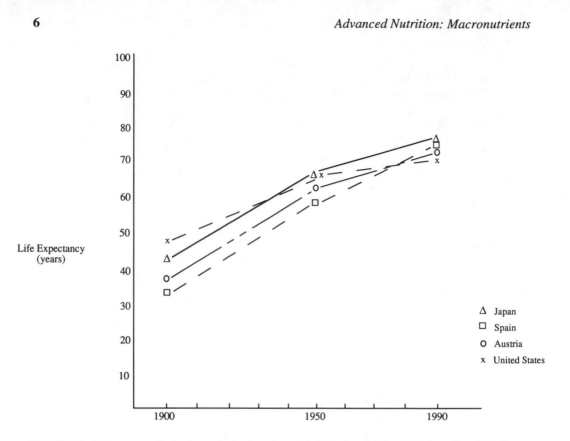

FIGURE 2.   Life expectancies in Japan, Spain, Austria, and the U.S. from 1900 to 1990. Data from U.S. Census Bureau.

develop. In 1900 the gender gap was 2.8 years; in 1990 it was 6.9 years. This gender gap may not continue to exist if females, in turn, adopt the same behaviors as males that affect their health. The rise in smoking by females is one such change that impacts health. In the last 25 years, more females adopted the smoking practice than in the prior 25 years. Over the last 25 years, premature death (death prior to age 65) from lung cancer has tripled for females. If the percentage of the female population that smokes increases further, one might anticipate a reduction in the gender gap in mortality and life expectancy. Other health behaviors likewise influence health and mortality. Among these are exercise, diet choice, willingness to accept medical advice and prophylactic measures, and willingness to change or adapt one's behavior in the face of need.

The strength of each of the many factors that influence human health and longevity is difficult to assess given the long life of the human and the complexity of that life. While population surveys and health and mortality statistics can *suggest* a relationship between one or more of these factors and the incidence of one or more diseases, *causality* cannot be shown. Causality means that if the human elects to smoke, for example, *that human will* die from lung cancer. Another example: if the human consumes a fat-rich/cholesterol-rich diet, *that human will* die from cardiovascular disease. These two statements are not necessarily true. There are very few absolutes when it comes to assessing the strength of a given behavioral attribute and disease development. Scientists are more certain about causal factors in infectious disease than in the chronic diseases which comprise the majority of reasons for death. This is because the chronic diseases may take many years to develop and the initial symptoms may be quite elusive. Furthermore, scientists cannot conduct cause and effect studies on humans. It would be unethical to cause a mortal disease. In addition, the time frame of degenerative diseases such as heart disease in humans is so long that the researcher may not live long enough to see the results of his or her work.

Nonetheless, population studies are valuable because they can suggest correlations between external variables such as diet choice and internal responses such as a disease process. These correlations are then converted into risk factors. Risk factors, therefore, are a public health expression of the correlation between a given characteristic and the presence of a given disease or death from a given disease. Risk factors are numerical expressions of chance. They give the individual an indication of whether a certain characteristic has a strong chance of eliciting an undesirable or desirable health outcome. Risk factors are not synonymous with causal factors. For example, consuming food heavily infested with active salmonella will result in symptoms of food poisoning. Diarrhea, vomiting, and enteric distress will result. In this example, the disease is food poisoning and the cause is the food burden of salmonella. In contrast, consider the risk factor of obesity. As men increase in body fatness, their risk of having a major coronary event increases twofold. This does not mean that excess body fat *causes* coronary disease, but rather that the two problems are related. The cause may not be known. Furthermore, it is also possible that an overly fat man may die of some other disease. Obesity, no doubt, is mathematically related to mortality. There is indeed a positive mathematical expression for this relationship, but a mathematical expression is just that. It is not synonymous with cause.

Shown in Table 3 are some of the risk factors that have been identified for heart disease, cancer, and stroke. No doubt other factors have been or will be identified. More risk factors have been identified for diseases of the heart than for cancer and stroke. Actually, stroke and the heart diseases are related disorders. As such, they share many of the same risk factors. Note that all three of the leading causes of death have smoking and family history as risk factors. One's family history may determine, to a large extent, the diseases to which a person is most susceptible. A family history of heart disease or cancer is strongly suggestive of a need to adopt behaviors that will forestall a repeat of this family history. While science has not developed sufficiently to provide tests that will definitively identify people whose genetics place them at risk, physicians are quite aware of the importance of the family's medical history.

In Table 3, the three leading causes of death in the U.S. are given. Diseases of the heart include congenital structural defects, damage to the heart secondary to infections, and degenerative changes in both the heart muscle and its vascular system. All forms of cancer are lumped together and stroke due to vascular aneurysm (rupture of blood vessel followed by hemorrhage) and ischemia (decreased blood supply due to atherosclerotic change in the brain's vascular system) are combined. The mortality statistics are not definitive because in many cases they are taken from the death certificate, rather than from an autopsy which gives a more definitive cause of death.

Note in this table that age is a risk factor for all of the diseases. This relates, in part, to the earlier discussion on mortality in different countries of the world. Obviously, if one escapes death from infectious disease, malnutrition, and childbirth, one lives long enough to die from heart disease, stroke, or cancer. The older the individual, the greater the risk of developing one of these diseases or developing one or more other diseases (diabetes or hypertension or renal disease) which, in turn, increases the risk for death due to heart disease and stroke. Some investigators have used factor analysis to age-adjust these risk factors. In other words, they acknowledge the fact that as one survives the more devastating infectious diseases and other life-threatening conditions, one is more likely to die of heart disease or cancer or stroke. Over the last decade, the age-adjusted mortality from heart disease has decreased in the developed nations of the world. While nutritionists would like to take credit for the decrease in mortality due to their efforts to educate the public about the value of low-fat diets, weight reduction, and exercise, in reality the decrease is probably due to a number of medical and nonmedical interventions. Such interventions include nutrition advice about food choices, advice and guidance on physical activity, medical management of elevated blood lipid levels, early diagnosis followed by appropriate medical management of hypertension, early diagnosis and

TABLE 3
Risk Factors for Heart Disease, Cancer, and Stroke

Heart disease	Cancer	Stroke
Excess body weight as fat	Excess body weight	Excess body weight
Hypertension	Family history	Hypertension
Hyperglycemia	Abdominal obesity	Diabetes mellitus
Diabetes mellitus	Smoking	Family history
Family history	High unsaturated fat intake	Age
Physical inactivity		Elevated blood cholesterol
Smoking		High saturated fat intake
Elevated blood cholesterol		Racial background
Elevated blood triglycerides		Smoking
Gender		
Age		
Abdominal obesity		
Repeated weight loss-regain		
High saturated fat intake		

treatment of vascular problems, and early diagnosis and management of diabetes. All together, these proactive practices retard disease development and lengthen life. This in turn, means that mortality from diseases of the heart occur at a later age. The same can also be said for cancer and stroke. Proactive diagnosis, treatment, and management extends the life span and delays death. Thus, age is indeed a risk factor in these diseases.

Human studies, using small groups of subjects with or without a definitive disease diagnosis, have provided support for the risk factors given for each of the groups of diseases listed in Table 3. However, as indicated earlier in this text, cause and effect human studies cannot be conducted. Nonetheless, scientists conducting diet studies, exercise studies, or family history studies have shown relationships between their treatments and changes in the relative risks for these diseases. For example, human subjects have been provided low-fat diets for periods of up to a year or in some instances longer. The investigators have been able to show that, as a result of these diets, serum lipids decreased. Similarly, other investigators have reduced the total energy value of the diet and have reported a decrease in body fat and serum lipids. These results do not mean that heart disease, if it existed in these subjects, has been "cured" or reversed or that the obesity has been corrected. What was shown was that certain features of the human which appear to be *associated* with heart disease can be attenuated through the use of special diets.

IV.   DIET AND DISEASE RELATIONSHIPS

Table 1 does not include the many health problems that have a diet component. It gives only the causes of death, not disability. Among the health disorders are the nutrient deficiency disorders, excess nutrient intake disorders, and a variety of degenerative and incapacitating disorders. Listed in Table 4 are diseases that fit into these categories.

Most of these disorders have a genetic component as well. The individual's genetic background dictates how much of each vitamin, mineral, or macronutrient is needed for optimal health. There can be considerable variation in these needs as will be discussed later. Nutrient deficiencies and toxemias will not be described in this volume as they pertain to the micronutrients. The details of some of the macronutrient influences on the degenerative disorders can be found in the units on energy, protein, carbohydrate, and lipid in this volume. These details would not have been sought and elucidated had not the epidemiologist suggested that such relationships existed, i.e., the risk factors described in the preceding section.

TABLE 4
Nutrition-Related Disorders

Deficiency disorders	Excess intake disorders	Degenerative disorders
Scurvy	Obesity	Cancer
Rickets	Alcoholism	Coronary vessel disease
Anemia	Mineral toxicities	Diabetes mellitus
Pellagra	Hypervitaminoses	Cirrhosis
Beriberi		Hypertension
		Renal disease

Diabetes is one such degenerative disease that has a profound influence on heart disease, renal disease, and neurological disease. Persons with diabetes have five times the risk of having a major coronary event as do persons without diabetes. More than 25% of all persons undergoing dialysis for renal disease are diabetics. The incidence of diabetes has increased dramatically with the discovery of insulin as the replacement hormone and with the development of effective management of the disorder. Early diagnosis of the non-insulin-dependent form of the disease is paramount to its management. Estimates of the number of people with diabetes vary from 1 in 14 to 1 in 20 in the general population. Certain populations have even larger numbers of affected individuals.

Despite the problems associated with studying humans, considerable progress has been made in understanding human disease processes. This progress has been possible because investigators have found similar problems in small laboratory animals. Especially valuable are small rodents that have short reproductive cycles and, compared to humans, a short life span. This is especially important to the study of genetic diseases in which the expression of the disease does not occur until midlife or late adulthood. Diseases that are degenerative in nature or that take several decades to become clinically observable are extremely difficult to understand. Needed are observations of subcell and cellular changes that precede tissue and organ changes that in turn develop into a clinical condition of note. With diseases such as cardiovascular disease, diabetes mellitus, or renal disease, diagnosis is possible only after clinical symptoms appear. Scientists seeking to understand how the disease developed and the sequence of biological changes that lead to the clinical state must study animals whose disease time frame is considerably shorter than that of the human. Some of these animal models are listed in the appendix. Fortunately, over the last century, considerable effort has been expended by animal breeders to provide scientists with a uniform animal for laboratory use. In an effort to provide this uniform animal, breeders have developed strains of rats, mice, chickens, rabbits, guinea pigs, and so forth that meet a well-defined standard of identity. Growth rate, hair color, health status, and nutrient needs are fairly similar within a given breeding group within a given strain and species. This is particularly true for mice and rats. For many breeders, the genetic history of every animal produced can be traced back many generations to a particular set of breeding animals.

In order to produce homogeneity within a breeding group, breeders select the traits they wish to preserve (and those they wish to delete) and plan their breedings accordingly, using brother-sister matings or backcrosses to strengthen the desired trait. If full sib matings of mice, for example, are used for 21 sequential generations, the colony of animals is considered inbred and should be homozygous at every gene locus. Producing an inbred animal is not without risk, however, since an unknown trait might appear that is lethal. If enough animals possess this trait, the colony dies. Hence, many breeders do not strive for full homozygosity at every locus. Instead, they are satisfied with homozygosity at only one, two, or three loci. The use of inbreeding to attain a specific trait(s) without full homozygosity has made possible the detection of several mutations that result in animals that spontaneously develop diabetes mellitus as well as some of its secondary complications. Not all of these mutations develop the same form of the disease. In this respect, these animals represent the variety of the disease seen in humans.

With respect to diseases of nutritional importance to humans, almost every micro- and macronutrient need has been established by using small animals. Almost every nutrient-related degenerative disease that afflicts humans likewise can be found in one or another form in one or more small animals. The choice of animals to be used for research depends wholly on the objective of the research. It would be folly to study heart disease development, for example, in a strain of rat that is not genetically susceptible to this problem or that is too young to develop it. The researcher must carefully define the problem before selecting the most appropriate animal model.

V.   FOOD INTAKE STUDIES IN HUMANS

As part of an epidemiological survey, the epidemiologist may ask about the food consumed by the population being studied. These data can be acquired in several ways. *Food disappearance* data are frequently used to assess the use of food by very large population groups. In the U.S., the Department of Agriculture (USDA) has since 1909 monitored the disappearance of foods from the marketplace. Knowing the population number (data from the Census Bureau), agricultural production, the processed food production by the food industry, the amount of food exported, and food not intended for human use directly, i.e., animal feed and the year-end inventory of food stocks, USDA experts can estimate the disappearance of food from the marketplace on a per capita basis. Specific nutrients and their availability or disappearance are calculated using the nutrient composition of food (*Handbook 8*, USDA). As can be seen, these are not direct measurements of individual food consumption. Instead, they are estimates of the food that is available and which disappears from the marketplace. As such they reveal overall trends in consumption while making no corrections for food loss in preparation, food not consumed, or for uses of food for non-food purposes. Shown in Figure 3 are moving averages for total energy fat, protein, and carbohydrate disappearance since 1909. These data are useful adjuncts to discrete studies of small population groups where detailed diet analysis or traditional food consumption patterns are studied.

The USDA, in addition to computing food disappearance based on the large data sets as described above, also collects data on the food consumed by households. This survey has also been conducted on a regular basis since the early 1900s. Representative householders participate in the survey by completing a questionnaire about the amounts of foods purchased and their cost. The early surveys used a food inventory method which requested that the person responsible for food preparation inventory their food supply over a set period of time. Corrections for initial and final food stocks were made. This method of assessing food consumption proved cumbersome. The participants in the survey lost interest and some provided records that were incomplete or not useful for other reasons. Realizing these problems, the food inventory sheets were replaced by a check list of foods used. This system is still in use today. It is frequently used by investigators interested in health problems as related to food consumption and often is used in conjunction with an interview of the respondent. The interview provides an opportunity for more in-depth questioning about the frequency of use of food items of interest. When coupled with a health status assessment and/or a nutritional status assessment, this food recall approach is very useful as it pertains to household food use. It does not include food consumed outside the home nor does it provide information about individual food consumption. For this kind of information, individuals must be questioned about their personal food choices and intake patterns.

Several techniques are available for obtaining individual food consumption data. The dietary recall method asks the participant to recall the amounts of all the food she/he consumed over the last 24 hours or the last 3 days. Sometimes a participant is very good at recalling the food consumed and sometimes not very good at all. Recall data are not very reliable when

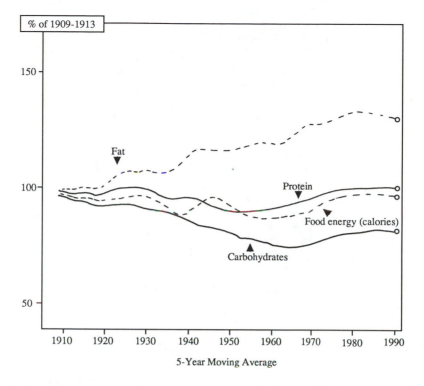

FIGURE 3. Food disappearance as indicators of food energy, protein, fat, and carbohydrate in the U.S. food supply. Data are shown as averages from 1909 to 1990. (USDA, Food Disappearance Studies).

obtained from children or the aged. Unreliability is also a problem if the participant believes that the choice of food will be criticized or if there is something to be gained or lost through truthful (or untruthful) answers. Some people honestly cannot remember what they ate or how much.

Another approach to this recall method is to ask the participant to indicate how often (daily, weekly, yearly) food items in a list are consumed. The frequency of consumption, together with simple measures of height and weight and questions about age and perhaps health status and medication use, can provide useful information about the amount of food consumed. When coupled with a physical examination and perhaps selected biochemical and physiological measurements, the nutritional status of the individual can be assessed. This kind of assessment is far more time consuming and more expensive than the simple recall method, but it has the advantage of providing a more reliable assessment of food intake and nutritional status.

Reliability can be further increased (with a consequence of further time and dollar expense) if the participant can be convinced to keep a food diary. In the diary, every morsel of every food consumed is described and quantified. The record is then used to compute the intake of nutrients from a table of food composition which gives the amounts of the major nutrients in most all foods. These tables are available in computer format such that the foods can be entered by code and the operator can quickly assess the daily nutrient intakes of the participant.

Results of the 1987 to 1988 survey are shown in Table 5. Which method a researcher or a government agency uses to obtain food intake data depends on the particular use for those data and the particular goals of the study. If all that is desired is an assessment of the food supply, individual consumption patterns are not needed. However, if one wishes to assess the health of a discrete population group in relation to the foods consumed, then obviously a different technique will be needed.

TABLE 5
Results of the 1987-1988 National Food Consumption Survey Conducted by the USDA-Human Nutrition Information Service

Nutrient	Males	Females
Energy (kcal)	2154	1497
Protein (g)	87.8	61.9
Fat (g)	90.7	61.1
Carbohydrates (g)	239.4	175.2
Vitamin A (IU)	6639	5690
Vitamin C (mg)	99	84
Thiamin (mg)	1.59	1.14
Riboflavin (mg)	1.98	1.46
Niacin (mg)	23.4	16.6
Vitamin B_6 (mg)	1.82	1.31
Vitamin B_{12} (μg)	5.95	5.02
Calcium (mg)	821	602
Magnesium (mg)	281	209
Iron (mg)	14.9	10.9

Source: HNIS, USDA, Hyattsville, MD.

Perhaps the most comprehensive survey of nutrient intakes and health status is the National Health and Nutrition Examination Survey (NHANES). The first survey (NHANES I) was conducted in the early 1970s (1971 to 1975) by the National Center for Health Statistics, a branch of the CDC of the U.S. Department of Health and Human Services. NHANES I consisted of a dietary intake (24-hour recall method and food frequency table), anthropometric measurements, clinical assessment for signs of nutrient deficiency(s), and a biochemical assessment of key blood and urine nutrients and metabolites. This was a cross-sectional survey which examined representative age and racial groups of both males and females. Approximately 29,000 (age 1 to 74 years) noninstitutionalized individuals from all parts of the country were examined. NHANES II followed NHANES I and examined a similar number of people. The lowest age group was 6 months. Ninety one percent were interviewed as in NHANES I, and 73% were clinically evaluated via a variety of biochemical tests, a glucose tolerance test, blood pressure measurement, electrocardiography, and radiography of the chest and spine. A survey with particular attention to Hispanics was conducted using these same methods during 1982 to 1984. This was called the HHANES. A third NHANES (NHANES III) is currently in progress. It should provide several important estimates of the nation's health as it relates to nutritional status. Estimates of compromised nutritional status, trends of nutrition-related diseases, prevalence of obesity, and data on growth and development of children are among the anticipated outcomes of these extensive and detailed surveys.

Shown in Table 6 are the various measurements made. The results of these surveys are available as computerized data sets and parts of these sets have been published in scientific journals. Note in Table 6 the blood measurements of vitamins and minerals. These blood values give only the amounts of these nutrients in transit, not the amount in storage. Tissue samples, such as a liver biopsy or a bone biopsy, would be required for the true assessment of stores, and hence, status. Biopsies are quite risky as well as being time and resource consuming. Unless there is a specific reason for harvesting such tissue samples, this is not done. In particular, tissue sampling was not done in any of the NHANES studies. The anthropometric measurements included weight, sitting, standing, and recumbent height, skinfold thickness at preselected sites, grip strength, bioelectrical impedance (an indirect measure of

TABLE 6
Measurements Made by NHANES

Hematology:	Sedimentation rate
	Differential white cell count
	Hemoglobin, carboxyhemoglobin, glycosylated hemoglobin
	Red cell number and distribution width
	Neutrophil hypersegmentation
	Mean cell volume
	Fibrinogen
Nutrition Profile:	Serum folacin, vitamins C, D, A, B_{12}, selenium, cholesterol, lipoprotein profile, calcium, zinc, copper, iron binding capacity, ferritin, chloride, phosphorus, sodium, potassium, lead
Biochemistry Profile:	Total carbon dioxide, blood urea nitrogen, total bilirubin, alkaline phosphatase, transaminase activities, lactate, dehydrogenase activity, total protein, albumin, creatinine, glucose
Disease Exposure Profile:	Carotenes, nicotine, bile salts, pesticides, syphilis serology, hepatitis A and B serology, tetanus, diphtheria, rubella, polio serology, herpes simples I and II, IgE, HIV, c-reactive protein, rheumatoid factor
Hormone Profile:	Follicle stimulating hormone, luteinizing hormone, thyroxine (T4), thyroid stimulating hormone, insulin, C-peptide, antithyroglobulin antibodies, antimicrosomal antibodies
Urinalysis:	Pesticides, vitamin metabolites, creatinine, albumin

body fat mass), head, chest, waist, hip, and thigh circumference, thickness at wrist and elbow, shoulder breadth, and breadth of hips. While participants of all ages were evaluated, not all measurements were made on all the subjects. Adults were more rigorously examined than infants and children. While the results of NHANES III are still being analyzed, HHANES and NHANES I and II data sets are available on computer discs. The laboratory methods have been carefully described in the NHANES manuals and, as well, can be found in the book by Lee and Nieman, *Nutritional Assessment.*

While federal agencies such as USDA and the U.S. Public Health Service are concerned with the nutritional status of the general population, there are numerous smaller scale studies either already published or in progress. These studies may involve only a few subjects by comparison to NHANES, and they may be very highly focused to answer one or two discrete questions. Many of these have been used as a basis for dietary recommendations for specific target groups. The book, *Diet and Health,* published by the National Academy of Sciences, is a compilation and summation of these studies.

VI. RECOMMENDED DAILY ALLOWANCES

Soon after it became apparent that certain components in the diet were necessary to prevent or cure endemic diseases such as scurvy, goiter, blindness, pellagra, and so forth, nutrition scientists set about determining how much of each of these nutrients was required to prevent the deficient state. Feeding studies using human subjects were conducted. These feeding studies were very time consuming, very expensive, and labor intensive. The preliminary work that established sensitive criteria for detecting the earliest possible indication of deficiency was conducted using small laboratory animals. Rats, mice, guinea pigs, chickens, and rabbits were frequently used. The species selected was critical since animals do differ in their nutrient needs. Most species synthesize ascorbic acid. The human and the guinea pig do not. Therefore, the study of scurvy, if not in humans, had to be conducted with the guinea pig, not the rat or mouse or rabbit. Choosing an appropriate animal with nutrient needs analogous to that of the human requires some knowledge about the species differences as well as the acknowledgment that human metabolism cannot always be duplicated in a single laboratory species.

Once sensitive criteria were developed, the feeding studies were conducted one by one by various investigators in the U.S. and elsewhere. They published the results of their work in the scientific literature. These results were then used as the basis for the recommended daily allowances (RDAs) for each nutrient. When the RDA table was first assembled in 1940, the data base was very small. In some instances, the members of the Food and Nutrition Board of the National Academy of Sciences (the group charged with setting the RDAs) had few or no data to use for specific age groups. The adolescent and preadolescent groups were least studied, yet the Board was charged with making recommendations for all age groups from infants to adults.

Because the Board recognized the fact that considerable variation in need can exist among individuals of the same age and gender, a safety factor was incorporated into the recommendations. The Board took the highest reported value for each nutrient need and doubled it for safety. Thus, if the highest reported need for riboflavin was 0.6 mg, the Board doubled it and recommended an intake of 1.2 mg. As the data base expanded through additional reports in the literature, the Board adjusted its recommendations. Hence, the RDA for protein has declined from 100 g per day for the adult man to 70 g and then to 55 g. The recommended intake for vitamin C likewise has been adjusted downward from 75 mg to 60 mg per day. Shown in Table 7 are the current RDAs published in 1990.

The RDAs should not be confused with the requirements for nutrients. They were devised as a means for planning adequate nutrition for the civilian population in the U.S. Recall that in 1941 the nation was involved in World War II and food rationing was being implemented. The nation's food planners had to have a guide in hand so that rationing could be implemented on as scientific a base as was possible given the level of knowledge at that time. Although the RDAs were developed in 1941, they were not officially published and publicly available until 1943. Every five years the data base is reviewed and, if needed, the RDAs are revised. The latest edition includes recommendations for 19 different nutrients, whereas the first edition included only 10. Table 7 is an abbreviated version of the 1989 revision. The sections on energy and protein may be found in Units 3 and 4.

Other countries also have developed similar tables. The recommendations are not always the same. The reasons for this may be various. The country's nutrition experts may use different criteria for adequacy of intake. The choice of criteria can range from absence of physical signs of deficiency to blood and tissue saturation of the nutrient in question. There may be political and economic pressures on the review panel that influence the choice of adequacy criteria. They may decide to set the value at a level sure to meet the needs of 75% of the people rather than the 96% called for in the U.S. This 96% figure reflects the concept of a Gaussian distribution (the typical bell-shaped curve of the statistician). The mean value of all the published data on the requirements for a particular nutrient plus 2 standard deviations is used to set the RDA for that nutrient. The mean plus 2 deviations is thus 95 to 96% of the total population. Of course, the more data one has to use to calculate the mean and its deviation, the better the estimate of real need and the closer one can predict an intake figure that will meet that need. Intercountry variation also could be due to interpopulation differences. Suffice it to say that no one country is "wrong" or "right" in their nutrient intake recommendations, simply that these guides are just that, guides. About 40 different nations in the world now have RDAs for their people.

Estimates of nutrient intakes for items not on the RDA table have also been made. This group of nutrients falls into the category of items for which there are insufficient data to use for making a recommended daily allowance but for which there are sufficient data to estimate a range of intake. Some of the micronutrients such as copper, manganese, fluorine, chromium, and molybdenum fall into this category. The Food and Nutrition Board gives a figure that is an estimate of an amount of that nutrient generally considered safe and adequate. For those nutrients, such as some of the minerals, this definition is especially important because intake

TABLE 7
Recommended Daily Allowances for Nutrients Needed by Humans of Different Ages

Category	Age	Weight lbs	Height inches	Protein g	Fat soluble vitamins A µgRE[a]	D µg	E mgαTE[b]	K µg	Water soluble vitamins C mg	Thiamin mg	Riboflavin mg	Niacin NE[c]	B6 mg	Folacin mg	B12 µg	Calcium mg	Phosphorus mg	Magnesium mg	Iron mg	Zinc mg	Iodine mg	Selenium µg
Infants	0-6 mo	13	24	13	375	7.5	3	5	30	0.3	0.4	5	0.3	25	0.3	400	300	40	6	5	40	10
	7-12 mo	20	28	14	375	10	4	10	35	0.4	0.5	6	0.6	35	0.5	600	500	60	10	5	50	15
Children	1-3 yr	29	35	16	400	10	6	15	40	0.7	0.8	9	1.0	50	0.7	800	800	80	10	10	70	20
	4-6	44	44	24	500	10	7	20	45	0.9	1.0	12	1.1	75	1.0	800	800	120	10	10	90	20
	7-10	62	52	28	700	10	7	30	45	1.0	1.2	13	1.4	100	1.4	800	800	170	10	10	120	30
Males	11-14	99	62	45	1000	10	10	45	50	1.3	1.5	17	1.7	150	2.0	1200	1200	270	12	15	150	40
	15-18	145	69	59	1000	10	10	65	60	1.5	1.8	20	2.0	200	2.0	1200	1200	400	12	15	150	50
	19-24	160	70	58	1000	10	10	70	60	1.5	1.7	19	2.0	200	2.0	1200	1200	350	10	15	150	70
	25-50	174	70	63	1000	5	10	80	60	1.5	1.7	19	2.0	200	2.0	800	800	350	10	15	150	70
	51 +	170	68	63	1000	5	10	80	60	1.2	1.4	15	2.0	200	2.0	800	800	350	10	15	150	70
Females	11-14	101	62	46	800	10	8	45	50	1.1	1.3	15	1.4	150	2.0	1200	1200	280	15	12	150	45
	15-18	120	64	44	800	10	8	55	60	1.1	1.3	15	1.5	180	2.0	1200	1200	300	15	12	150	50
	19-24	128	65	46	800	10	8	60	60	1.1	1.3	15	1.6	180	2.0	1200	1200	280	15	12	150	55
	25-50	138	64	50	800	5	8	65	60	1.1	1.3	15	1.6	180	2.0	800	800	280	15	12	150	55
	51 +	143	63	50	800	5	8	65	60	1.0	1.2	13	1.6	180	2.0	800	800	280	10	12	150	55
Pregnancy				60	800	10	10	65	70	1.5	1.6	17	2.2	400	2.2	1200	1200	320	30	15	175	65
Lactation	0-6 mo			65	1300	10	12	65	95	1.6	1.8	20	2.1	280	2.6	1200	1200	355	15	19	200	75
	7-12 mo			62	1200	10	11	65	90	1.6	1.7	20	2.1	260	2.6	1200	1200	340	15	16	200	75

[a] RE = retinol equivalent; 1 µg retinol = 6 µg β carotene.
[b] αTE = 1 mg dα tocopherol.
[c] NE = niacin equivalents; 1 mg niacin = 60 mg tryptophane.

Data from Food and Nutrition Board, National Academy of Sciences - National Research Council, 1989.

in excess of this recommendation could be toxic. The range of safety with some of the minerals is relatively small. A two- to threefold increase in intake could elicit a toxic response.

The RDAs are not requirements, yet there is the tendency to view them as such when populations are studied with respect to nutrition and health. Individuals differ so much that identifying persons at risk for nutrient deficiency using the RDA as the standard of comparison is invalid. Rather, one must use clinically established biochemical/physiological criteria of adequacy before such risk can be established. The usual food intake pattern can be assessed using the composition of the food data base, but whether that food sufficiently nourishes the *individual* can only be determined from a detailed assessment of that individual. Furthermore, although one can now easily evaluate the nutrient intake of a person's usual food consumption, the investigator should realize that (1) people typically underestimate the quantities of food consumed, and (2) the handbooks of food composition may not be completely accurate. Just as individuals differ in their needs for and use of the foods they consume because of their genetic make-up, so too do foods differ in the nutrients they contain. While the differences may not be large, they nonetheless exist.

Efforts to circumvent the concept that the RDA is synonymous with the requirement has led to the development of additional terms. The Food and Drug Agency (FDA) developed the term *minimum daily requirement* (MDA), a misnomer that implied knowledge about an individual's absolute need for a given nutrient. The MDA later was called the USRDA (Table 8). This term was developed for use in regulating the labeling of the nutrient content of food. It was based on the RDA. Note the differences between Tables 7 and 8. The FDA has included those nutrients for which an RDA has not been set. The rationale for FDA to do this is to protect the consumer from overdosing on potentially toxic nutrients. The other main difference between the tables is the compression of the categories of consumers. The FDA recognized infants, children, adults, and pregnant or lactating women, whereas the Food and Nutrition Board subdivided these categories into age groups.

In 1992 the FDA established further labeling regulations for processed foods. It established reference values that were based not only on RDA, but also on the Surgeon General's Report on Nutrition and Health and on the recommendations for diet and health made by the Food and Nutrition Board of the National Research Council. Two terms were devised: the Reference Daily Intake (RDI) and the Daily Reference Values (DRV). These values are to be used as the basis for nutrition foundation labels and are used for regulatory purposes. A typical food label format is one which gives information about the nutrients which most concern the consumer. This information is presented as a percentage of the total recommended intake. On the label the consumer might see that the product contained 10% of the recommended daily intake of energy if the consumer needed to consume 2000 kcal/day. Again, just as the RDA does not provide individual values, the DRV and the RDI do not either. The FDA attempted to provide the consumer with a way of comparing products. The consumer could read the label and learn that product A provided 10% of the daily allowance for protein while product B provided 15%. The consumer can then make a judgment about the relative nutritional value vis à vis protein of the two products.

Devices to help the consumer understand how to select foods that provide the appropriate amounts of the different nutrients likewise have been based on the RDA. The USDA Nutrition Information Service has put forth the Food Pyramid. The American Dietetics Association has developed a food exchange system which has many applications in planning meals for both normal persons and persons needing to control their intakes of a certain nutrient, such as sodium, protein, fat, or total energy. All of these devices are consumer oriented and are directed toward educating consumers about food choices that will assist them in maintaining good health.

Students of nutrition science should be aware of the need to conduct research that can ultimately be applied to humans. While the majority of the research is conducted in lower

TABLE 8
U.S. Recommended Daily Allowances (USRDAs)

	Infant	Children 4 and under	Adults	Pregnant/lactating women
Vitamin A, IU	1500	2500	5000	8000
Vitamin D, IU	400	400	400	400
Vitamin E, IU	5	10	30	30
Ascorbic acid, mg	35	40	60	60
Folacin, mg	0.1	0.2	0.4	0.8
Thiamin, mg	0.5	0.7	1.5	1.7
Riboflavin, mg	0.6	0.8	1.7	2.0
Niacin, mg	8	9	20	20
Pyridoxine, mg	0.4	0.7	2	2.5
Vitamin B_{12}, µg	2	3	6	8
Biotin, mg	0.05	0.15	0.30	0.30
Pantothenic acid, mg	3	5	10	10
Calcium, g	0.6	0.8	1	1
Phosphorous, g	0.6	0.8	1	1
Iodine, µg	45	70	150	150
Iron, mg	15	10	18	18
Magnesium, mg	70	200	400	450
Copper, mg	0.6	1	2	2
Zinc, mg	5	8	15	15

species (and usually in rodents), the justification for doing so must, in the final analysis, provide an increased understanding of how nutrients are used and why the diet must provide them.

SUPPLEMENTAL READINGS

ARTICLES
Kinsella, K. G. (1992) Changes in life expectancy, *Am. J. Clin. Nutr.,* 55:1196S–1202S.
Kirkwood, T. B. L. (1992) Comparative life spans of species: Why do species have the life spans they do?, *Am. J. Clin. Nutr.,* 55:1191S–1195S.

BOOKS
Berg, F. M. (1993) *Health Risks of Obesity,* Healthy Living Institute, 402 South 14th Street, Hettinger, ND, 58639.
Anon. (1989) Diet and Health. Implications for Reducing Chronic Disease Risk, National Research Council-National Academy of Sciences, Washington, D.C.
Lee, R. D. and Nieman, D. C. (1993) *Nutritional Assessment,* W.C.B. Brown and Benchmark Press, Madison, WI, 407 pages.
Anon. (1990) U.S. Recommended Daily Allowances, *Federal Register,* July 19, 1990, 55:29477.

Unit 2

WATER

TABLE OF CONTENTS

I. INTRODUCTION

Of the macronutrients mammals need, water is by far the most important. Deprived of water, humans can live only three to four days. However, survival is much longer than this if deprived only of food. If deprived of food and water, the sensation of hunger abates after a short time whereas the sensation of thirst tenaciously persists.

Water as a nutrient is essential because of its unique function as a solvent and as an important component of the temperature regulation system. Water is present throughout the body, yet is in constant flux between the various body compartments and between the internal and external environment. Water flux is so closely controlled that the total water content in the fat-free body remains constant in normal adults. In this unit, water as an essential nutrient will be discussed.

II.   CHEMICAL AND PHYSICAL PROPERTIES OF WATER

The functions of water in the body relate directly to its unique chemical and physical properties. When compared to other common solvents such as ethanol, ether, acetone, methanol, or toluene, water has a higher freezing point, a higher boiling point, a higher specific heat of vaporization, a higher heat of fusion, and considerable surface tension. These unique properties are related to the great internal cohesion of the water molecules, which is due to the presence of relatively strong intermolecular forces. These forces are the result of an unequal sharing of electrons by the oxygen and hydrogen ions which comprise the water molecule. Oxygen has a stronger affinity for electrons than does hydrogen (oxygen is more electronnegative) and thus, hydrogen tends to develop a partial positive charge while oxygen develops a partial negative charge. Just as oppositely charged magnets strongly attract each other, so too do the hydrogen and oxygen atoms in different water molecules attract each other, creating strong intermolecular forces. This electrostatic attraction keeps the oxygen and hydrogen from separate molecules in close proximity and is called the hydrogen bond.

The electrons are arranged around the oxygen atom in a nearly tetrahedral array. As a result, each water molecule is able to bond to four neighboring water molecules (see Figure 1). Through this kind of an interaction among many water molecules a lattice is formed. Hydrogen bonding exists in ice, liquid water, and water vapor. As the phase changes from solid to liquid to vapor, the average number of water molecules which associate decrease and the distance through which a hydrogen bond can be formed increases. This means a decrease in the intermolecular forces of attraction as heat is applied and, thus, the water changes its physical state. Water is a solid at temperatures below 0°C and vaporizes at temperatures above 100°C. Water must be heated to 600°C to completely dissipate the intermolecular forces described above. While the intermolecular forces are great, the hydrogen bonds themselves are not very stable. They form and reform with great ease and speed. The half life of the hydrogen bond in water is about 10^{-10} to 10^{-11} seconds. For this reason, water can be viewed as both fluid and rigid. The lattice-like structure of water, because it is constantly changing, has been aptly described as a flickering cluster.

As a result of its dipolar nature, water dissolves or disperses many substances. It will form ionic solutions with salts such as sodium chloride, and it will form solutions with such polar compounds as ketones, sugars, and alcohols. It can dissolve these latter compounds because it will form hydrogen bonds with the polar groups of these substances. It will not form true solutions with large molecules such as proteins; instead, small particles of these proteins (1 to 100 nm) form colloidal solutions. Finally, as discussed in the unit on lipids, water is involved in the formation of emulsions. Emulsions are suspensions of particles in water with diameters in the range of 1 to 100 μm. Homogenized milk is an example of an emulsion of fat globules, protein particles and other solutes in an aqueous medium. It is not a true solution.

III.   FUNCTIONS OF WATER

Water serves many functions in the body. It participates in the heat economy of the animal due to its low thermal conductivity and its high specific heat. Metabolic reactions in the cell produce heat. This heat can be absorbed by the water in the cell with no appreciable rise in temperature. The heat can then be transferred to the body surface and, through the vaporization process, the body is cooled. Because of its high heat of vaporization (586 cal/g water evaporated at 0°C), evaporative water losses can account for 25% of the total heat emission of the adult under nonstress conditions. This principle has been used to calculate the basal heat loss of animals (see Unit 3). Under the stress of an environment incapable of receiving heat by radiation, convection, or conduction, the total heat produced by the adult human may dissipate entirely as the latent heat from the vaporization of water. This is especially true if

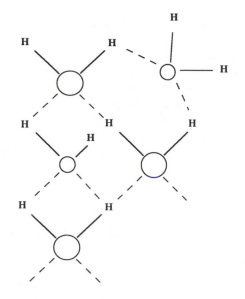

FIGURE 1. Schematic representation of water, showing transient hydrogen bonding.

profuse sweating occurs and the relative humidity of the environment is low. Thus, the properties of water, high specific heat and high heat of vaporization, help maintain a relatively constant body temperature even though the environmental temperature may vary over a wide range. If the body temperature was not to remain at or near 37°C (98.6°F), such processes as enzymatic reactions would be seriously impaired.

Because of its dipolar nature, water is an excellent solvent. Both true and colloidal solutions are formed in the body, thus making possible the transport of large and small molecules throughout. Truly, it is said that in the body water is the "medium of exchange." Water is an essential constituent of all tissues. Many (but not all) enzymes are soluble in or suspended in water, and most enzymes function best in an aqueous medium.

The high dielectric constant of water promotes the ionization of solutes, particularly the inorganic salts, thus facilitating their function as co-factors in a variety of metabolic processes. In metabolism, water participates in a number of reactions. It enters into compounds undergoing hydrolysis (addition of water) and is removed when other compounds are made. An example of the latter is the removal of one molecule of water when a peptide bond is formed during protein synthesis or when two monosaccharides are joined to form a disaccharide. Water also participates in the regulation of the acid/base balance.

Another important function of water is that of a lubricant. Water in conjunction with a variety of proteins lubricates the joints and protects, through its lubricating action, a variety of important organs such as the heart, the intestines, the eyes, and the lungs. Water is the major component of the pericardial sac, the peritoneum, the conjunctive tissue, and the pleural sacs. The secretions of the salivary glands, the respiratory tract, and the gastrointestinal tract are primarily water, and amongst the functions of these secretions is that of lubrication.

IV.   BODY WATER

Water is ubiquitous and abundant in all living things. A living cell is approximately 80% water. Frequently, the amount of water in the body is given in terms of the lean body mass. Lean body mass refers to the weight of the body less its fat content. It includes the muscle, bone, internal organs, and essential structural lipids. Fat free body mass, on the other hand, is not equivalent to lean body mass; it refers to the weight of the body less its fat content, including structural lipids. Because of the differences in the definition of lipid, i.e., the inclusion of structural lipids, the percentage of the total body weight that is lean body mass is slightly higher than that for fat-free body mass.

While body protein and body mineral content are fairly constant as a percent of the body weight, body lipid and body water fluctuate in an inverse relationship to each other; that is, as the percent body lipid increases, the percent body water decreases and vice versa. However, if one were to exclude the lipid content and refer only to the lean body weight, then the percent water remains relatively constant. For the normal adult, approximately two thirds of the lean body weight is water. As a constituent of the body, it is the most abundant. The constancy of the body protein, minerals, and water in the lean body mass allows investigators to express values which relate to these components on a lean body weight basis. For example, the protein intake required for maintenance can be expressed as grams protein required per gram lean body weight under the assumption that the maintenance of the fat depots is a function of the energy intake and requires little or no protein. Expressing protein intake requirements in this fashion allows one to compare the protein nutritive need of animals of different body sizes or weights.

A. WATER COMPARTMENTS

Total body water (TBW) is distributed into two main compartments or spaces, the intracellular space and the extracellular space. The water contained in the intracellular space, the intracellular water (ICW), is that portion of the TBW that is contained within the cells. In normal healthy adults, 55% of the TBW is found in the cells. Females tend to have equal quantities of water within and around the cells, whereas trained young male athletes, who have a relatively large skeletal muscle mass, have a higher percentage of the TBW in the intracellular compartment.

Extracellular water (ECW) is distributed into several subcompartments (plasma, interstitial and lymph fluids, fluids of connective tissue, cartilage and bone, and transcellular fluids) which are not clearly defined. About 45% of the TBW is found in the extracellular compartments.

Plasma is the fluid within the heart and blood vessels. The interstitial and lymph fluids are an approximation of the fluid surrounding the cells. There is an active exchange of fluids between the cells and the fluid surrounding them and between this fluid and the plasma. Dense connective tissue, cartilage and bone, and the transcellular fluids, however, do not participate to any great extent in this exchange. The transcellular water includes such fluids as the spinal fluid, the ocular fluids, the synovial fluid that lubricates joints, the fluids in the mucous secretions of the linings of the gastrointestinal tract, the respiratory tract, and the genitourinary tract, and the fluids found in the pancreas, liver and biliary tree, thyroid and skin.

Accurate determination of ECW is difficult. Ideally, it requires a substance that does not penetrate into the cell, that is nontoxic in the required dose, that does not participate appreciably in metabolic reactions, and is distributed rapidly and evenly in all of the extracellular fluid. A tracer substance such as this has not been found. Certain saccharides, mannitol and inulin, give a reasonably accurate measure of the interstitial and lymph fluid. Plasma volume may be measured by injection of Evans blue dye into the bloodstream. Estimates of the volume of the remaining components of the extracellular fluid can be obtained from direct chemical analysis of representative samples of the individual tissues. The transcellular water volume is usually not determined experimentally. It is assumed to be the difference between the total body water and the measurable extracellular and intracellular water.

B. COMPOSITION OF EXTRACELLULAR AND INTRACELLULAR FLUIDS

An important difference exists between the chemical composition of the fluids within the cells and those of the extracellular compartment. Intracellular fluid contains primarily potassium cations with phosphate, protein, and bicarbonate anions. Extracellular fluid is primarily a solution of sodium chloride. The composition of plasma is more precisely known than is that of interstitial or intracellular water. Figure 2 illustrates the approximate composition of the plasma and the intracellular fluid.

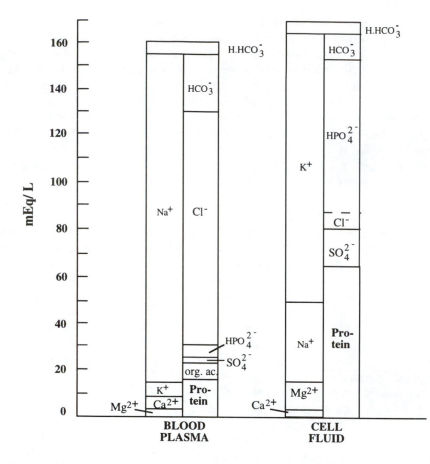

FIGURE 2. Comparison of composition of plasma and intracellular fluid. (From *Biological Handbooks, Blood and Other Fluids,* FASEB, Bethesda, MD, 1961. With permission.)

Water exchanges rapidly between the plasma, lymph, and interstitial fluids and between the interstitial and intracellular fluids. For instance, the water found in the capillaries will exchange with that found in the interstitial space several times a second. The direction and rate of exchange are regulated by diffusion, osmotic pressure, and hydrostatic pressure.

Diffusion is the result of random motion of the molecules. Because of this motion, water molecules pass from one fluid compartment to another. Osmosis is the passage of a solvent across a semipermeable membrane from an area of high concentration to an area of low concentration. By this process, the concentrations of the solutes on each side of the semipermeable membrane approach equal values. The osmotic pressure is that pressure which must be applied to prevent the flow of solvent. Only those particles which do not pass through the semipermeable membrane contribute to osmotic pressure. The osmotic pressure does not depend upon the nature of the solvent particles; it depends, instead, on their number. A solution of NaCl, which completely dissociates to sodium ions and chloride ions, will have twice the osmotic pressure of an equimolar solution of glucose which does not dissociate.

A specialized form of osmotic pressure is oncotic pressure or colloid osmotic pressure. The dissolved proteins of the plasma do not pass through the capillary membrane, the point at which most of the exchange between plasma and the interstitial space occurs; hence, a concentration gradient and its associated osmotic pressure exist at this membrane. The term colloid is applied to this type of osmotic pressure because the solute is a large protein molecule and is held in the solution (plasma) as a colloid.

Hydrostatic pressure is that pressure which is caused by the weight of a column of water. In a large chamber of water, the pressure on the surface of the water is equal to atmospheric pressure. For each 13.6 mm below the surface of the water, there is a corresponding increase of 1 mm mercury. Hydrostatic pressure also occurs in the vascular system of the human being; the pressure of the fluids in the arteries descending to the feet is greater than that in the neck. Hydrostatic pressure will push fluid out of the capillaries into the interstitial space and hence into the intercellular fluids. The various pressures—osmotic, hydrostatic, and that exerted by the pumping action of the heart—serve to regulate the volume of the water in each of the water compartments. Should any of these regulatory mechanisms become compromised, then water will not move as easily between the compartments and will accumulate. When water accumulates, the clinical condition known as edema develops.

C. CELL STRUCTURE AND FUNCTION

The typical cell (Figure 3) consists of a nucleus, mitochondria, lysosomes, endoplasmic reticulum, Golgi apparatus, and microsomes surrounded by the cell sap or cytosol. Membranes surround each of these organelles as well as the cell itself. Each segment or organelle has a particular function and is characterized by specific reactions and metabolic pathways. These are listed in Table 1. Although all nucleated cells possess the genes coded for all metabolic processes, some genes are not transcribed nor translated. If translated, some gene products are not very active. Thus, not all cells have the same processes with the same degree of activity. Cellular differentiation has taken place such that muscle cells differ from fat cells, which differ from brain cells, and so forth. In each cell type there are processes and metabolic pathways that may be unique to that cell type. An example is the great lipid storage capacity of the adipocyte, a feature not found in a bone cell or a brain cell or a muscle cell. Similarly, the capacity to form and retain a mineral appetite (an amalgam of different minerals) is characteristic of a bone cell, and the synthesis of contractile proteins by muscle cells are also examples of cell uniqueness. Cells differ in their choice of metabolic fuel. Hepatic and muscle cells make, store, and use significant amounts of glycogen. Adipocytes and hepatocytes make, store, and sometimes use triacylglycerols. All of these special features have an impact on the composition of specific organs and tissues in the body that collectively comprise and contribute to body composition.

Analysis of the composition of specific organs and tissues does not necessarily reflect the whole-body composition. One must consider the function of each organ and tissue in the context of the whole-body. Similarly, determination of the activity of a single process in a single cell type or organ may not necessarily predict the activity (and cumulative result) of that process in the whole-body. However, some processes are unique to certain tissues so some exceptions to the above rules are possible. For example, one can measure glycogenesis in samples of liver and muscle and be fairly confident that these measures will represent whole-body glycogen synthesis.

With respect to cell function and its contribution to the body's metabolic processes, mention should be made of the differing rates of cell renewal. Cells differ in their life span depending on their location and function. Skin cells (epithelial cells) are short lived compared to brain cells. The turnover time for an epithelial cell in humans is of the order of 7 days. Brain cells cannot be regenerated, and renewal of neural tissue is fragmented; that is, there is turnover of individual cellular components such as the lipid component but the cell, once formed, is not replaced as an entity as are the epithelial cells. Shown in Table 2 are some estimates of the life span of several sources of epithelial cells in humans and in the rat. While the average life span of the human is on the order of 70 years, that of the rat is between 2 and 3 years. Despite this species difference in whole-body life span, the life span of epithelial cells is surprisingly similar.

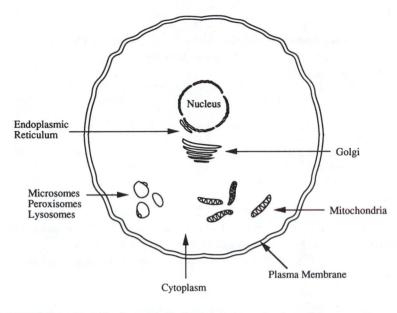

FIGURE 3. Typical eukaryotic cell showing representative intracellular structures.

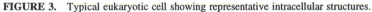

TABLE 1
Functions of the Organelles/Cell Fractions that Comprise the Typical Eukaryotic Cell

Organelle/cell fraction	Role in cell	Processes found
Plasma membrane	Cell boundary holds receptors for a variety of hormones	Processes, exports and imports substrates, ions, etc., binds hormones to their respective receptors
Cytosol	Medium for a variety of enzymes, substrates, products, ions	Glycolysis, glycogenesis, glycogenolysis, lipogenesis, pentose shunt, urea synthesis (part) protein synthesis (part)
Nucleus	Contains DNA, RNA	Protein synthesis starts here with DNA transcription
Endoplasmic reticulum	Ca^{++} stored here for use in signal transduction	Has role in many synthetic processes
Golgi apparatus	Sequesters and releases proteins	Export mechanism for release of macromolecules
Mitochondria	Powerhouse of cell	Krebs cycle, respiratory chain, ATP synthesis, fatty acid oxidation, first step of urea synthesis
Ribosomes	Site for completion of protein synthesis	Protein synthesis
Lysosomes	Intracellular digestion	Protein and macromolecule degradation
Peroxisomes	Suppression of oxygen free radicals	Antioxidant enzymes
Microsomes	Drug detoxification	Detoxification

V. BODY COMPOSITION

Of the four major body constituents, fat, protein, water, and ash (minerals), water is by far the most abundant. Normal bodies usually consist of 16 to 20% protein, 3 to 5% ash (mineral matter), 10 to 12% fat, and 60 to 70% water. Age, diet, genetic background, physical activity, hormonal status, and gender can affect not only the proximate composition of the whole body, that is, the magnitude of each of these components, but also their distribution.

Regardless of the methods used to estimate lean body mass, total body water, and percent body lipid, it is generally agreed that the composition of the human body, as well as the bodies of other species, can vary. Age, sex, degree of physical activity, and diet have all been shown

TABLE 2
Life Span of Epithelial Cells From Different Organs
in Humans and Rat

Cell type	Human (days)	Rat
Cells lining the gastrointestinal tract	2 to 8	1.4 to 1.6
Cells lining the cervix	5.7	5.5
Skin cells	13 to 100	19.1
Corneal epithelial cells	7	6.9

to affect body composition. For example, a 175-g fetus contains 154 g of water (88%), a 3.5-kg baby contains 2.4 kg water (69%), and a 70-kg man contains 42 kg water (60%). As the human progresses from conception to birth to maturity, the percent water decreases and, as mentioned previously, the percent fat increases. Actively growing tissue has a high water content and very little fat.

Differences in water content on the basis of sex have also been observed in adults. Females tend to have less water and more fat than do males. These differences can be attributed in part to the effects of the female sex hormones on fat synthesis and deposition and, in part, due to the tendency of young adult males to engage in more strenuous physical activities which increase their muscle mass and hence their body water content.

Diets, particularly energy rich diets which increase fat deposition, affect body composition. For example, Brozek and Keys found that in overfed men who gained weight, 14% of the weight gain was due to an increase in extracellular fluid, 24% was an increase in cellular components, and 62% was an increase in fat. When humans are fed energy poor diets, changes in body composition can also be observed. One such subject was followed for 60 days and, as might be anticipated, showed a loss in body weight, body fat, and body water. The pattern of loss is shown in Figure 4. Weight loss and regain (weight cycling) alter body composition, particularly the distribution of the body fat. There is a tendency to accumulate subcutaneous fat at the expense of visceral fat by obese people who lose weight and then regain it, yet their total body fat following regain is not different from that prior to weight loss.

While each cell type has a unique composition and organization, all together, they comprise the whole-body. Frequently, nutritionists wish to know whether dietary and nondietary factors affect body composition. Researchers might want to know, for example, whether changes in dietary protein can affect the protein content of the whole body, or whether a certain exercise routine affects the body fat content, or how age affects bone mineral content. In small animals, body composition can be determined directly. The fat content is the difference in body weight before and after extraction with a fat solvent. Typically a 2:1 mixture of chloroform:methanol is used.

$$\% \text{ fat} = \frac{\text{body weight} - \text{extracted body weight}}{\text{body weight}}$$

Similarly, % body water can be determined as the difference in body weight before and after drying.

$$\% \text{ body water} = \frac{\text{body weight} - \text{dried body weight}}{\text{body weight}}$$

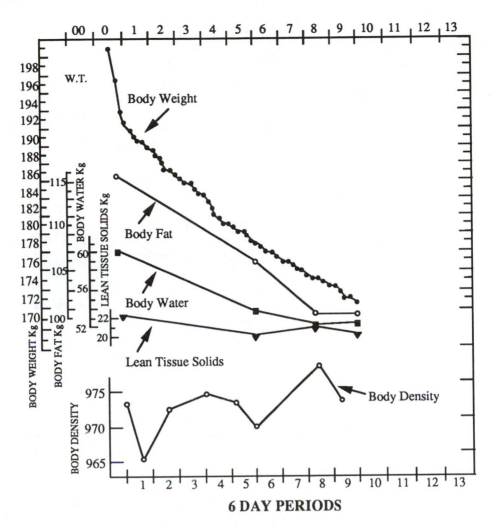

FIGURE 4. Changes in body weight, total body water and body density, and calculated fat and lean tissue solids in a subject consuming 800 calories/day. (From Berlin et al., *Metabolism,* 11:302, 1963. With permission.)

The percent of the body that is mineral (ash) is determined as the difference in body weight before and after all the organic matter is oxidized using a muffle furnace. This furnace can achieve heat up to 3000° and will oxidize everything except the mineral matter.

$$\% \text{ body ash} = \frac{\text{body weight after complete oxidation}}{\text{body weight}}$$

Lastly, the protein content of the body is determined by measuring the nitrogen content and multiplying by 6.25 to convert to protein and then calculating % as above:

$$\% \text{ body protein} = \frac{\text{nitrogen content} \times 6.25}{\text{body weight}}$$

Needless to say, one does not measure body composition directly using the *whole* body, but rather uses a sample taken from a homogenate of the whole body. That way one can determine all components (water, ash, fat, protein) in the same body using a small sample size.

It is not always practical, however, to determine the body composition in this fashion. The animal under study may be too large for convenient handling, or one may wish to make sequential measurements in the same body, i.e., to study changes in body composition in response to dietary or nondietary (e.g., exercise) treatments, or one may wish to work with humans. In the latter instance, direct measurements would be out of the question.

A limited amount of data are available (Table 3) on the body composition of the adult human as determined through direct measurements; however, most of the data in the literature on humans are based on indirect or derived values for each of the major body components. Sequential estimates of body fat or bone density or body water or protein content are possible using sophisticated instrumentation together with established methods for estimating the magnitude of the fat store and the lean body mass.

The data in this table were collected in the early 1950s from persons who had donated their bodies for scientific research. The cause of death and age varied widely. Four of the ten patients had died from heart disease and two were accident victims. The other patients died from a variety of degenerative diseases. The values were obtained from many very small samples of tissues taken as representative of each tissue type.

Lean body mass (LBM) can be calculated if one assumes that the fat-free body has a constant water content (72%) and that the neutral fat is stored dry. Thus, the formula

$$\text{LBM (kg)} = \frac{\text{total body water (kg)}}{0.72}$$

can be used. The figure 72% is an average figure derived from careful direct measurements of the water content of lean tissue. It may not be applicable to all situations. To confirm the usefulness of the 0.72 figure, one must obtain a biopsy of the lean tissue and determine its water content. This may not be practical, so one generally assumes that 0.72 can be used. One must also determine the total body water (TBW) and the body fat. Total body water can be measured by infusing heavy water (deuterium), allowing this to equilibrate within the body, and then withdrawing a sample of blood. This method is called the Water Dilution Method. Knowing the level of deuterated water, the volume that was infused, and the concentration in the blood sample withdrawn, one can calculate the volume of dilution of the infused labeled water. This will provide a value for the TBW.

The calculation of TBW is as follows:

$$\frac{C_1}{C_2} = \frac{V_2}{V_1}$$

where V_2 is the volume in which the solute is distributed or the TBW. Dividing TBW by 0.72 (as per the above equation) gives an estimate of the LBM. LBM is also equal to the total body mass minus its fat content.

Lean body mass can also be predicted from skeletal measurements and from bone weight. Sophisticated techniques using ultrasound, neutron activation analysis, infrared interactance, dual energy X-ray absorptiometry, computer assisted tomography, magnetic resonance imaging, or bioelectrical impedance are available, and as the instrumentation improves, these methods may become practical in the clinical setting. Presently, considerable efforts are being expended to validate these methods because they are noninvasive and allow for the sequential determination of changes in one or more of the major body components as a result of dietary change, activity change, age, or a change in endocrine status. In addition, these noninvasive methods could be useful in assessing population groups vis à vis fat mass or bone density, or adipose tissue distribution. For example, Sohlström et al. used magnetic resonance. They compared these estimates to those obtained from underwater weighing and from body water

TABLE 3
Proximate Composition of
Adult Humans

% Water	50 to 70
% Fat	4 to 27
% Protein	14 to 23
% Ash	4.9 to 6

dilution studies. The three methods gave similar results with magnetic resonance imaging (MRI) and body water dilution providing $1.4 \pm 2.9\%$ less and $4.7 \pm 4.0\%$ more, respectively, than underwater weighing for total body fat. However, because MRI can provide information about where this fat is found, this method is superior to the other methods. In MRI, images are created by a combination of electromagnetic radiation and a magnetic field. Individual body segments such as shoulders, chest, hips, thighs, etc., can be examined as discrete entities. Thus, the amount and distribution of fat can be detailed.

Dual energy X-ray absorptiometry (DEXA) is another of the newer methods being developed. It has been used to estimate bone density and soft tissue composition. The advantage of this method is that it eliminates the need to use the assumption that the body exists as a two-pool system. The one pool is the fat and the other is the fat-free mass (or lean body mass). Bone density as a fraction of the fat-free mass can be distinguished and quantitated using DEXA. The result is that bone mass and density can be quantitated as can the fat mass, and the remaining tissue is more legitimately the lean body mass. One can then distinguish and quantitate the muscle mass using its creatine content.

If one assumes that the major component of the lean is the muscle, one could determine the muscle mass using the dilution of radioactive creatine or creatine labelled with a heavy nonradioactive isotope. This has been used successfully in rats and may be applicable to humans because creatine is almost exclusively located in the muscle. Labelled creatine must be infused and, after a set interval, a muscle biopsy obtained. The total muscle mass can be calculated using the $C_1/C_2 = V_2/V_1$ equation as follows:

$$\frac{\text{Total } ^{14}\text{C creatine infused}}{\left[^{14}\text{C creatine} \right] \text{in sample}} = \frac{\text{Muscle sample size}}{\text{Total muscle mass}}$$

On the assumption that lean body mass has a constant potassium content and that neutral fat does not bind the electrolyte, lean body mass can be estimated by measuring the body content of the heavy potassium isotope K^{40} or by measuring the dilution of K^{42} (the radioactive isotope) in the body cells. The former requires a whole-body scintillation counter whereas the latter can be determined in a small tissue (muscle biopsy) sample. The formula for calculating lean body mass is as follows:

$$\text{LBM} = \frac{\text{Total K content}}{\text{Concentration of K/kg tissue}}$$

Either of these methods may underestimate the lean body mass because of the lack of corrections for the small amounts of potassium in the extracellular fluids.

Lean body mass and percent fat can be estimated using measures of body density or specific gravity of the individual. The fat-free body will have a specific gravity of 1.1000. This will decrease as the body increases its fat content since fat has a lower (~0.92) specific gravity than the fat-free body mass. Thus, the fatter the subject, the lower the specific gravity or density. The body density can be determined in the adult using Archimede's principle. The subject is weighed in air and again when immersed in water. The difference in the two body weights is the weight of the body which is water. Since water has a density of 1 (1 ml of water weighs 1 g), the volume of the water displaced represents both the volume of the body immersed and its density. The immersion weight/unit volume of water displaced then is diluted by the air weight/unit volume of water displaced which, in turn, is the specific gravity of the subject. Corrections for the residual air in the lungs and intestines must be made. There are a number of reports on body density and body fat using this technique. Age affects body density and percent body fat. In one study of women of different ages, it was found that young (16 to 40 years of age) women had body densities of 1.0342 to 1.0343 g/ml and percent body fats of 28.69 to 28.75. Older women (50 to 70 years of age) had body densities which ranged from 1.0095 to 1.0050 g/ml and percent body fats of 41.88 to 44.56. Body fat can be estimated using the following equation from Siri et al.:

$$\text{fat \%} = \frac{2.118}{\text{density}} - 1.354 - 0.78 \left(\frac{\text{\% TBW}}{\text{body weight}} \right)$$

where 2.118, 1.354, and 0.78 are constants and the density (g/cc), body weight (Kg), and TBW (Kg) are determined. One can calculate the lean body mass from the following formula

$$\text{LBM} = \text{body weight} - \text{fat weight}$$

$$\text{fat weight} = (\text{body weight} \times \text{\% of the body that is fat})$$

Other prediction equations for percent fat from specific gravity are available: % fat = 100 $\frac{(5.548 - 5.044)}{\text{specific gravity}}$ (Siri); and % fat = $100 - \frac{\text{TBW}}{0.732}$ (Pace and Rathbun) have been used. The Pace-Rathbun method is based on TBW only and compensates for the structural lipids (those in cell membranes, etc., as contrasted to the depot lipids) by adding 3%. This gives a lean body mass that is somewhat different from that of Siri et al.

Underwater weighing as described above is a method used by researchers and is based on the difference in density of the different body components. Estimating fat stores in this way is cumbersome and/or not feasible in many clinical settings or under conditions of field surveys. Researchers using this method have made some correlations between this estimate and estimates of body fatness using the measurements of skinfold thicknesses at key locations. These locations are places where subcutaneous fat can be assessed using calipers to estimate the skinfold thickness. The fold below the upper arm (triceps fold) and the fold at the iliac crest are frequently used locations. Other locations include the abdominal fold and the thigh fold. Equations (Table 4) have been derived to calculate body fatness using these measurements.

For population surveys where close estimates of body fat, protein, lean body mass, etc., are not critical, simpler estimates of body fatness can be derived. Using the patient's body weight and height one can compare these values to those considered desirable for men and women. The first such tables were developed by the Metropolitan Life Insurance Company. This company made the assumption that young (age 20 to 30) people applying for life insurance (and found insurable) were healthy. They then took the body weights of these people and their heights and arranged these weights according to height for both males and females. They called these weights "desirable" weights because they were associated with the lowest mortality due to disease. Because the weight range for each height was so large, they later subdivided each weight for height range into thirds and presented these thirds as being representative of small, medium, and large frame sizes. This table has been found useful by many in estimating desirable body weight, but the user must remember that this table was not based on actual measurements of

TABLE 4
General Formulas for Calculating Body Fatness From Skinfold Measurements

Males:

$\%$ Body Fat $= 29.288 \cdot 10^{-2}(X) - 5 \cdot 10^{-4}(X)^2 + 15.845 \cdot 10^{-2}(Age)$

Females:

$\%$ Body Fat $= 29.699 \cdot 10^{-2}(X) - 43 \cdot 10^{-5}(X)^2 + 29.63 \cdot 10^{-3}(Age) + 1.4072$

Note: X = sum of abdomen, suprailiac, triceps, and thigh skinfolds and age is in years.

skeletal size. The table was based only on heights and weights of individuals in the third decade of life who wanted (and could afford) life insurance. In this respect there is a bias in the table. The heights and weights were from those individuals wealthy enough to want and obtain life insurance. Minority groups were largely underrepresented in the data base used for these tables.

A broader data base using subjects of all ages, economic status, both sexes, and from minority and majority cultural/ethnic groups was obtained by the National Health and Nutrition Examination Survey (NHANES) that has been conducted at intervals by the Center for Disease Control of the U.S. Public Health Service. These surveys have collected data not only from young adult men and women but also from children and aging adults. These weights and heights have been used to create tables giving desirable weight ranges for males and females. In addition, NHANES made more detailed measurements of skinfold thickness, skeletal size and density, and a variety of biochemical and physiological features using a representative subset of the population assessed. The NHANES tables therefore have a broader data base than the Metropolitan Life Insurance tables. Despite the difference in data bases used to construct the tables, both are useful in evaluating the patient in terms of desirable body weight.

Perhaps more popular now is the use of body mass index (BMI). This is a useful term in that it is an index of the body weight (kilograms) divided by the height (meters) squared (wt/ht^2). BMI correlates with body fatness and with the risk of obesity related disease or diseases for which obesity is a compounding factor. Overweight is defined as a BMI between 25 and 30 and obesity is a BMI over 30. The BMI varies with age. A desirable BMI for people age 19 to 24 is between 19 and 24, while that for people age 55 to 64 is between 23 and 28. While simple in concept, this term does not assess body composition per se. It only provides a basis for assessing the health risks associated or presumed to be associated with excess body fatness. BMI applies only to normal individuals, not the super athlete or the body builder who may be quite heavy yet have little body fat.

While total body fatness is an important risk factor for several degenerative diseases, the distribution of the stored fat may impact upon these disease states as well. Males and females differ in the pattern of body fat stores. Males tend to deposit fat in the abdominal area while females tend to deposit fat in the gluteal area. Measuring the waist and hip circumference allows one to compute the waist to hip ratio (WHR) and as this ratio increases so too does the risk for cardiovascular disease, diabetes mellitus, and hypertension. In men, if the WHR is greater than 0.90 and in women if the WHR is greater than 0.80, the risk for cardiovascular disease increases significantly.

VI. WATER BALANCE

The existence of several body compartments and the knowledge of the importance of water in the body, as well as the fact that water has an average half-life of 3.3 days in the body, gives a clear indication that both water intake and excretion must be closely regulated. Numerous investigators have been involved in the study of thirst regulation and the regulation of water excretion.

The quantitative features of water balance are presented in Tables 5 and 6. As can be seen, water is obtained through the beverages consumed, as a component of food, and as an end product of metabolism. Foods vary in their water content: lettuce, for example, is 96% water; beef steak, 60%; and table sugar, 0.5% water. Typically, a mixed diet providing 2000 kcal will provide 500 to 800 g of water. The water consumed as such, that available from food, that lost in the urine, feces, and by evaporation, can be determined directly. Metabolic water, preformed water, insensible water, and respirative losses must be estimated.

The term metabolic water refers to that amount of water liberated through the metabolism of carbohydrates, lipids, and proteins. In addition to metabolic water, when polysaccharides, triglycerides, or proteins are formed one molecule of water is produced when each interglycosidic linkage, each glyceride bond, and each peptide bond formed. This water is referred to as the preformed water and is sometimes separated from the water that is produced when fats, carbohydrates, and proteins are oxidized (see Table 6).

One can calculate the amount of metabolic water available to the subject if one knows the amount of carbohydrate, fat, and protein consumed and the respiratory quotient. The respiratory quotient (RQ) is the ratio of carbon dioxide released to oxygen consumed. The typical RQ of an individual consuming a mixed diet is 0.85. The water produced by the combustion of carbohydrate, fat, and protein is 0.60, 1.07, and 0.41 g/g nutrient, respectively, or 15.8, 11.5, and 10.3 g water/100 calories of the nutrient. This assumes that the individual is in energy and protein balance. If the individual is gaining weight, then a correction for the gain in weight as fat must be made. If the weight gain results in a positive nitrogen balance, then a correction for the gain in protein must also be made. Similar corrections must be made if the subject is losing weight since more fat and protein will be oxidized than can be accounted for by these respective components in the diet. This oxidation will contribute additional water to the metabolic water category. For example, Newburgh's subject (Table 6) consumed 69 g protein, 83 g fat, and 267 g carbohydrate. Newburgh calculated that this subject had an average heat production of 1907 kcal per day and, based on nitrogen balance data, a daily destruction of 11.9 g of tissue protein. If one subtracts 1907 kcal (the heat produced by the subject) from the kilocalories of the diet plus the available kilocalories of the tissue protein (11.9 × 4), one finds that 232 kcal were stored. This means that 26 g (232 ÷ 9) of fat were stored. Now then, applying all the correction factors, one finds that Newburgh's subject was oxidizing 80.9 g (69 + 11.9) of protein, 267 g of carbohydrate (assuming all the carbohydrate was oxidized), and 57 g (83 − 26) of fat. Newburgh separated the preformed water from the metabolic water. He assumed that the destruction of 11.9 g of tissue protein would release approximately 36 g of water since tissue protein is associated with about 3 times its weight in water. This 36 g was corrected for the storage of 26 g of fat, which he estimated would hold about 3 g of water. Thus, 33 g of preformed water was available to the subject described in Table 6.

Heat production by an animal represents the energy lost from the body as heat. This energy loss is the result of its metabolism (see next section on energy). It can be calculated from the insensible water loss. Insensible water loss is defined as the loss in body weight attributable to the vaporization of water from the body surface. This is not to be confused with the water and heat loss due to profuse sweating. Insensible water loss is just that: the insensible water lost by the body when it is at equilibrium with its environment in its zone of thermic neutrality — that is, an environmental temperature and humidity which induces neither shivering nor sweating. The insensible water loss can be determined by careful weighing of the fasting (but not starving) subject during short periods of time. The difference in the body weights corrected for any loss in weight through the urine and feces is then the insensible weight loss. In the fed

TABLE 5
Typical Water Balance in Adult Humans

Sources of water (g)		Water losses (g)	
Liquid[a]	1100–1200	Urine	1000–1300
Solid food	500–800	Feces	80–100
Metabolic water	300–500	Evaporative losses	550–600
		Lungs	375–400
Total	1900–2500	Total	2000–2400

[a] Water, beverages, soup, etc.

TABLE 6
Water Balance in Human Subject Consuming
a Liquid Diet

Water intake (g)		Water excretion (g)	
Water	268	Urine	1482
Liquid diet	2018	Feces	105
Metabolic water	254	Insensible water	1102
Preformed water	33	Sweat	0
Total	2573	Total	2689

Data selected from Newburgh, L. H., et al., *J. Clin. Invest.,*
8:161, 1930.

subject, a correction for the weight of the food and drink consumed must be made. Thus, insensible weight loss (IW) is equal to the difference between the initial weight (Wi) corrected for intake (I) and the final weight (Wf) corrected for loss of excreta (E).

$$IW = (Wi - I) - (Wf - E)$$

The insensible weight loss (IW) must then be converted to the insensible water loss (IWL). This is possible if one knows the weight of the carbon dioxide exhaled and the oxygen consumed. Thus, $IWL = IW - (CO_2 - O_2)$. If, for example, the IWL were 1213 g and the difference between the carbon dioxide produced and oxygen consumed was 111 g, then the insensible water loss would be 1102 g. The heat produced by the IWL, which is the heat production by the animal as a result of its metabolism, can be calculated if one assumes that 1 g of water will absorb 0.58 kcal of heat at skin temperature. For example, heat production (HP) of a human consuming a low carbohydrate diet will equal the IWL times 0.58 divided by the vapor heat ratio (24.5).

$$HP = IWL \times 0.58 \times (100/24.5)$$

The vapor heat ratio can vary depending on diet, clothing, and environmental temperature. Likewise, the IWL can vary depending on the environment and on age. As humans approach old age there is an impairment in their ability to regulate the evaporative heat loss from the skin. The reasons for this decrease in ability to regulate evaporative heat loss are not fully understood; however, older persons frequently tolerate cold or very hot environments less well than younger persons.

There are other methods available for the calculation of metabolic water. One, devised by Morrison, uses the respiratory exchange, the urinary nitrogen production, and the energy production. This formula is as follows:

$$W = \frac{[K(0.1998 + 0.4692R) - N(3.3352 + 0.2443R)]}{(3.840 + 1.195R)}$$

where W = metabolic water in grams
       K = energy production in kilocalories
       N = total urinary production in grams
       R = respiratory quotient

This method is useful when one does not know the composition of the diet consumed but can measure both respiratory quotient and urinary nitrogen. As indicated earlier, heat production can be calculated or measured indirectly.

As for the other components of the water balance sheet (Tables 4 and 5) the water in the food, beverages, urine, and feces can be determined directly. The water lost through respiration can be estimated. Respired air is fully water saturated and if one can measure the volume of air expired and the number of respirations, one can then calculate the grams of water lost in this manner. Newburgh (Table 6), in his calculations of water balance, did not correct for water loss by this route; however, others generally agree that humans lose 350 to 400 g of water/day through the lungs. Newburgh and others lump the respiratory water loss in with the insensible water loss because it is an unavoidable loss and meets the criteria of being insensible.

As mentioned earlier, urine and fecal losses are determined directly. Typically, the urine is 97% water; its normal level of excretion is 1 to 2 L per day. Fluid is filtered through the kidney tubule at a rate of 125 ml per minute. An amount sufficient to maintain blood volume is resorbed; the rest is excreted. If the fluid intake is low, more of the water is resorbed than normal; this results in a more concentrated urine. If it is high, the urine is less concentrated. The regulation of water resorption by the kidney is under the control of the hormone ADH (antidiuretic hormone, also called vasopressin). When ADH is high, water resorption is high; when ADH is low, water resorption is low. There is a continuous secretion of water in the form of digestive juices into the alimentary canal. As much as 7 to 10 L per day can be secreted. The majority of this liquid is resorbed along with the water from food and drink; only about 100 to 200 ml will be excreted in the feces.

VII.   REGULATION OF WATER BALANCE

Thirst, like hunger, is a basic physiological drive. The urge to drink as a factor in the overall control of body fluid homeostasis has been studied both by psychologists and physiologists alike. In contrast to a number of species, a person's urge to drink is not directly related to his/her water requirement. While thirst is a factor in the overall control of body fluid requirements, other factors play important roles as well. The concentration of Na^+ in the extracellular fluid, ADH (vasopressin), and the angiotensin-renin-aldosterone system are all involved in the regulation of water balance.

A. VASOPRESSIN (ADH)
Vasopressin, the antidiuretic hormone, is synthesized by the supraoptic and paraventricular neurons of the posterior pituitary. The synthesis of vasopressin occurs in the ribosomes and proceeds via the formation of a macromolecular precursor or prohormone. This precursor or propressophysin has a molecular weight of about 20,000 Da. The prohormone contains

several subunits, each of which has a biological function. One of these, vasopressin, is preceded by a signal peptide. When the osmoreceptors located in the anterolateral hypothalamus perceive a change in the osmolarity of the blood (normal range: 275 to 290 mOsm/kg) ADH release is altered via this signal peptide. When osmoreceptors are stimulated, ADH is released and binds to receptors in the glomerulus and renal convoluted tubules, with the result that water is reabsorbed. The exact mechanism by which this system operates is not known. However, it is known that the sensitivity of the system can be affected by the physiological status of the individual. For example, the phase of the menstrual cycle in females affects the sensitivity to the action of ADH such that water balance (water retention) varies through the cycle.

The osmoregulatory mechanism is not equally sensitive to all plasma solutes. Sodium and its anions (which contribute roughly 95% of the osmotic pressure of the plasma) are the most potent solutes with respect to the stimulation of the osmoreceptors. Certain sugars such as sucrose and mannitol have been shown to stimulate these receptors *in vitro*, but these sugars do not normally appear in the plasma. Urea concentrations above 2 pg/ml stimulate ADH release, as does sustained hyperglycemia.

Uncontrolled diabetes and end stage renal disease both are characterized by abnormal water balance. Uncontrolled diabetics are polyuric (excess urine production) and very thirsty. In severe hyperglycemia the solute load in the blood is increased. ADH functions retain water to dilute these solutes. In principle, the same thing happens in the early phase of renal disease. In this instance, the solutes are not excreted because of the disease state of the kidney and ADH functions to retain water so as to dilute these solutes. Later, with end stage renal disease the patients are thirsty and polyuric because their disease renders them less able to reabsorb water via the convoluted tubules. They may have the signals to release ADH but the target tissue (the renal convoluted tubules) is not able to respond. Other stimuli for vasopressin release include emesis (vomiting), changes in blood volume or pressure, excessive sweating, hemorrhage, diarrhea, drugs that act as diuretics or that are antihypertensive agents, hyperinsulinemia, and other hormones related to water balance, i.e., angiotensin.

B. ATRIAL NATRIURETIC HORMONE

The action of ADH in retaining water is counteracted by a peptide hormone, the atrial natruiretic hormone (ANH), that induces water, sodium, and potassium loss, decreases blood pressure, and increases the glomerular filtration rate. ANH interferes with the renin-angiotensin system by decreasing the release of renin and aldosterone. It also antagonizes the action of such vasoconstrictors as angiotensin II and norepinephrine.

C. RENIN, ANGIOTENSIN II, AND ALDOSTERONE

A cascade system, shown in Figure 5, is comprised of renin, angiotensin II, and aldosterone. It exerts effects not only on blood pressure but also on water balance. Renin is a protease that catalyzes the conversion of angiotensin I (the inactive hormone) to angiotensin II. Renin is produced by the juxtaglomerular cells of the kidney. Its release is controlled by neurons in the sympathetic nervous system, negative feedback by angiotensin II, prostaglandin E, calcium, potassium, arginine, vasopressin, and a number of other factors whose effects are not well understood. In turn, angiotensin II affects a wide variety of physiological processes, but the one of importance in this discussion is its effect on water excretion. Through its effects on sodium balance, it affects vasopressin release. At low serum sodium levels it conserves sodium by increasing its reabsorption. At high sodium levels, it has the reverse effect. Through its effect on vasoconstriction, it reduces the glomerular filtration rate and decreases water loss. Lastly, through effects on aldosterone, an adrenal cortical steroid hormone responsible for electrolyte conservation, it also indirectly affects serum sodium levels, vasopressin release, and water retention. If any aspect of this intricate system for controlling water balance is disturbed, excessive thirst and/or excessive urination will result.

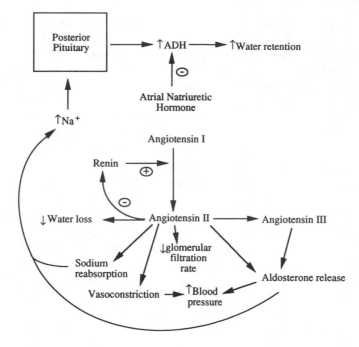

FIGURE 5.   Hormones that affect water balance.

Infusion of epinephrine, acetylcholine, or other monoamines into the third ventricular cavity has been shown to elicit thirst and ADH release in the goat and rat. These effects have generally been regarded as being due to their transmitter action at the various synapses in the ventricular cavity, especially by acting directly on the juxtaventricular receptors involved in the control of water balance. Angiotensin II, norepinephrine, and prostaglandin E have all been found to elicit ADH and thirst and, in addition, have been shown to activate the Na^+-K^+ ATPase in cerebral as well as other tissues. This activation would then allow one to relate Na^+ concentration to thirst (since Na^+ activates this ATPase) and suggests that this enzyme may be essential to receptor excitation. This suggestion is not new. Several years ago it was shown that an inhibitor of transmembrane Na^+ transport, hydrochlorothiazide, markedly reduced drinking in sodium loaded nephrectomized rats. Inhibition of drinking can also be shown with ouabain, an inhibitor of Na^+-K^+ ATPase, and with glycerol. Glycerol suppresses the thirst induced by dehydration.

D. SATIATION OF THIRST

It is evident that thirst does not become satiated until enough water has been absorbed to offset those factors responding to Na^+ concentration, osmolarity, and volume changes in the body fluids. The mechanism for this satiation is unknown. In fact, more is known about the initiation of drinking than about its cessation. Work with the monkey has provided evidence for the existence of pre- and postabsorptive signals elicited from the intestine which play important roles in the cessation of drinking. When water was drained from the stomach via a gastric cannula, the monkeys drank several times their normal intake of water. When a duodenal cannula was used, water intake was increased above normal but was not as great as when the stomach was drained. In monkeys having a gastric drainage, if water was reintroduced into the intestine the monkeys ceased drinking. Whatever the ultimate mechanism is which counterbalances the initiation of water intake, water consumption is closely regulated so that under wide variations in activity, diet, and environmental conditions, normal individuals are able to maintain fluid balance.

VIII. WATER NEEDS

The needs of humans for water vary with the kinds of foods consumed, level of physical activity, environmental temperature, and age. The water need is dictated by the water loss as can be seen in Table 5. Obviously, the variability is great. While there is no minimum requirement for adults it has been recommended that infants be given 1.5 ml water/kcal of food. As discussed in an earlier section in this unit, if excess protein is oxidized for fuel, this will increase water needs since water assists in the elimination of the nitrogenous end products of protein catabolism. This increase has been termed the protein overload effect on water needs.

A. ABNORMALITIES IN WATER BALANCE

As indicated in the preceding sections, the regulation of both water intake and excretion is extremely important to the regulation of water balance and, indeed, to survival itself. A variety of clinical conditions have been described which have as one of their characteristics a change in the normal pattern of intake and/or excretion of water. Only rarely does the primary disorder reside with the regulation of water balance itself. The disorder diabetes insipidus develops in the absence of vasopressin. The disease is characterized by extreme urinary water loss (up to 30 L/day) and extreme thirst.

In this disorder, the posterior pituitary may be diseased or have a tumor which interferes with the production of vasopressin. In this disease, the resorption of water by the renal tubules is not stimulated and the patient excretes a large volume of very dilute urine. Patients with diabetes insipidus can be successfully treated. Interestingly, their treatment consists of providing the hormone in an aerosol which allows the patient to inhale the hormone through the nose.

An even rarer disease of water balance is a form of diabetes insipidus which does not involve the production and release of vasopressin by the posterior pituitary but is primarily of renal origin. In this disorder, the kidney is unresponsive to the hormone. The reasons for this unresponsiveness are not known nor has a suitable treatment been devised.

B. EDEMA

Of the conditions where a disordered water balance is secondary to the primary disease, edema is perhaps the most common. In this condition, water is accumulated in the tissues distal to the kidneys. Urine volume is very low and highly concentrated. As the fluids in the extracellular compartment increase, the functionality of the patient decreases. At first, the edema is noted in the extremities. Feet, ankles, legs, and hands become swollen, then, noticeably, there is an accumulation of fluid in the abdominal cavity and in the pericardial sac. This fluid accumulation makes it difficult for the patient to walk, and eventually interferes with the vital functions of the internal organs such as the heart. Depending on the primary disorder, edema can be treated. If due to inadequate protein or thiamin intakes, these nutrients can be supplied and the edema will subside as the patient's nutritional status improves. If, however, the edema is due to heart disease characterized by an impaired ability to pump the blood throughout the body, a loss in the pressure differential needed for peripheral fluid exchange and circulation through the renal tubules will occur. In this instance, the treatment is much more difficult since it depends on the successful treatment of the diseased heart. Edema can also result from a loss of vascular elasticity which characterizes high blood pressure (hypertension). Hypertension occurs when the vascular system is continually stimulated to constrict. In this disorder, the pressure of the blood is so high in the peripheral tissues that water cannot flow from the tissues to the blood in response to the usual pressure differential between the arteries, arterioles, capillaries, venules, and veins and the tissues they serve. However, if the blood pressure can be reduced through antivasoconstrictor medication, sodium intake restriction, and, if needed, weight reduction, then the edema will also be reduced.

While these disorders are all related to the excretion of water through the kidneys, disturbances in other routes of water loss can also result in an abnormal water balance. Excess environmental temperatures can result in excessive water losses (as well as electrolyte losses) through the skin as sweat. Unless compensated for by an increase in fluid and electrolyte intake and a decrease in urine output, dehydration results. The extracellular fluid becomes concentrated and hypertonic to the cells. Water then shifts from the intracellular compartment to the extracellular compartment. The obvious result of this shift is cell death and unless water is provided, death of the patient is imminent.

C. DIARRHEA

Excess water loss can also occur through the intestine. Large watery stools characterize diarrhea and can arise as a result of a variety of disorders. Perhaps the most common of these is that associated with food contamination. Various organisms such as those from the Salmonella family or the *Vibrio* cholerae can cause massive diarrhea and fluid loss. In the case of the latter, the cholera-causing organism produces a toxin which binds to specific receptors on the intestinal cell wall. The toxin activates adenylate cyclase by causing ADP-ribosylation of the GαS protein (Figure 6) involved in regulating the cyclase. This results in an elevation in cAMP levels which turns on electrolyte secretion and thereby inhibits the active transport processes necessary for the absorption of nutrients (and water) from the gut. While the water can pass freely from the intestine, other materials cannot and, as such, create an osmotic pull on the water. In turn, the water and unabsorbed nutrients fill the intestine, stimulating peristalsis and evacuation of the colon. If the massive fluid and electrolyte losses are not replaced, the cholera victim does not survive and recover. Cholera victims can be given an oral solution rich in glucose (~110 mM), sodium (99 mM), chloride (74 mM), bicarbonate (39 mM), and potassium 4 mM). This solution takes advantage of the fact that the cholera toxin does not "poison" the sodium dependent ATP dependent glucose uptake system. By giving excess glucose, sodium is "pushed" into the cell and electrolyte balance is restored. If the victim cannot swallow, an intravenous replenishment must be followed. If untreated, the victim becomes severely dehydrated and death ensues. In countries where fresh human excreta is used as fertilizer for the fields, epidemics of cholera occur frequently. Epidemics are particularly evident in very warm climates since the cholera organisms multiply very rapidly under these conditions. Food contamination by organisms other than *Vibrio* cholerae is also common in areas where both animal and human excreta are used in the untreated state. If the excreta is allowed to ferment, the heat generated by the fermentation process will kill most of the organisms likely to cause diarrhea.

Diarrhea can also result if the individual develops an irritable colon. A hyperirritable intestine may be the result of a particular medication or it may be permanent due to a genetic error. Genetic errors resulting in the absence of a particular digestive enzyme will result in an accumulation of that substrate in the gut. This in turn will "pull" water into the intestine and diarrhea will result. Lactose intolerance due to the absence of the enzyme lactase is an example of a genetic disorder characterized by diarrhea. Gluten-induced enteropathy is another example. In this instance the patient is unable to digest the wheat protein gluten. Diarrhea is characteristic of this condition and if allowed to continue untreated, the intestinal villi will be abraided and the absorption of nutrients in addition to the gluten will be seriously impaired. Treatment for these types of diarrhea is fairly straightforward. If the offending nutrient is eliminated from the diet, the patient will gradually rebuild the absorptive surface of the intestine and will recover.

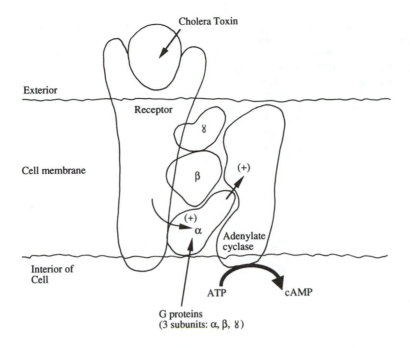

FIGURE 6. Schematic of inhibited active transport processes caused by the cholera toxin.

SUPPLEMENTAL READINGS

ARTICLES

Adreoli, T. E. and Schafer, J. A. (1979) External solution driving forces for isotonic fluid absorption in proximal tubules, *Fed. Proc.,* 38:154–160.

Andersson, B. (1978) Regulation of water intake, *Physiol. Rev.,* 58:582–603.

Berlin, N. I., Watkin, D. M., and Gevirtz, N. R. (1962) Measurement of changes in gross body composition during controlled weight reduction in obesity and body density — body water technics, *Metabolism,* 11:302–314.

Brosek, J. Ed. (1963) Body composition, *Ann. N.Y. Acad. Sci.,* 110:1–1018.

Brozek, J. and Keys, A. (1955) Composition of tissues accounting for individual differences in body density, *Fed. Proc.,* 14:22–27.

Christian, J. E., Combs, L. W., and Kessler, W. V. (1963) Body composition. Relative in vivo determinations from potassium-40 measurements, *Science,* 140:480–490.

Clark, R. R., Kuta, J. M., and Sullivan, J. C. (1993) Prediction of percent body fat in adult males using dual energy X-ray absorptiometry, skinfolds and hydrostatic weighing, *Med. Sci. Sports Exer.,* 25:528–535.

Cote, K. D. and Adams, W. C. (1993) Effect of bone density on body composition estimates in young adult black and white women, *Med. Sci. Sports Exer.,* 25:290–296.

Dibona, D. R. and Mills, J. W. (1979) Distribution of Na^+-pump sites in transporting epithelia, *Fed. Proc.,* 38:134–143.

Fishman, P. A. and Atikkan, E. E. (1980) Mechanism of action of cholera toxin. Effect of receptor density and multivalent binding on activation of adenylate cyclase, *J. Membrane Biol.,* 54:51–60.

Forbes, R. M., Cooper, A. R., and Mitchell, H. H. (1953) The composition of the adult human body as determined by chemical analysis, *J. Biol. Chem.,* 203:359–366.

Forbes, R. M., Mitchel, H. H., and Cooper, A. R. (1956) Further studies on the gross composition and mineral elements of the adult human body, *J. Biol. Chem.,* 223:969–975.

Fuller, M. F., Fowler, P. A., McNeille, G., and Foster, M. A. (1990) Body composition. The precision and accuracy of new methods and their suitability for longitudinal studies, *Proc. Nutr. Soc.,* 49:423–426.

Kreitzman, S. N. (1992) Factors influencing body composition during very low calorie diets, *Am. J. Clin. Nutr.,* 56:2175–2235.

McCargar, L. J., Baracos, V. E., and Clandinin, M. T. (1989) Influence of dietary carbohydrate to fat ratio on whole-body nitrogen retention and body composition in adult rats, *J. Nutr.,* 119:1240–1245.

Meador, C. K., Kreisberg, R. A., Friday, J. P., Jr., Bowdoin, B., Coan, P., Armstrong, J., and Hazelrig, J. B. (1968) Muscle mass determination by isotopic dilution of creatinine-[14], *Metabolism,* 17:1104–1108.

Pace, N. and Rathbun, E. N. (1945) Studies on body composition; body water and chemically combined nitrogen content in relation to fat content, *J. Biol. Chem.,* 158:685–691.

Reeds, P. J. and Fiorotto, M. L. (1990) Growth in perspective, *Proc. Nutr. Soc.,* 49:411–420.

Schafer, J. A. (1979) Water transport in epithelia, *Fed. Proc.,* 38:119–120.

Siri, W. E. (1956) The gross composition of the body, *Adv. Biol. M. Physics,* 4:239–280.

Smalley, K. J., Kneer, A. N., Kendric, Z. V., Colliver, J. A., and Owen, O. E. (1990) Reassessment of body mass indices, *Am. J. Clin. Nutr.,* 52:402–408.

Sohlström, A., Wahlund, L.-0., and Forsum, E. (1993) Adipose tissue distribution as assessed by magnetic resonance imaging and total body fat by magnetic resonance imaging, underwater weighing and body water dilution in healthy women, *Am. J. Clin. Nutr.,* 58:830–838.

Van der Kooy, K., Leenen, R., Serdell, J. C., Dourenberg, P., and Hautvast, J. G. A. J. (1993) Effect of weight cycling on visceral fat accumulation, *Am. J. Clin. Nutr.,* 58:853–857.

Young, C. M., Martin, M. E. K., Chihan, M., McCarthy, M., Manniello, M. J., Harmuth, E. H., and Fryer, J. H. (1961) Body composition of young women. Some preliminary findings, *J. Am. Diet. Assoc.,* 38:332–344.

BOOKS

Lee, R. D. and Nieman, D. C. (1993) Chapter 6: Anthropometry, pg. 121–163. In: *Nutritional Assessment,* Wm. C. Brown Publishers, Dubuque, IA.

Mitchell, H. H. (1962) *Comparative Nutrition of Man and Domestic Animals,* Academic Press, New York.

Unit 3

ENERGY

TABLE OF CONTENTS

I. OVERVIEW

After water, the most important requirement to sustain life is the need for energy. It is expressed in heat units known as calories or joules. No other nutrient requirement can be met if the energy intake is insufficient to meet the body's need for energy.

Classical nutritionists use the term Calorie or kilocalorie (kcal) to represent the amount of heat required to raise the temperature of 1 kg of water 1°C. The international unit of energy is the joule. One Calorie or kilocalorie is equal to 4.184 kilojoules (kJ) or 4.2 kJ. There are cogent reasons to express energy in terms of kilojoules. Nutritionists have realized that the energy provided by food is used for more than heat production. It is also used for mechanical work (muscle movement) and for electrical signaling (vision, neuronal messages) and is stored as chemical energy. The joule is 10^7 ergs where 1 erg is the amount of energy expended in accelerating a mass of 1 g by 1 cm/s. The international joule is defined as the energy liberated by one international ampere flowing through a resistance of one international ohm in one second. Even though the use of joules or kilojoules is being urged by international scientists as a means to ease the confusion in discussions about energy, the student will still find the term Calorie or kcal in many texts and references. In some texts, the term calorie is spelled with an upper case "C". Physicists use the term calorie to represent the amount of heat required to raise the temperature of 1 g of water 1°C. Note that this definition uses one <u>gram</u>, not one <u>kilogram</u> as stated above. Even though it is not correct, the term calorie is used in some nutrition literature when in fact Calorie or kcal is intended.

When foodstuffs are burned in the presence of oxygen, heat is produced. The quantity of heat produced can be measured in a bomb calorimeter and used as an estimate of the energy value of the food. The bomb calorimeter is an instrument used to measure heat production when a known amount of food is completely oxidized. It is a highly insulated, box-like container. All the heat produced during the oxidation of a dried sample of food is absorbed by a weighed amount of water surrounding the combustion chamber. A thermometer registers the change in the chamber temperature. The instrument's name is derived from the design of the combustion chamber: it is a small bomb. The energy value of protein foods obtained in this manner is higher than the actual biologic value, for in biologic systems, the end products of oxidation must be excreted as urea, a process which costs energy. For instance, in a bomb calorimeter (Figure 1), the combustion or oxidation of protein yields 5.6 Calories/gram; the energy yield from the oxidation of protein after correction for urea formation and digestive loss by the body is about 4 Calories/gram. Corrections for digestive losses are also applied to the values obtained for the combustion of lipids and carbohydrates. The value of 4.1 Calories/gram is rounded off to 4 for carbohydrates and the value of 9.4 for lipids is rounded off to 9. Listed in Table 1 are some common foods and their energy values.

The objectives of digestion, absorption, and metabolism in the animal system is to convert the chemicals in the foods to the chemicals in the body. The conversion of food chemicals to body chemicals is stepwise and not 100% efficient. Energy exchange and conversion is an integral part of the process which converts the food chemicals to the body chemicals. Some of the chemical energy from the food is trapped in high-energy storage compounds, but at each step of the conversion process some of the energy escapes as heat. This heat, generated by the body in the course of oxidizing various food components or converting these food components to body components, serves to maintain the body temperature. However, because this heat is also lost from the body through radiation as well as through the various excretory processes, these losses must be replaced. Hence, the daily need for food and its associated energy value. Figure 2 illustrates the continuity of energy losses and gains by the living system. Energy is gained from the oxidation of the fats, carbohydrates, and proteins consumed as food. This energy is transmitted via ATP (and other high-energy transfer compounds) to a variety of essential macro- and micromolecules in the body which in turn are needed to sustain its optimal function. As these functions also consume and release energy more must be provided by the diet. Over and over this cycling occurs, and this is the nature of the dynamic state of the living body. No reaction or process ever goes to completion and stops because it is done. The only time this happens is at death.

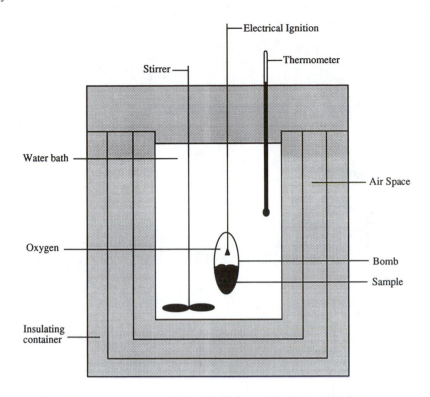

FIGURE 1. Cross section of a bomb calorimeter showing essential features.

TABLE 1
Energy Content of Selected Human Food

Item	Amount	Food energy (kcal)
Milk (3.3% fat)	8 oz	150
Skim milk	8 oz	85
Butter	1 oz (~25 g)	204
Egg	50 g	80
Bacon	2 slices (15 g)	85
Hamburger, lean	3 oz	185
Apple	138 g	80
Avocado	216 g	370
Banana	119 g	100
Grapefruit	241 g	50
Orange	131 g	65
Bread, white	25 g (slice)	70
Brownie with nuts	20 g	95
Peanut butter	16 g	95
Green beans	1 cup, 125 g	30
Corn	1/2 cup, 83 g	65
Tomato, raw	135 g	25

II. ENERGY NEED

Although the Food and Nutrition Board of the National Academy of Sciences have made recommendations for the energy intake (Table 2) for people of different ages, these figures should not be considered immutable. The energy need is so variable that the intake which would result in obesity in one person would be totally inadequate for another. Genetics and

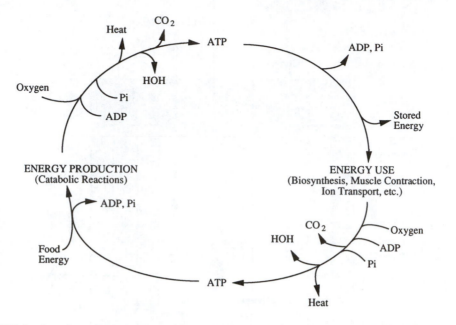

FIGURE 2. Overview of energy gains and losses showing the high-energy compound ATP as the medium of exchange. Other high-energy compounds also participate in bioenergetics.

TABLE 2
Recommended Energy Intakes for Infants, Children, and Adults Based on Weight and Height

Category	Age	Weight (lb)	Height (in.)	Average energy allowance (kcal)
Infants	0–6 mo	13	24	650
	6–12 mo	20	28	850
Children	1–3 yrs	29	35	1300
	4–6	44	44	1800
	7–10	62	52	2000
Males	11–14	99	62	2500
	15–18	145	69	3000
	19-24	160	70	2900
	25–50	174	70	2900
	51+	170	68	2300
Females	11–14	101	62	2200
	15–18	120	64	2200
	19–24	128	65	2200
	25–50	138	64	2200
	51+	143	63	1900
Pregnant	1st trimester:	No change		
	2nd trimester			+300
	3rd trimester			+300
Lactation	1–6 mo			+500
	7–12 mo			+500

lifestyle choices have profound effects on energy balance and energy need. Perhaps the best way of understanding the dimensions of the energy requirement is to examine what happens to the energy provided by the food when it is consumed.

The energy provided by the food can be determined in a bomb calorimeter as described in the first segment of this unit. As mentioned, not all of this energy is available to the consumer. Some is lost in the preparation of the food and some is lost through digestion (the digestion energy lost, DE). When the deduction for preparative and digestive losses are made, the energy available to the body is the metabolizable energy (ME). Metabolizable energy is the gross energy minus the energy lost in feces and urine and the food preparative losses. Most tables of food composition giving the gross energy value of specific foods make the correction for preparative loss. In some instances, corrections for digestive energy lost are also made. Metabolizable energy consists of the energy needed to keep the body warm (the heat increment) and to run the body processes. Each of these major divisions are subdivided as illustrated in Figure 3. The heat increment (HI) is composed of the heat released through body work, for example, muscle contraction, and the heat released as food is oxidized and converted to usable body components. The latter is sometimes referred to as the specific dynamic action of food or diet induced thermogenesis (DIT), while the former is called the utilizable energy (UE). Utilizable energy is that which is used for body work. The net energy (NE) likewise has two components. One is the basal energy (BE) or the absolute minimum amount of energy that is needed to keep the body alive, while the other is the energy that is either available for storage or is withdrawn from storage (EB).

A. DIGESTIVE ENERGY

The energy lost through digestion can be measured by collecting the feces and urine and determining its energy content. Some of the fecal energy is due to the desquamated intestinal cells and intestinal flora (and its end products) and some from the undigested portion of the food. However, for the purposes of determining the energy balance of the individual, all of these components of the fecal energy can be grouped together because they represent energy lost from the body.

B. BASAL ENERGY

By definition the basal energy reflects the energy used to sustain life. It is the sum of the energy lost as heat or used by anabolic and catabolic processes that are involved in body maintenance. It excludes the energy used for growth, production/reproduction, lactation, movement, or work. The clinical definition for the basal energy is the amount of energy used by the body at rest (not asleep), in the post absorptive state (not starving), at sexual repose, and in a comfortable environment where neither shivering nor sweating occurs.

The measurement of energy need based on energy lost as heat or based on the consumption of oxygen needed to oxidize fats, carbohydrates, and proteins to provide energy has been well studied and several methods are available. The energy need is additive. That is, energy is needed to maintain the body (the basal energy) and sustain its various activities such as voluntary movement, work, or growth. Methods developed for estimating the basal energy requirement are listed in Table 3. The methods vary from very simplistic ones based on height and weight to those based on actual measures of heat production or estimates of heat production based on the heat needed to evaporate water lost by the body. Each method has its advantages and disadvantages. In those methods where actual measurements are made, the basal energy need must be measured in the post absorptive state and the energy needed for growth and activity added to it. The post absorptive state occurs after the consumed food is digested and absorbed but before the state of starvation ensues. Starvation involves a series of hormonal responses that can affect the fuel used by the different tissues. In the human, the post absorptive state is about 12 to 14 hours after the last meal. In the mouse it is 10 hours, the rat 17 hours, guinea pig 22 hours, rabbit 60 hours, pig 96 hours, and the ruminant 5 to 6 days. The time needed to achieve the post absorptive state depends on the length of the digestive tract and whether the animal is a ruminant or has a sizeable "fermentation vat" within the gastrointestinal tract. In some species the cecum serves this function while in other species

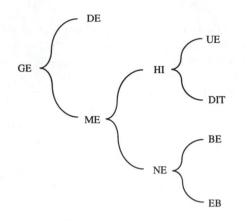

FIGURE 3. Energy losses from food consumed. GE = gross energy in food; DE = energy lost through digestion; ME = metabolizable energy; HI = heat increment; UE = utilizable energy; DIT = diet induced thermogenesis; NE = net energy; BE = basal energy; EB = energy balance (energy either stored or mobilized from stores).

TABLE 3
Methods and Equations Used for Calculating Basal Energy Need

Method	Equation
1. Heat production, direct calorimetry	kcal (kJ)/m^2 (surface area)
2. Oxygen consumption; indirect	O_2 cons/w$^{0.75}$
3. Heat production; indirect	Insensible Weight Loss (IW) = Insensitive water loss (IWL) + (CO_2 exhaled − O_2 inhaled)
	Heat production $= IWL \times 0.58 \times \dfrac{100}{25}$
	(0.58 = kcal to evaporate 1 g water)
4. Energy used; indirect	$BE = \dfrac{\text{Creatinine N (mg/day)}}{0.00482 \ (W)}$
5. Estimate (energy need not measured)	BE = 66.4730 + 13.751W + 5.0033L − 6.550A (men)
	BE = 655.0955 + 9.563W + 1.8496 L − 4.6756A (women)
6. Estimate (energy need not measured)	$BE = 71.2W^{0.75}\left[1+0.004\,(30\text{-}A)+0.010\left(\dfrac{L}{W^{0.33}}-43.4\right)\right]$ *(men)*
	$BE = 65.8W^{0.75}\left[1+0.004\,(30\text{-}A)+0.018\left(\dfrac{L}{W^{0.33}}-42.1\right)\right]$ (women)

Note: Abbreviations are as follows: W = weight in kg; L = height in cm; A = age in years; BE = Basal Energy.

an enlarged intestinal tract has this function. At any rate, the post absorptive state is characterized by a respiratory quotient of 0.8, indicating that a mixture of fat and carbohydrate is being oxidized. If only fat was being oxidized, the respiratory quotient would be about 0.7. If only carbohydrate was being oxidized, the RQ would be 1.0. If energy need was being assessed by measuring heat production, the post absorptive state would be that heat released at the point (in a continuous measurement) where the slope of the line changes, as shown in Figure 4.

The energy released as heat can be determined directly using a calorimeter. This instrument is nothing more than a large insulated box with sensors that can detect very small differences in temperature. Using a calorimeter is extremely tedious and the instrumentation is very expensive. Subjects are placed in the box, kept at a comfortable temperature, and the heat transfer from the body to the chamber measured. The food energy available to the subject is carefully measured, as is the weight of the subject (before and after the period in the box) and

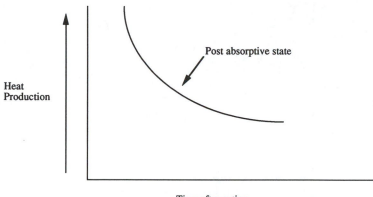

FIGURE 4. Changes in heat production mark the postabsorptive state.

the energy content of the feces and urine. Usually 24 hours must elapse to acquire good measurements of heat production. The basal energy is presumed to be that heat produced by the subject upon waking. Smaller time intervals can be used to assess heat production as a result of specific treatments, such as the responses to hormone treatments or specific dietary ingredients or as a result of physical activity. The box is kept at a temperature that elicits neither sweating nor shivering. This temperature range is called the *zone of thermic neutrality*. Both sweating and shivering are energy using processes. Sweating allows the individual to lose heat energy through water evaporation and loss. Shivering generates heat gain through surface muscle contraction and relaxation. Both processes are important to body heat regulation at environmental temperatures above and below the zone of thermic neutrality. If one were to measure energy loss above, at, and below this zone, increased energy loss would be observed at each extreme, as shown in Figure 5.

The temperatures that mark the limits of the zone of thermic neutrality can vary between species as well as between individuals within a species. The zone of thermic neutrality is influenced by body covering. The winter coat of many species is longer and thicker than the summer coat. The winter coat can trap a layer of air around the body which insulates it against the lowered environmental temperature. Humans do the same thing with their clothing choices. Heavier, more insulating clothing is selected for winter wear and this clothing affects the temperature at which shivering as a heat generating mechanism begins. In the summer, the reverse occurs to allow heat dissipation without the need for sweating to facilitate body heat loss. Heated houses and social behaviors such as huddling also work to decrease the need to generate heat via shivering. Air conditioning has the reverse effect. For humans, these environmental controls (heating/air conditioning) serve to decrease energy wasting and this, in turn, affects energy balance, adding to the amount of energy available for storage as fat and for use to maintain the body's metabolism.

Measuring directly the energy lost as heat from the body is not always convenient or possible. Few clinical settings can afford the time and expense to assess energy needs in this way. There is an alternative. Metabolic processes not only produce heat but also consume oxygen. The consumption of oxygen and heat production are direct correlates of each other. Oxygen consumption can thus be measured as an indirect method of assessing energy use and need. The oxidation of energy-providing nutrients (detailed in Units 4, 5, and 6) requires oxygen. This oxygen is used to make water and carbon dioxide. For every molecule of oxygen used to make water, there is an associated release of energy that is trapped in the high-energy bond of ATP and an associated release of energy as heat. The process whereby water and ATP is synthesized simultaneously is called oxidative phosphorylation. Actually, there are two processes: one, respiration, joins hydrogen and oxygen ions to make water, and the other, ATP

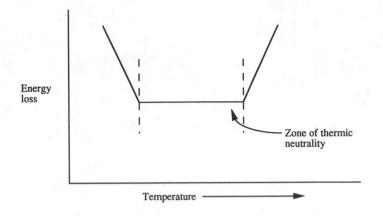

FIGURE 5.   Energy is lost when the environmental temperature is below or above the zone of thermic neutrality.

synthesis, uses some of the energy so released to synthesize ATP. These coupled processes occur in the mitochondria of the cell.

1.   Mitochondrial Structure and Function

The number and size of mitochondria within the cell are influenced by many factors: age, genotype, diet, hormones, and nutritional state. However, within a given cell type, within the same animal, the number is relatively constant. For example, rat liver cells taken from a young, well-nourished, nonstressed, normal animal contain about 800 mitochondria/cell. These mitochondria are scattered throughout the cytosol and are in close proximity to other organelles that have a high ATP requirement. Thus, electronmicrographs of cell cross sections often show mitochondria in close proximity to the nucleus and ribosomes where protein synthesis is taking place. High rates of protein synthesis demand large amounts of ATP, since every amino acid incorporated into the protein macromolecule must first be activated by ATP. Thus, if the protein being synthesized contains 300 amino acid residues, 300 molecules of ATP will be required. Similarly, one will find large numbers of mitochondria in muscle located in close proximity to the contracting muscle fibrils. The ATP molecules produced by the mitochondria need diffuse only a very short distance to where they are used. Mitochondria are frequently located near fat droplets which serve as sources of metabolic fuel. Stored triacylglycerides are hydrolyzed in the cytosol to glycerol and fatty acids. The fatty acids are then transferred, via the acylcarnitine transferase mechanism, into the mitochondria and oxidized. Unit 6 gives the details of fatty acid oxidation. Mitochondria are of many sizes and shapes. In the brown fat cell, they are spherical, in hepatocytes they are oval-shaped, in the kidney they are cylindrical, and in fibroblasts they are thread-like. The organelle consists of two membranes. The outer membrane surrounds the inner one which is highly convoluted. Within the inner membrane is the matrix. This matrix can change in volume and organization as it changes its respiratory activity. The matrix contains, in addition to its enzymes, some DNA and ribosomes with which it synthesizes approximately one third of its complement of respiratory chain enzymes.

The membranes of the mitochondria differ not only in appearance but in function as well. The outer membrane is smooth and somewhat elastic whereas the inner membrane, as mentioned, is convoluted. These convolutions serve to increase the surface area of the inner membrane. The inner membrane is covered with regularly spaced spheres on stalks called inner membrane spheres. These spheres are not present on the outer membrane. The two membranes have been separated and their functional components studied.

2.   Respiration

Respiration is the process by which aerobic cells obtain energy from the oxidation of fuel. Carbon dioxide, water, heat, and ATP are the products of this process.

Glycolysis, as well as fatty acid and amino acid oxidation, results in the production of an activated two-carbon residue, acetyl CoA. This common metabolic intermediate is joined to oxalacetate to form citrate and is then processed by the citric acid cycle. This cyclic sequence of reactions is found in every cell type that possesses mitochondria. The cycle is catalyzed by a series of enzymes and yields reducing equivalents (H') and carbon dioxide. It is illustrated in Figure 6. Reducing equivalents are produced when α-ketoglutarate is produced from isocitrate, when α-ketoglutarate is decarboxylated to produce succinyl CoA, when succinate is converted to fumarate, and when malate is converted to oxalacetate. These reducing equivalents, one pair for each step, are carried to the respiratory chain by way of either NAD or FAD. Reducing equivalents from succinate are carried by FAD while those produced by the oxidation of the other substrates are carried by NAD. Once oxalacetate is formed, it can then pick up another acetate group from acetyl CoA and begin the cycle once again by forming citrate. Thus, for every turn of the cycle, two carbon dioxide molecules and eight pairs of reducing equivalents are produced. As long as there is sufficient oxalacetate to pick up the incoming acetate the cycle will continue to turn and reducing equivalents will continue to be produced, and these, in turn, will be joined with molecular oxygen to produce water, the end product (with carbon dioxide) of the catabolic process.

The above simplistic description of the citric acid cycle implies that it is free of controls and proceeds unhindered given adequate supplies of substrates, enzymes, and molecular oxygen. This is not true. There are numerous controls in place that regulate the cycle. The citric acid cycle produces the reducing equivalents needed by the respiratory chain and the respiratory chain must transfer these hydrogen ions and their associated electrons to the oxygen ion to produce water. In doing so, it generates the electrochemical gradient necessary for the formation of the high-energy bonds of ATP. Obviously, then—these processes, citric acid cycle, respiratory chain, and ATP synthesis—are regulated coordinately.

3. Respiratory Chain

The pairs of electrons produced at the four steps described above in the citric acid cycle, as well as electrons transferred into the mitochondria via other processes, are passed down the respiratory chain to the ultimate acceptor, molecular oxygen. The respiratory chain is shown in Figure 7.

The enzymes of the respiratory chain are particularly complex. They are embedded in the mitochondrial inner membrane and are difficult to extract and study. They catalyze the series of oxidation-reduction reactions which comprise the respiratory chain. Each reaction is characterized by a redox potential which can be calculated using the Nernst equation:

$$Eh = E_0^1 + 2.30 \text{ PRT} \log n \left(\frac{[\text{electron acceptor}]}{[\text{electron donor}]} \right)$$

where Eh = observed potential, E_0^1 = standard redox potential (pH = 7.0, T = 25°, 1.0 M concentration), R = gas constant (8.31 J deg^{-1} mol^{-1}), T = Temperature (°K), N = Number of electrons being transferred, P = Faraday (23,062 cal, V^{-1} = 96,406 J V^{-1}).

The more positive the potential, the greater the affinity of the negatively charged acceptor for the positively charged electrons. It is this potential that drives the respiratory chain reactions forward toward the formation of water. Each succeeding acceptor donor pair has a higher affinity for the electrons than the preceding pair until the point in the chain where the product, water, is formed. By comparison to the preceding pairs, water itself has little tendency to give up its electrons and unless this water is immediately removed, the chain reaction will stop. Of course, water does not accumulate in the mitochondria; it leaves as quickly as it is formed and thus does not feed back to inhibit the chain. If it did accumulate, it would change

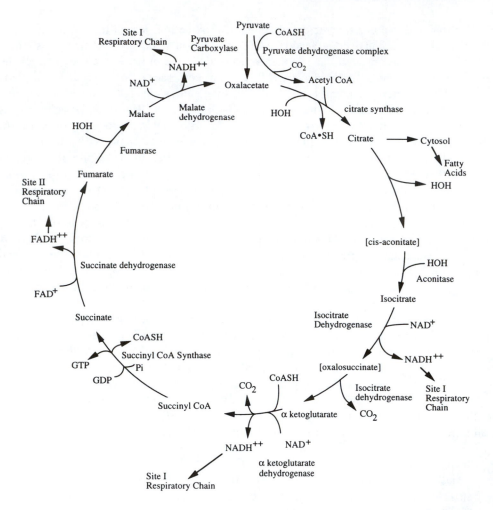

FIGURE 6. Krebs citric acid cycle in the mitochondria. This cycle is also called the tricarboxylate cycle.

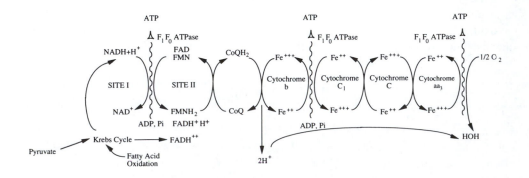

FIGURE 7. The respiratory chain showing the steps where a sufficient proton gradient is developed to make possible the formation of ATP.

the concentration of the chain components by diluting them. When water accumulates, the mitochondrion swells; if in excess, the mitochondrion bursts and dies. Obviously, then, water must exit the organelle as soon as it is formed so as to maintain optimal osmotic conditions.

Although the respiratory chain usually proceeds in the forward direction (toward the formation of water) due to the exergonic nature of the reaction cascade, it should be realized that except for the final reaction, all of these steps are fully reversible. In order to be reversed, sufficient energy must be provided to drive the reaction in the reverse direction. For example, the reducing equivalents derived from succinate are usually carried by FAD (as $FADH^+H^+$). These can be transferred to NAD (as $NADH^+H^+$) with the concomitant hydrolysis of ATP. Electron transport across the other two phosphorylation sites can also be reversed, again, only if sufficient energy is provided.

Overall regulation of respiration or the activity of the intact respiratory chain is vested in the availability of the phosphate acceptor, ADP. A rapid influx of ADP into the mitochondrial compartment is what is needed to ensure a rapid respiratory rate. For example, the working muscle uses the energy provided by the hydrolysis of ATP and creatine phosphate. ATP is hydrolyzed to ADP and Pi and the ADP travels into the mitochondria and stimulates respiration and thence ATP synthesis. The energy of the creatine phosphate is likewise transferred to the ADP to remake ATP.

4. ATP Synthesis

As electrons pass down the respiratory chain, ATP is synthesized. The sequential reactions of the respiratory chain generate an electrochemical gradient of H^+ ions across the inner mitochondrial membrane. This gradient serves as the means for coupling the energy flow from electron transport and water formation to the formation of ATP. The inner and outer mitochondrial membranes are integral parts of the mechanism which couples the energy gradient of the electron flow in the respiratory chain to the synthesis of ATP. In order to do this, the membrane must be intact and in the form of a continuous closed vesicle. If the membranes are disrupted, coupling will not occur. Respiration may occur but ATP synthesis will not. The enzymes of the respiratory chain are arranged so as to transport hydrogen ions from the matrix across the inner membrane such that the gradients will develop in close proximity to the $F_1F_0ATPase$ (ATP synthase) complex and provide a proton gradient sufficient to drive ATP synthesis by causing a dehydration of ADP and Pi.

The components of oxidative phosphorylation are divided into five complexes. Complexes I through IV plus ubiquinone (Q) and cytochrome C comprise the respiratory chain. Complex V is the $F_1F_0ATPase$. The electron carriers are the quinoid structures (FMN, FAD, Q) and the transition metabolic complexes. At three stages in the chain, oxidative energy is conserved (Figure 7) via coupled vectorial proton translocations and the creation of a membrane proton gradient ($\Delta\mu H^+$). This protonic energy is what drives the synthesis of ATP. Should this energy be dissipated, as happens when agents such as dinitrophenol are present, ATP synthesis does not occur or occurs to a very limited extent. Uncoupling occurs because protons are transported through the membrane from the intramembrane space to the matrix. This "short circuits" the normal flow of protons through complex V. In such a circumstance, electrons continue down the respiratory chain but the protonic energy thus generated is not captured in the high-energy phosphate bond. Instead, this energy is released as heat. There are variations or degrees of protonic energy capture *in vivo* which are related to the presence or graded absence of naturally occurring agents which serve to either inhibit the action of complex V or uncouple the respiratory chain energy generation process from the energy capture process of ATP synthesis.

Long-chain fatty acids can act as uncoupling agents as can a specific protein made in the brown fat, called brown fat uncoupling protein or thermogenin. Other compounds may also serve in this way so as to reduce energetic efficiency and increase body heat production. This is an important defense reaction to invading pathogens. Increased body heat (fever) serves to reduce the viability of these pathogens. Some of the catabolic hormones affect coupling as well. These include the thyroid hormones, glucocorticoids, sex hormones, catecholamines, insulin, glucagon, parathyroid hormone, and growth hormone. Some of these hormones have direct effects on mitochondrial respiration and coupling through affecting the synthesis and activation of the various protein constituents of the five complexes. These effects are listed in Table 4. Other hormones have their effects on the exchange of divalent ions, notably calcium, and/or on the phospholipid fatty acid composition of the inner mitochondrial membrane. Some hormones, thyroid hormones for example, influence enzyme synthesis/activation, calcium flux, and membrane lipid composition. Clearly, Mother Nature intended to create a very carefully regulated system with checks and balances to ensure the continuity of life. Without this careful control, survival during times of energy stress could not be assured.

Recently, there have been reports that some degenerative diseases are due to mutations in the genes which encode the protein components of the respiratory chain or the various subunits of the $F_1F_0ATPase$. Deletions in these codes or point mutations could result in proteins with abnormal function which, in turn, would affect the activity of the respiratory chain and/or its coupling to ATP synthesis. Diseases attributed to mutations in the codes for the components of oxidative phosphorylation include diabetes mellitus, heart disease, several neurological diseases, and several neuromuscular diseases. The genetic codes for the chain and the $F_1F_0ATPase$ are found primarily in the nuclear DNA. Some, however, are found in the mitochondrial DNA (mt DNA). These include complex I NADH dehydrogenase, cytochrome b, several subunits of the ATPase, and cytochrome c. The discovery that an organelle other than the nucleus contained DNA was rather remarkable. There are some distinct characteristics of mt DNA. It is circular rather than linear and codes for only a few proteins compared to the many encoded by the nuclear DNA. The mt DNA for many species has been completely sequenced and mapped. The codes present in the mt DNA all come from the female, because during fertilization of the egg only the head of the sperm penetrates the coating of the egg. The mitochondria in the sperm is located in its tail. Thus, the sperm cannot contribute its mitochondria to the fertilized egg.

Errors in mt DNA can be inherent ones (point mutations) or due to oxidative stress. Mitchondria are rich in lipids and consume ~90% of the oxygen used by the cell. Free oxygen radicals and fatty acid radicals can form in these organelles, attacking the mt DNA, and these attacks can result in deletions of portions of the code. Intermittent anoxia followed by reperfusion of oxygen-rich blood can set the stage for such a free radical attack. Because the mt DNA has no self repair mechanism, the code error (damage) would be sustained. Luckily, the cell has many mitochondria and not all would be affected. The cell can survive but may be somewhat compromised in function. With age, there may be cumulative assaults on the mt DNA and scientists have reported that there is an age-related decline in mitochondrial function.

5. Metabolic Control: Oxidative Phosphorylation

Changes in the dietary or hormonal status of the individual result in large changes in the cytosolic pathways for glucose and fatty acid use as well as changes in protein turnover. All of these are orchestrated by changes in oxidative phosphorylation which, in turn, is orchestrated by these changes in cytosolic activity. Starvation and diabetes, for example, result in decreased cytosolic glycolytic activity and lipogenesis while increasing lipolytic and gluconeogenic activity. These coordinated decreases and increases have in common a change in compartment redox state (ratio of oxidized to reduced metabolites) and phosphorylation state (ratio of ATP to ADP). Reducing equivalents generated in the cytosol and carried by NAD^+ or $NADP^+$ must be transferred to the mitochondria for use by the respiratory chain. Through transhydrogenation (Figure 8), reducing equivalents generated in the cytosol through NADP-linked enzymatic reactions are transferred to NAD. In turn, since NAD cannot traverse the mitochondrial membrane, these reducing equivalents must be carried on suitable metabolites into the mitochondrial compartment. Several shuttle systems exist. The malate-aspartate shuttle (Figure 9) is thought to be the most important shuttle. The shuttle requires a stoichiometric influx of malate and glutamate and efflux of aspartate and α-ketoglutarate from the

TABLE 4
Effects of Hormones on the Coupling of Respiration to ATP Synthesis

Hormone	Effect
Thyroxine	Increase
Triiodothyronine	Increase/decrease; dose dependent
Epinephrine	Decrease
Norepinephrine	Decrease
Insulin	Increase
Glucocorticoid	Increase/decrease; dose dependent
Glucagon	Increase
Parathyroid hormone	Increase; dose dependent
Growth hormone	Increase

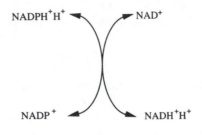

FIGURE 8. Transfer of reducing equivalents from NADPH+H+ to NAD+ via transhydrogenation.

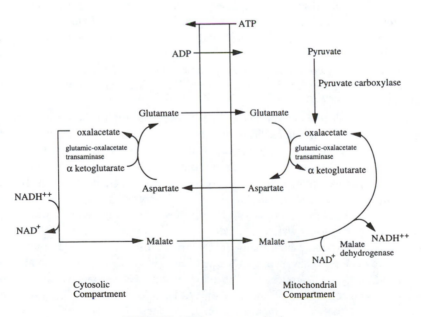

FIGURE 9. Malate-aspartate shuttle.

mitochondria. Alterations in the rate of efflux of α-ketoglutarate can significantly alter the shuttle activity in terms of the rate of cytosolic NADH utilization. α-Ketoglutarate efflux is dependent on mitochondrial ATP/ADP ratio and on the concentration of cytosolic malate. Shuttle activity is controlled by cytosolic ADP levels, malate levels, and availability of NADH.

Malate can also be exchanged for citrate (Figure 10) or for phosphate. The malate-citrate exchange involves transport of malate into the mitochondria where it is converted to citrate via oxalacetate. The citrate is then transported out of the mitochondria and the reactions reversed. This exchange is thought to be particularly active in lipogenic states since it provides citrate to the cytosol for citrate cleavage. Because the cleavage of citrate provides the starting acetate for fatty acid synthesis, this exchange plays a key role in lipogenesis. As shown in Figure 10, other exchanges also take place to varying degrees. One can recognize the components of the malate shuttle among these exchange systems as well as identify the system for the exchange of adenine nucleotides. When the activity of the malate-aspartate is increased, the redox state of the cytosol is decreased as is lipogenesis, whereas gluconeogenesis is increased. All of these exchanges of metabolites are related to each other via a coordinated control exerted by the phosphorylation state, the latter in turn being controlled by ADP/ATP exchange.

Of importance to the control of glycolysis (see Unit 5) is the α-glycerophosphate shuttle (Figure 11). This shuttle is located at the outer side of the mitochondrial inner membrane. Transport of α-glycerophosphate and dihydroxyacetone phosphate across the mitochondrial inner membrane is not required. The activity of the shuttle is related to the availability of α-glycerophosphate and the activity of the mitochondrial α-glycerophosphate dehydrogenase. It is particularly responsive to thyroid hormone. Thyroid hormone is thought to act by increasing the synthesis and activity of the mitochondrial α-glycerophosphate dehydrogenase.

Adenine nucleotide translocation or the exchange of adenine nucleotides across the mitochondrial membrane (Figure 10) also plays a role in the regulation of oxidative phosphorylation. Although any one of the adenine nucleotides could theoretically exchange for any other one, this does not happen. AMP movement is very slow (if it occurs at all). Under certain conditions, ADP influx into the mitochondria is many times faster than ATP efflux. This occurs when the need for ATP within the mitochondria exceeds that of the cytosol. An example of this occurs in starvation, where ATP is needed to initiate urea synthesis and fatty acid oxidation and to support gluconeogenesis.

Under normal dietary conditions, however, the exchange of ADP for ATP is very nearly equal. For every 100 molecules of ADP that enters the mitochondrial compartment, about 87 molecules of ATP exit.

The number of molecules of ATP produced by the coupling of the respiratory chain to ATP synthesis depends on where the reducing equivalents enter the chain. If they enter carried by NAD, they are said to enter at site I. If they enter carried by FAD they are said to enter at site II. Site I substrates are those that are oxidized via NAD-linked dehydrogenases. Pyruvate, for example, is a site I substrate while succinate is a site II substrate. Reducing equivalents entering at site I will generate the energy for the synthesis of three molecules of ATP. Those entering at site II will generate enough energy to result in two molecules of ATP. Knowing which substrate provides their reducing equivalents to which site allows one to determine how many ATPs will be produced by a particular reaction sequence. Since each ATP has an energy value of 36.8 kJ or 7.6 kcal one can also estimate the amount of energy each sequence will produce or use. Going one step further, one can measure the oxygen consumed and calculate or estimate the amount of energy released. This then is the basis for the indirect measure of energy expenditure through the measurement of oxygen consumed. The basal oxygen consumption can be measured as can the increase in oxygen consumption with activity. The difference between growing and nongrowing animals can be obtained such that the energy cost of growth can be estimated. Similarly, if a person or animal is either gaining or losing weight, the energy cost of this weight gain (or energy provided by the loss) can be estimated.

The details of each of the major metabolic pathways are given in Units 4, 5, and 6. Each pathway is characterized by the number of ATPs it uses and/or produces. Not all of the ATPs are produced by the mitochondrial oxidative phosphorylation process. Some are produced as

Carrier System

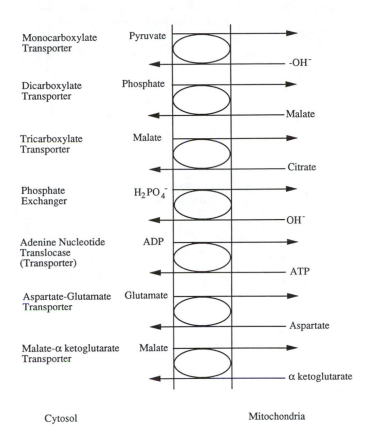

FIGURE 10. Metabolite exchanges across the mitochondrial membranes.

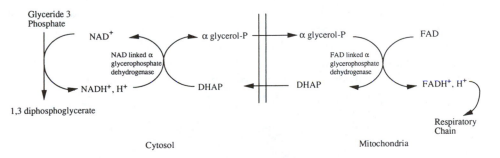

FIGURE 11. The α-glycerophosphate shuttle.

a product of substrate oxidation. Shown in Table 4 are the number of ATPs used or produced by these pathways.

As can be noted in Table 5, if one knew the metabolic mixture consumed and oxidized one could calculate the energy change. Rarely can one do this. Usually, one can measure the oxygen consumed and the carbon dioxide produced and can determine whether the subject is gaining or losing weight and whether the subject is in nitrogen balance. Nitrogen balance means that the nitrogen from the protein in the food is replacing that of the proteins being degraded in the body. The nitrogen balance concept is discussed in greater detail in Unit 4. Energy balance has a similar meaning. The energy used by the body is replaced by the energy

TABLE 5
ATP Produced or Used and Oxygen Consumed by the Major
Metabolic Pathways

Pathway	Number ATP	Moles oxygen
Glycolysis		
Gluco or hexokinase	−1	0
Phosphofructokinase	−1	0
Glyceraldehyde-3-phosphate dehydrogenase-(2-NADH$^+$H$^+$) produced	−6	3
Phosphoglycerate kinase	+2	0
Pyruvate kinase	+2	0
Krebs Cycle		
Pyruvate dehydrogenase (2NADH$^+$H$^+$)	6	3
Isocitrate dehydrogenase (2NADH$^+$H$^+$)	6	3
α-Ketoglutarate (2NADH$^+$H$^+$)	6	3
Succinate thiokinase	2	0
Succinate dehydrogenase (2FADH$^+$H$^+$)	4	2
Malate dehydrogenase (2NADH$^+$H$^+$)	6	3
Urea Synthesis		
Carbamyl synthetase	−4	0
Protein Synthesis		
Amino acid-tRNA binding	−2/amino acid	0
Amino acid-tRNA bound to ribosome	−1/amino acid	0
Amino acid chain formation	0	
RNA degradation	−2	
Fatty Acid Synthesis		
Formation of methyl malonyl CoA	−1	
Fatty Acid Oxidation		
Activation of fatty acid (thiokinase)	−1	
Acyl CoA dehydrogenase (FADH)	2/acetyl unit	1
L(+), β-hydroxyacyl CoA dehydrogenase (NADH$^+$H$^+$)	3	1
Krebs cycle	24/acetyl unit	12

provided by the diet. A subject in energy and nitrogen balance is neither losing nor gaining weight. By measuring the respiratory gases one can calculate the respiratory quotient (RQ). RQ is the ratio of carbon dioxide produced to oxygen consumed.

When glucose is the sole substrate being oxidized, then the RQ is 1 since the oxidation of glucose uses and releases equal amounts of oxygen and carbon dioxide. $C_6H_{12}O_6$ is glucose.

$$C_6H_{12}O_6 + 6O_2 \rightarrow 6CO_2 + 6HOH$$

$$RQ = \frac{6CO_2}{6O_2} = 1.0$$

When fatty acids are being oxidized, the RQ is close to 0.7. This is because fatty acids require far more oxygen for their oxidation than they produce as carbon dioxide. $C_{16}H_{32}O_2$ is palmitic acid.

$$C_{16}H_{32}O_2 + 23O_2 \rightarrow 16CO_2 + 16HOH$$

$$RQ = \frac{16CO_2}{23O_2} =\sim 0.7$$

When one considers that the fatty acids are mobilized from the stored triacylglycerols and one computes the RQ on this basis, a slightly higher RQ results. For example, by using a theoretical triacylglycerol consisting of two molecules of stearic acid and one of palmitic acid attached to a glycerol backbone the equation is as follows;

$$C_{55}H_{106}O_6 + 76.5O_2 \rightarrow 55CO_2 + 53HOH$$

$$RQ = \frac{55CO_2}{76.5O_2} = 0.701$$

A molecule of glucose will, when oxidized, yield a net of 38 molecules of ATP (2 molecules of ATP are needed for glycolysis), whereas a fatty acid such as palmitate will yield a net of 129 molecules of ATP (2 molecules of ATP are needed for activation). When related to oxygen consumption, glucose produces 2 molecules of ATP for each molecule of oxygen consumed while palmitate produces ~5.6 molecules of ATP per molecule of oxygen consumed. If each ATP has an energy value of 7.6 kcal/high-energy bond, then *in vivo* glucose oxidation will yield 7.6 kcal × 38 ATP or 294.8 kcal per molecule, while palmitate will yield 7.6 kcal × 129 ATP or 980.4 kcal trapped in the high-energy bond of ATP. When palmitate is oxidized in a bomb calorimeter, 2609 kcal of heat is released per molecule. The difference in the energy released as heat in the bomb calorimeter and that captured in the high-energy bonds of the ATP is the energy lost as heat in the body plus that amount of energy captured in the bonds of CO_2 and water. If one were to make a ratio of the amount of energy captured in the ATP to that totally available (980:2609) one would find that about 38% of the total inherent energy of palmitate can be captured in the chemical bonds of ATP vs. ~62% that is released as heat and used to make CO_2 and water. Note that palmitate oxidation produces more than three times the amount of ATP than does glucose. This is the reason why fats are more dense energetically than carbohydrates. Per gram, fat provides 9 kcal and carbohydrate 4.

The ratio of glucose to fatty acids being oxidized will be reflected in the measured RQ. Most humans consuming a mixed diet will have an average RQ of about 0.87. It will vary throughout the typical feeding-fasting day-night cycle followed by most people who work during the day and sleep at night. Just before breakfast the RQ will be at its lowest while after the evening meal it will likely be at its highest. This, of course, is dependent on the composition of the meals consumed as well as on their spacing. As mentioned in the beginning of this section, the basal heat production or oxygen consumption is usually measured in the post absorptive state. This usually means a measurement made before breakfast and it also usually means that the metabolic fuel mix is that of glucose (from glycogen) plus fatty acids (from the fat depots).

C. ENERGY RETAINED

After heat production due to thermogenesis by brown fat cells and exercising muscles and the inefficiency of energy capture as described above are accounted for, two other components must be included. These are the energy that is either stored in the fat and glycogen depots or needed to sustain growth or production. This is quite straightforward. If weight is neither gained nor lost, then the energy balance (energy retained) is zero. If weight is gained as fat, the energy value of that fat must be accounted for. If the fat is deposited as preformed fat, that is, the fat in the diet is hydrolyzed at the gut, transported to the depot and reesterified for storage, the energy cost of this storage is minimal. This is a very efficient way to accumulate body fat stores. On the other hand, if glucose is used to make the stored triacylglycerols, the process is quite inefficient. In order to make one molecule of tripalmitin (palmitate is a 16-carbon fatty acid), you would need 12 molecules of glucose and 45 molecules of ATP to make 3 molecules of palmitoyl CoA. You would need another half molecule of glucose and 4 ATPs to make the glycerol phosphate. All together you would need 12.5 moles of glucose plus 49 moles of ATP to make 1 mole of tripalmitin. In order to generate the ATP in this synthesis you would have to completely oxidize 1.3 moles of glucose since one mole would only give you 38 ATPs and 49 are needed. Thus, the efficiency of energy storage as fatty acids synthesized from glucose is much less than if you stored the dietary fat in the depot and used the dietary carbohydrate to supply whatever ATP is needed. Humans consuming a mixed diet will have RQ closer to 1 than to 0.7 because these humans will oxidize glucose in preference to fatty acids. Table 6 illustrates these calculations.

Using protein for energy is even more costly and less efficient. Each amino acid that is incorporated into a polypeptide chain requires an ATP for its activation. In a protein containing several hundred amino acids the requirement for ATP is enormous. ATP is also required for the synthesis of the RNA coded for the protein being synthesized. Because protein synthesis is so energy dependent, the energy requirement to support growth (protein synthesis) can be quite large. If instead of using the amino acids from the dietary protein to synthesize body protein, they are used to provide energy, the cost of this energy must be corrected for the costs of synthesizing urea from the amino groups liberated prior to the oxidation of the amino acid carbon skeleton for energy. Approximately 20% of the gross energy of a typical protein is lost because of the need to synthesize urea.

Using dietary protein for body protein synthesis can be very efficient or very inefficient depending on the amino acid content of the diet and the body proteins being synthesized. This aspect of metabolism will be described in Unit 4. However, the energetics of protein deposition using dietary protein is quite straightforward.

TABLE 6
Efficiency of Storing Energy From Dietary Fat vs. That Using Glucose Triglyceride Synthesis (Tripalmitin) from Palmitate

Cost

6 ATP	3 pal + 3 ATP + 3 CoASH → 3 palCoA + 3 AMP (2 ATP/palmitate → pal CoA)
+4 ATP	4 ATP + 0.5 glucose → αGP + 4 ADP
	3 pal CoA + αGP → tripalmitin
10 ATP	10 ATP/38 ATP per mole glu = 0.26 moles glucose
	0.5 + 0.26 = 0.76 moles glucose + 3 moles palmitate + 10 moles ATP → 1 mole tripalmitin.

The energy cost is therefore 10 ATP, each with a value of 7.6 kcal. The total cost would be 76 kcal. If the total energy value of tripalmitin was 7597, then the efficiency of storing preformed fat would be (7597–76) ÷ 7597 or ~98%. Tripalmitin synthesis from glucose is energetically more expensive because only four of the six glucose carbons are used to make the 16-carbon fatty acid, palmitate. It will take 4 glucoses to make 1 palmitate and 12 glucoses to make 3 palmitates.

$$12 \text{ glucose} + 45 \text{ ATP} + O_2 \rightarrow 3 \text{ palmityl CoA} + 24 \text{ CO}_2$$

$$0.5 \text{ glucose} \frac{+4 \text{ ATP}}{49 \text{ ATP}} \rightarrow \alpha\text{-glycerophosphate} + \text{ADP}$$

$$3 \text{ palmityl CoA} + \alpha\text{-glycerophosphate} \rightarrow \text{tripalmitin}$$

1 mol of glucose, completely oxidized, yields 38 ATP. 49 are needed ∴ 49/38 = 1.3 mol of glucose are needed to provide the ATP or 1.3 × 294.8 = 383.24; 12 + 0.5 + 1.3 = 13.8 mol of glucose needed to produce 1 mol of tripalmitin; each glucose has a value of 294.8 kcal.

The cost of making tripalmitin would be 383.24 kcal. The efficiency would therefore be $(7597 - 383.24) \div 7597 = {\sim}95\%$. However, if you computed this cost using the energy value of tripalmitin (7597 kcal) corrected for the energy value of all the glucose needed to make the palmityl CoA and all the ATP used, the cost would be $(7597 - 4068 - 383.24) \div 7597$ or 41% of the total energy value of the tripalmitin.

Disregarding amino acid oxidation and urea formation and the growth process, if one examines the energetic efficiency of protein turnover, one finds an efficiency of about 82%. This figure is arrived at using the assumption that the dietary protein is used completely *and exclusively* to replace degraded body protein. For the sake of ease of description, the amount of protein degraded and replaced is 100 g. This 100 g would have a gross energy value of 570 kcal or ${\sim}2383$ kJ. For every amino acid incorporated into this protein, 5 ATPs would be used plus 1.2 ATPs for rearrangements of the structure. This would mean an energy cost of about 694 kcal or ${\sim}2902$ kJ. Dividing the energy value of the protein produced by the cost of its production $\left(\dfrac{570}{694} \text{ or } \dfrac{2383}{2902} \right)$ we have an efficiency of about 82%. Practically speaking, for the average human adult in the U.S., the energy efficiency of protein turnover is of little importance. The typical U.S. diet is not limiting with respect to protein or energy.

D. ENERGETIC EFFICIENCY

The food which provides the energy does so by providing fuel for oxidation to provide heat, ATP, CO_2, and water. The heat which is produced through this oxidation is needed to keep the body warm, but it is also a measure of the energy need. That is, the heat that is produced (and which can be measured) is the energy that is lost from the body and must be replaced. For example, if a molecule of palmitate is oxidized in a bomb calorimeter, the amount of heat released is 2609 kcal. However, when oxidized in the body, it yields 130 ATPs, 146 molecules of water, and 1384 kcal of heat—38% of the inherent energy of palmitate is trapped by the body when this fuel is used and 62% is released as heat. This 40/60 (rounded figures) distribution of energy available to the body vs. that released as heat is an average distribution. More or less in each category can occur. The pattern of distribution is influenced by the composition of the diet and the genetics of the consumer. An example of the former occurs when an essential fatty acid deficient diet is fed. This deficiency state is characterized by a decrease in the use of food for body weight gain.

Feed efficiency is a term used to designate the efficiency with which an animal (or human) uses the food it consumes to build new tissue as it grows or rebuild body tissue that is lost through the normal conditions of life. Those animals that can gain more body weight on less food are more efficient than those animals that require more food for the same gain. Meat animal production research has been devoted to increasing energetic efficiency using dietary and nondietary techniques. Selective breeding, for example, of beef animals has resulted in bovines that grow rapidly and consume less food per pound of weight gained than animals used for this purpose a century ago. Whereas it used to take three years to produce a bovine of a size suitable for use, it now takes two years or less to produce a meat animal ready for market. Furthermore, the meat produced today is of high quality in terms of tenderness, flavor, and nutrient content compared to that produced 100 years ago. Other meat animals (sheep, pigs, chickens, goats) likewise have been selectively bred to produce a rapidly growing energetically efficient animal. With the growing emphasis today on the production of meat with a lower fat content, animal scientists are continuing to use genetics and dietary maneuvers to produce an animal that meets the consumers' demands.

Just as the diet and genetics of the meat animal determine its energetic efficiency, so too can one expect these same effects in humans. Genetic and dietary factors interact and, in so doing, determine the rate and extent of longitudinal growth as well as the development of muscle mass and fat mass. At present, the segregation of humans by genotype is not possible. However, genes that appear to be important in the development of obesity (excess fat mass) are being identified. How diet, particularly the sources of energy, can affect the phenotypic expression of these obesity related genes is not known.

E. UTILIZABLE ENERGY

The energy expended to do the body's work is referred to as utilizable energy. This is the energy used by muscles as they contract in the course of voluntary activity or work. This energy is sometimes referred to as the activity increment. That is, it is energy cost associated with body movement which is added to the basal energy need when the energy requirement is calculated. For sedentary persons only a small increment is needed, but for very active persons a large increment will be needed to sustain their activity. As much as a 200% increment above basal energy need may be required to sustain a high level of activity and maintain body weight. Shown in Table 7 are some representative activities and their associated energy cost given as heat units per kilogram body weight per hour. In the course of muscle contraction, oxygen is used for the oxidation of metabolic fuels by the working muscle. Heat is released and water plus carbon dioxide is produced. The more active a person is, the more oxygen is needed for the oxidation of metabolic fuel by the muscle.

Trained athletes are more efficient in their use of metabolic fuels than are untrained, sedentary individuals. Training involves an increase in use of specific muscle groups as well as an increase in lung and heart action. Muscle contraction, which is usually supported by the oxidation of glucose (from blood glucose or glycogen breakdown) in the sedentary person, can use fatty acids as fuel after training. During exercise, the respiratory quotient (RQ) in the trained individual decreases. This means that fat is being oxidized since the oxidation of fatty acids results in a lower RQ than the oxidation of glucose. Fatty acid oxidation by working muscle will spare glucose and will decrease the rate of lactate production. The muscle does not store large amount of lipid for use during work but it can use the fatty acids liberated from the fat depots through the action of the catabolic hormones. Part of training is to increase muscle fatty acid oxidation while also increasing the glycogen-glucose reserve in the muscle. The so-called glycogen loading technique dictates the exhaustion of the muscle glycogen store, followed by rest and glycogen repletion just prior to the competitive event. During the rest/repletion period a high carbohydrate diet is consumed. This exhaustion/repletion routine results in an increased supply of glucose from glycogen within the muscle. Since the first phase of glycolysis is anaerobic, an enlarged supply of glucose from glycogen can be oxidized in the absence of oxygen and thus exhaustion which is characterized by an oxygen debt is delayed. Training or adaptation to exercise or work is thus characterized by a decrease in RQ due to both an increase in the oxidation of fatty acids and an increase in the anaerobic use of glucose from glycogen. Table 8 summarizes the effects of exercise on metabolism while Table 9 gives some typical results of a comparison of trained and untrained subjects with respect to their oxygen and glucose use during a bout of exercise. Note that the untrained and trained subjects consumed the same amount of oxygen, but the trained subjects had a lower RQ. This means that the trained subjects were oxidizing some fatty acids. That fatty acids were used is seen in the last column showing that the trained subjects consumed less glucose per minute than did the untrained subjects.

F. DIET-INDUCED THERMOGENESIS

Another way energy is lost from the body as heat is the heat associated with the oxidation of food (diet-induced thermogenesis). Formerly, it was thought that this heat was associated with the degradation of the food components in preparation for its use by the body for its maintenance. Now, however, there seems to be another explanation having to do with a special tissue in the body called brown fat.

TABLE 7
Energy Cost of Activities Exclusive of Basal Metabolism and Influence of Food

Activity	kcal/kg/hr	Activity	kcal/kg/hr
Bedmaking	3.0	Playing cards	0.5
Bicycling (racing)	7.6	Playing ping pong	4.4
Bicycling (moderate speed)	2.5	Piano playing (Mendelssohn's *Song Without Words*)	0.8
Boxing	11.4	Piano playing (Beethoven's *Appassionata*)	1.4
Carpentry (heavy)	2.3	Piano playing (Liszt's *Tarantella*)	2.0
Cello playing	1.3	Reading aloud	0.4
Cleaning windows	2.6	Rowing	9.8
Crocheting	0.4	Rowing in race	16.0
Dancing, waltz	3.0	Running	7.0
Dishwashing	1.0	Sawing wood	5.7
Dressing and undressing	0.7	Sewing, hand	0.4
Driving car	0.9	Sewing, electric machine	0.4
Eating	0.4	Singing in loud voice	0.8
Exercise, very light	0.9	Sitting quietly	0.4
Light	1.4	Skating	3.5
Moderate	3.1	Skiing (moderate speed)	10.3
Severe	5.4	Standing at attention	0.6
Very severe	7.6	Standing relaxed	0.5
Fencing	7.3	Sweeping with broom, bare floor	1.4
Football	6.8	Sweeping with carpet sweeper	1.6
Gardening, weeding	3.9	Sweeping with vacuum sweeper	2.7
Golf	1.5	Swimming (2 mi per hr)	7.9
Horseback riding, walk	1.4	Tailoring	0.9
Horseback riding, trot	4.3	Tennis	5.0
Horseback riding, gallop	6.7	Typing, rapidly	1.0
Ironing (5-lb iron)	1.0	Typing, electric typewriter	0.5
Knitting sweater	0.7	Violin playing	0.6
Laboratory work	2.1	Walking (3 mi per hr)	2.0
Laundry, light	1.3	Walking rapidly (4 mi per hr)	3.4
Lying still, awake	0.1	Walking at high speed (5.3 mi per hr)	8.3
Office work, standing	0.6	Washing floors	1.2
Organ playing (1/3 handwork)	1.5	Writing	0.4
Painting furniture	1.5		
Paring potatoes	0.6		

TABLE 8
Summary of the Effects of Training on Metabolism and Body Composition

Decreased RQ during exercise
Decreased fat mass
Increased muscle mass[a]
Increased fatty acid mobilization during exercise
Increased glucose synthesis by the liver
Increased aerobic capacity of muscle
Improved glucose tolerance
Decreased need for insulin to facilitate glucose use

[a]   May be localized; depends on the types of muscles used for the activity.

TABLE 9
Effect of Training on Oxygen Uptake
and Fuel Use

Subject	O₂ (L)	RQ $\dfrac{[CO_2]}{[O_2]}$	Glucose used (mmol/min)
Trained	3.0	0.90	10.6
Untrained	3.0	0.95	13.3

Brown fat depots are located at the base of the neck, along the backbone and, in males, across the shoulders. Males and females differ in the distribution of these depots, as shown in Figure 12.

The brown fat cell differs from the white fat cell in that it contains many more mitochondria in the cytosol than does the white cell. Both cell types have stored lipid droplets which, if sufficiently large, can push all of the other organelles off to the sides of the cell. In contrast to the white cell depots, the brown fat depots are highly innervated and vascularized, as shown in Figure 13. This increase in vascularization gives the depot its brownish color and name, brown fat.

As described above, much of the structure of the white cell is similar to that of the brown fat cell. Both cell types can store lipid that can be readily mobilized in times of energy deficit. However, the brown fat when it mobilizes its stored lipid, oxidizes its lipid *in situ* rather than releasing it for utilization by other tissues. Furthermore, because the brown fat cell has many more mitochondria than the white fat cell, it produces more heat during metabolism than does the white fat cell. This process is called thermogenesis. In addition to the larger number of mitochondria in the brown fat cell, the fat in the brown fat cell is in smaller discrete droplets.

Whereas white depots are distributed throughout the body, brown depots are found in just a few locations (Figure 12). More brown fat can be observed in newborns than in adults and it is thought that thermoregulation in the immature animal is dependent on the activity of the brown fat depot with respect to its ability to generate heat. Brown fat cells, if allowed to accumulate lipid, may change in appearance and look like white fat as the lipid droplets enlarge. Histochemical studies have failed to reveal any qualitative differences between the two cell types.

In the newborn, brown adipose tissue has the function of generating heat as part of the body's thermoregulatory process. This is particularly important at this age because newborns lack the insulation provided by the subcutaneous fat store. This fat layer helps conserve body heat. In addition, the newborn's metabolic processes are relatively immature with respect to energy conservation. Heat loss from these processes can be quite large. Thermoregulation therefore is quite dependent on the thermogenic capacity of the brown fat. Brown fat thermogenesis (BAT) is also thought to be a means for ridding the body of excess intake energy. It has been proposed that one of the ways a body maintains a constancy in body weight in the face of inconsistent food energy intake is through this process. On days where intake energy exceeds need, the surplus energy is released as heat via brown fat thermogenesis.

It has been suggested that genetically obese individuals become obese because they are unable to increase their heat production when overfed or when suddenly thrust into a cold environment. It has been hypothesized further that the genetically obese animal develops the subcutaneous fat pads as insulation against heat loss or gain, thereby circumventing their relative inability to thermoregulate. In order to increase their insulation layer, they must overeat in order to provide the requisite substrates for lipogenesis. Such an hypothesis has some elements of validity. The ob/ob mouse, for example, is unusually sensitive to cold and

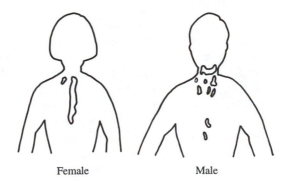

Female   Male

FIGURE 12. Location of the brown fat depots.

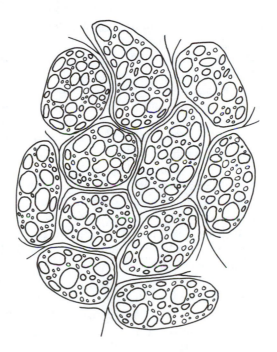

FIGURE 13. High vascularization of brown fat depots.

is incapable of increasing its heat production when exposed to cold or injected with epineph-rine. These features of the ob/ob mouse precede the development of both hyperphagia (overeating) and obesity. Since the mobilization of body fuel (induction of lipolysis and glycogenolysis) is not abnormal in the obese ob/ob mouse, it would appear that only the release of heat when these fuels are oxidized is defective. In other words, more energy is trapped in the chemical bonds of high-energy compounds than is released as heat. This, of course, is related to the increased energetic efficiency of these animals as well, since they also gain more fat per unit food consumed (and release less heat) than lean animals.

Impaired thermoregulation has been reported in genetically obese Zucker rats. Lower body temperatures in the neonates and an impaired ability to increase thermogenesis in response to overeating, cold exposure, or to epinephrine has been reported in a variety of genetically obese animal models. Several scientists have suggested that obese humans may also have this defect. When stimulated by cold or infusions of epinephrine, normal weight subjects increased their heat production while obese subjects did not. Normal weight humans appear to regulate their body fat mass by increasing their brown fat heat production when overfed. Stock and Rothwell developed an animal model to study the effects of overfeeding on brown fat thermogenesis. They showed that when offered a variety of energy-rich snack foods, normal animals increased their heat production to maintain a normal weight. However, this mechanism is far from perfect in that, over time, these overfed animals did become fatter than did their control-fed littermates. Nonetheless, the observation that brown fat can adjust its heat production in response to fluctuations in the energy intake is a very interesting facet of its function within the body. The mechanism whereby its heat production is increased involves the synthesis and release of an uncoupling protein called UCP or thermogenin. This protein is unique to the mitochondria of brown fat cells. It is not found in any other cell type. This protein is not always present and active. In the starved animal, for example, it cannot be found. This means that heat production by the brown fat, or brown fat thermogenesis (BAT), can be switched on and off. Thermogenin synthesis is rapid. Exposure to cold or hyperthyroidism or birth or starvation-refeeding triggers a rapid and marked increase of messenger RNA for this protein as well as a marked increase in the level of the protein. In most animals, the increase in the level of thermogenin parallels an increase in nonshivering thermogenesis. In lean animals, surplus food intake seems to signal thermogenin synthesis. The regulation of thermogenin synthesis occurs at the level of messenger RNA transcription.

Thermogenin is a small protein having 306 amino acid residues. The gene which codes for its synthesis has been isolated and sequenced. The protein completely traverses the inner mitochondrial membrane and has a C-terminal region that projects from the outer surface of the membrane. It works by dissipating the proton gradient that is developed when pairs of reducing equivalents are passed down the respiratory chain to make water. The energy that is developed by the respiratory chain is not captured in the high-energy bond of ATP, but instead is released as heat. The control of its uncoupling function is through the external C-terminal region that contains the nucleotide (ADP) binding site. If the thermogenin binds the nucleotide, it is not available to the F_1F_0 ATP synthase for ATP synthesis. Fatty acids interact with the nucleotide binding site such that ADP binding is increased. These fatty acids are released from the stored triacylglycerols via a hormone-stimulated cyclic AMP mechanism. This explains how epinephrine can stimulate BAT. Epinephrine works by increasing the cAMP levels in the cytosol. This, in turn, stimulates the activity of the cytosolic lipoprotein lipase which serves to release the fatty acids from the stored lipid. Norepinephrine is particularly effective with respect to intracellular fatty acid release in the brown fat. Other lipolytic hormones that work through increasing adenylate cyclase activity and cAMP levels also work to increase BAT. Diets rich in polyunsaturated fatty acids potentiate these hormone effects on BAT.

While insulin is not thought of as a lipolytic hormone, it too has a role in regulating the synthesis and activity of thermogenin and BAT. Both the synthesis of the uncoupling protein and the ability of brown adipose tissue to assist in the regulation of body temperature and dissipate the energy provided by excess food intake is impaired in the insulin-deficient animal. Once insulin is restored, the impairment is corrected. Of interest is the observation that many genetically obese rats and mice are hyperinsulinemic, yet they have impaired BAT.

III. ABNORMAL ENERGY STATES

A. STARVATION AND UNDERNUTRITION

The basic metabolic response of an otherwise healthy individual to starvation is conservation. As the gut receives less food, it slowly empties. First the stomach, then the duodenum, the jejunum, the ileum, and the large intestine lose their contents and shrink in size. Simple mono- and disaccharides are the first to disappear followed by the products of the progressively more complex nutrients: polysaccharides, proteins, and lipids. As the sugars disappear, there is less stimulus for insulin release and basal insulin levels are approached. As glucose is less available from the gut the body begins to mobilize its glycogen stores, and when they are close to being depleted the body will begin to mobilize its stores of triacylglycerol and, to a lesser extent, its body protein. It can use certain of the amino acids and glycerol from the triacylglycerols to synthesize glucose via gluconeogenesis and utilize the carbon skeletons of deaminated amino acids plus the fatty acids liberated from the triacylglycerols for fuel. In 1915, Benedict, in an extensive monograph on the metabolic responses to starvation, reported that the body carbohydrate (glycogen and glucose) provided only a small fraction of the total fuel needed for maintenance. Cahill later estimated that a 70-kg man had approximately 75 g of glycogen stored in the muscle and liver which provides approximately 300 Calories during the initial 24 hours of starvation. The glycogen plus the glucose synthesized via gluconeogenesis thus provide only a small percentage of the 2000 to 2500 calories needed per day for maintenance. Benedict estimated that mobilizable body protein could provide about 15% of the body's fuel needs and that the fat stores of the adipose tissue provided the rest. Although Benedict did not have today's sophisticated technology at his disposal, his estimates were remarkably close to those of Cahill. Cahill estimated that a "normal" 70-kg man required about 2000 calories per day to maintain his body and that he had sufficient fuel stores to sustain life for about 80 days. As shown in Figure 14, adapted from Cahill's paper, most of the energy comes from the lipid stored in the adipose tissue.

These lipids, primarily triacylglycerols, are hydrolyzed to fatty acids and glycerol through the action of hormone-sensitive lipase. This enzyme, located on the interior aspect of the fat cell membrane, is activated by the catabolic hormones, epinephrine and glucocorticoid, and its activity is increased when glucagon is high and insulin is low. The glycerol is converted to glucose via gluconeogenesis in the liver and kidney. The fatty acids are oxidized to ketones and then to carbon dioxide and water. Whereas the liver can oxidize the fatty acids completely to carbon dioxide and water, the muscle is unable to do so and thus ketones, the end products of muscle fatty acid oxidation, rise. These ketones can be used by the brain as a fuel when the supply of glucose becomes more limited. After about 40 days of starvation, the brain has been shown to obtain nearly 65% of its energy from the ketones. These fuel fluxes are diagrammed in Figure 15. Under normal (i.e., fed) conditions, the central nervous system uses 115 g of glucose/day while erythrocytes, bone marrow, renal medulla and peripheral nerves use about 36 g of glucose/day. Most of this glucose can be synthesized through gluconeogenesis from glycerol, lactate, and selected amino acids during the early phase of starvation. However, as the starvation continues, the body attempts to protect its protein component and the amino acid substrates for gluconeogenesis become less available. This, coupled with the rising ketone level (ketones can cross the blood-brain barrier), serves to induce the utilization of the ketones by the brain as a metabolic fuel.

Proteolysis, initially increased, after 48 hours of starvation is suppressed by rising levels of growth hormone as the body attempts to conserve its body proteins. The initial proteolysis, however, serves to provide the needed amino acids for the synthesis of enzymes needed for survival (enzymes needed for energy mobilization and conservation). Once these mechanisms are established, body protein is conserved. The temporal relationship of fuels and the hormones which control their availability is diagrammed in Figure16.

B. PROTEIN ENERGY MALNUTRITION

Starvation is the extreme state of malnutrition that occurs when the individual is provided little or no food to nourish the body. Between starvation and the state of adequate nourishment to meet nutrient needs there are graded levels of inadequate nutrient intake. Although infants and children of third-world nations come to mind when malnutrition is pictured, people of all ages in all countries are vulnerable. Where the intake of macronutrients is inadequate the syndrome is called protein-calorie malnutrition or more correctly, protein energy malnutrition.

Chronic malnutrition is characterized not only by energy deficit (energy need exceeding energy intake) but also by a deficit in the protein intake and the intake of micronutrients. The needs for these nutrients and energy are determined by the age and health status of the individual.

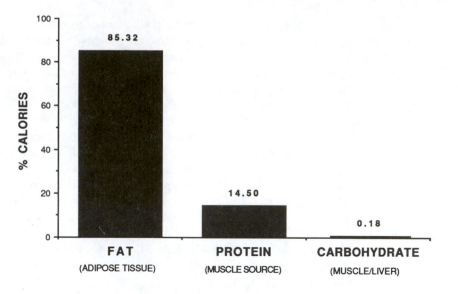

FIGURE 14. Sources of metabolic fuel for a starving human. The lipid utilized is primarily the fatty acids released from triacylglycerol by the adipose tissue depots. The protein is mainly that raided from the muscle. And the carbohydrate utilized is that released by the liver and muscle glycogen and that synthesized by the kidney and liver via gluconeogenesis.

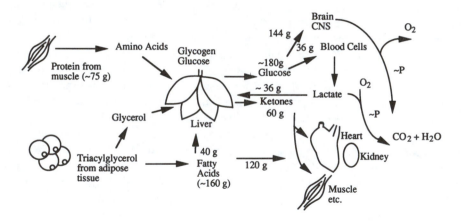

FIGURE 15. Intertissue fuel fluxes after 24 hours of starvation. Note the central position of the liver. This organ uses glycerol, lactate, fatty acids, and amino acids to produce ketones and glucose which serve as fuel sources for blood cells, the brain and central nervous system, heart, kidney, and muscle. These fuels are oxidized to carbon dioxide and water, requiring only the presence of molecular oxygen and energy from the high-energy phosphate bonds as provided by adenine and guanine nucleotides.

Rapid growth, infection, injury, and chronic debilitating disease can drive up the need for food and the nutrients it contains. Infants and young children have been described as having protein-calorie malnutrition, abbreviated as PCM. The characteristics of PCM are described in Unit 4.

Just as infection or trauma potentiates the needs for protein, energy, and micronutrients in third-world children, so too do these conditions increase the need for nutrients in developed nations. Injury and sepsis both increase energy needs. Suffice it to say that both adults and children may have increased nutrient needs under these circumstances and if these needs are not met varying degrees of malnutrition or PCM will be observed. Malnutrition has been documented in hospitalized patients in the U.S. and this malnutrition may have a negative effect on the time course of recovery as well as on mortality.

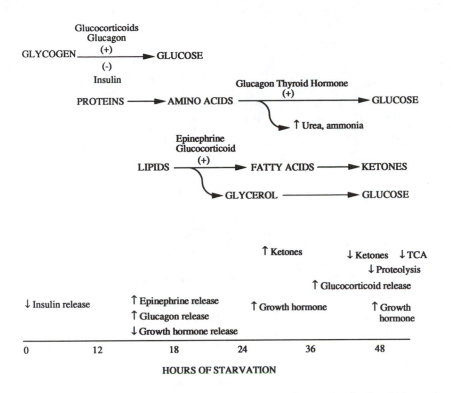

FIGURE 16. Temporal relations of fuel and hormones during starvation. During the first 24 hours there is a decrease in blood glucose levels and an increase in proteolysis. After 18 hours, measurable increases in gluconeogenesis due to glucose production from glycerol can be observed. There is a rise in lipolysis initially stimulated by epinephrine, but then maintained by rising glucocorticoid, glucagon, and lastly, by growth hormone levels. As the levels of these hormones rise, they serve to decrease peripheral tissue sensitivity to insulin and decreased glucose tolerance can be observed. With rising growth hormone levels, proteolysis is decreased and the body attempts to conserve body protein. By 48 hours, ketosis, having been high, now begins to decline as the body adapts to using ketones and fatty acids as its metabolic fuel.

C. TRAUMA AND ENERGY NEEDS

Since Cuthbertson first described the body's disproportionate catabolic response to trauma, physicians, nutritionists, and physiologists alike have accepted this response as an obligatory and necessary response to illness or injury. With the advent of parenteral and enteral feeding techniques it has been possible to show that this loss, formerly thought to be obligatory, is not. Indeed, losses due to surgery, infection, or burn have been shown to be minimized and even reversed (in some cases) with the provision of adequate nutritional support. This implies, then, that the catabolic response to trauma or illness is more a response to inadequate nutrition in the face of a greatly increased set of nutrient requirements than to the trauma or illness itself.

The endocrine and metabolic responses to injury are closely related (Figure 17). Increased production of some hormones and the inhibited release of other hormones are integral parts of the body's basic defense mechanisms. The primary function of this mechanism is to provide a continuous fuel supply to the central nervous system and the required substrates for the repair of body tissue. While the body may respond to trauma with an increased release of the hormones that regulate metabolism through cAMP or through the phosphatidyl inositol cycle, this response, in comparison with the overall metabolic response to injury or illness, is relatively short lived. It appears, therefore, that the hormonal responses to injury serve as initiators or inducers of metabolic events that must occur if recovery is to proceed. As relief from the trauma occurs, these hormonal responses recede and other metabolic control mechanisms assume command. These, in turn, give way to the normal metabolic control mechanisms

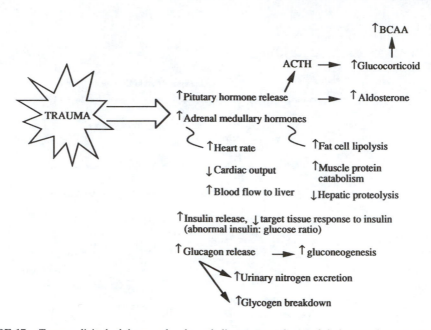

FIGURE 17. Trauma elicits both hormonal and metabolic responses that result in increased energy need.

as recovery proceeds. Aging patients and children likely will have an exaggerated metabolic response to trauma compared to young, otherwise healthy adults. Although the sequence of hormonal and metabolic response may be similar, the time frame and intensity of response will differ. Sometimes these differences can be life threatening if close monitoring is not practiced. The elderly may already have peripheral tissue insulin resistance which is made worse by the trauma. The child may be more likely to quickly exhaust energy stores and have little reserve. In each instance the difference between death and survival may rest with the provision of adequate nutrition support in terms of amounts of energy, glucose, and amino acids, plus appropriate amounts of insulin to facilitate the return to normal fuel homeostasis.

The temporal changes in the choice of metabolic fuels are characterized by subtle transitions from one fuel source to another. These are orchestrated by the hormonal response to the trauma or infection which in turn may be influenced by the pre-injury nutritional status of the patient and the nutrients provided during the recovery period.

Basal energy requirements can increase by as much as 200% in traumatized patients. Part of this increase in energy requirements can be attributed to the thermogenic effects of the catecholamines released in response to injury. In addition, increases in the energy requirement may be due to the increased energy needed to support protein synthesis. Protein synthesis is highly dependent on energy intake. New proteins are needed for tissue repair and for the inflammatory and immunologic responses of the body to infection or injury or both. If the diet is inadequate, the synthesis of these proteins occurs at the expense of muscle protein. The amino acids not used for protein synthesis are deaminated and the resulting ammonia is converted to urea. Urea production, likewise, is energetically expensive. Thus, large increases in both protein synthesis and ureogenesis represent an increase in the basal energy requirement and an increase in the protein requirement in the traumatized or severely ill individual. Unless this additional energy and protein is provided, weight loss will occur.

D. OBESITY

Although excess body fat stores, or obesity, is considered a risk factor in a number of diseases, we have no permanent cure for the disorder. Research on the genetic basis for excess body fatness is very active. Several investigators have shown that the familial trait for body fatness has a much stronger influence on body size than environmental influences such as culture, socioeconomic status, or food intake patterns. Studies of monozygotic and dizygotic twins reared by their biological parents or by adoptive parents have been conducted. In one study, adopted children and their biological and adoptive parents were compared with respect to body weight and body fatness while in other studies twins reared together or apart were compared. All these studies showed that the genetic influence far outweighed the environmental influence. Further, a number of genetically obese rats, mice, dogs, and desert animals have been described. In the rodent species, the mode of inheritance and, in some instances, the chromosomal location of genes for obesity have been identified. Obesity can be inherited via an autosomal recessive or dominant or sex-linked trait. There are several mutations that are phenotypically expressed as obesity. In each of these mutations, an error occurs that affects energy balance. Errors in the perception of hunger and/or satiety by the brain can explain the excess food intake (hyperphagia) that characterizes several of these mutants. Both inappropriate hunger signals and satiety signals have been implicated. Higher than normal food intake may also characterize the genetically obese human. Yet, there are many overly fat people who are not hyperphagic. There are those who cannot dissipate their surplus intake energy as heat, i.e., thermogenesis (see Section II.F). These individuals do not tolerate cold well, either. The common thread to these two conditions is the apparent inability of the brown fat to uncouple its mitochondria so as to release heat rather than synthesize ATP, which in turn transfers its energy to the synthesis of fat. It has also been attributed to a failure of the brown fat cell to respond to the stimulatory effects of epinephrine and is associated with an anomalous central regulation of the sympathetic input to this tissue.

As mentioned in the section on anorexia (Section III.A), hormonal balance is important to the regulation of energy balance and normal body weight. Hypercortisolism and hyperinsulinism are associated with obesity. Cortisol and its related compounds, corticosterone and cortisone, play an important role in the regulation of lipogenesis. While these hormones are usually catabolic hormones, there are circumstances when they stimulate anabolic processes, such as fat synthesis.

Lastly, there are social and cultural influences that can ensure or potentiate genetic tendencies to develop obesity. Anthropologists and medical historians have identified examples of cultural groups that consider excess body fat as a mark of beauty as well as an indication of economic status within their society. Examples of this are the various statuary of different ages all the way from the upper Paleolithic period through the Renaissance to the 18th and 19th century. Women have been represented with large bellies and breasts; they are to the eye of the contemporary observer, overfat. Men too, are of ample proportions. In fact, there is an old German expression that indicates the desire of men to have, as wives, overweight women: "A fat wife and a full barn never did a man harm." Even today there are cultures, notably in Africa, that have customs that include preparing girls for marriage by fattening them. Malcom, for example, described this practice for elite Efik girls in traditional Nigeria as well as the custom in Kenya of demanding high bride prices for fat brides. In these cultures, female fatness may not only be a testament to the families' wealth, it may also be a symbol of maternity and nurturance. This is important to the woman if the only way she gains status is through motherhood. A fat woman is thus assumed to be very maternal and nurturing.

With respect to societally determined fatness and the values of fatness, it can be assumed that the fatter a person is in a society that values fatness, the more likely that person will be married and produce children carrying genetic tendencies to be fat and who will be similarly taught to eat enough to be fat also. Lean people will be less likely to contribute to the gene pool because they will be considered as less desirable mates. While people in the U.S. as well as other developed nations may not have these values, there is no doubt that eating behaviors can be taught. If young children are constantly reminded and coached to overeat, there may be a continuing stimulus to overconsume food. Added to this may be cultural and social dictates with respect to physical activity. A decrease in energy expenditure ensures a positive energy balance which, in turn, may well result in excess body fatness.

Frequently, those who are overfat are told that they could become lean if they would reduce their food intake. However, simply restricting one's food intake does not cure the problem; it merely treats the result of the positive energy balance: excess body fat. Once this fat is lost, the formerly obese person frequently abandons the restricted diet and returns to his/her previous eating habits, and as a result returns to his/her prior weight. In some, there may also be an increase in body fatness, not just a return to the prior body weight.

1. Set Point Theory in Body Weight Regulation

The idea that each body has its own unique size and weight has been discussed, denied, and supported by a wide variety of researchers. The hypothesis that adult body weight is closely regulated at its own unique level developed from observations of both humans and animals. The mechanism(s) that serve to regulate this steady-state body weight are not fully known.

Healthy adult humans vary very little over the years in their body weight. They may be overweight and/or overfat but, for most humans, that weight is maintained for years until some event occurs that results in a body weight change. In women, pregnancy, a perfectly normal physiological event, may perturb the system sufficiently to establish a new steady-state body weight (or new set point) which, again, will be defended tenaciously. A change in the endocrine system, an insult to the body, or a conscious decision to eat more (or less) over a prolonged period (months to years) are other examples of events which might perturb the system sufficiently to result in a new set point — a new body weight which is maintained from that time on.

Similarly, animals appear to regulate their body weight within fairly tight limits. Much of the research on the set point hypothesis had used rats and mice. Studies using rats that were either overfed or underfed revealed that these rats had a body weight that was related to their food intake. That is, if they were forced to consume more calories than they would voluntarily consume, they would become overfat. If they were underfed, they would be leaner than normal. After these feeding treatments were discontinued, the rats that were overfed significantly reduced their food intake and used their fat stores to provide their energy needs, while those rats that were underfed dramatically increased their voluntary food intake until they gained the weight they would have gained had they not been food restricted. When both these groups of rats attained the weight of their untreated controls they resumed normal feeding behavior.

Although the body weight returned to normal in these overfed or underfed rats after the treatment was terminated, the composition of the body was not the same as their untreated counterparts. The percent of the body that was fat was affected. Those rats that were underfed recovered by significantly increasing the synthesis and deposition of body fat. This recovery was faster than the recovery of body protein. In the overfed rats, the carcass protein normalized within days of cessation of the overfeeding yet the carcass fat content remained elevated weeks after overfeeding ended.

Other studies have used parabiotic rats or mice to study the consequences of overfeeding or underfeeding on body weight and composition. Parabiosis is a technique where two weanling animals are joined together surgically at the skin so that they have a common circulation. Hervey, Harris, and others have used this technique to answer the question of whether there are blood-borne factors that are involved in the regulation of feeding and body weight. Genetically obese animals have been joined to genetically lean ones, as have normal weight partners in which one partner was either overfed or underfed or was lesioned in either the feeding center of the hypothalamus or the satiety center. In each of these instances, the feeding behavior of both as well as their body weight and composition were monitored. In each instance where the one partner overate and became obese, the other underate or starved and subsequently lost its body fat as well as its lean body tissue. These results were interpreted as indications that there are blood-borne factors generated by the fat store that signal the feeding behavior. In addition, there are a number of rodents (as well as other species) that carry a mutation in their genetic material that expresses itself as obesity. A number of mutations have been identified. Some are characterized by hyperphagia (abnormally increased food intake) and some are diabetic as well as obese. Still others are hypertensive and obese. Some develop renal disease while others do not. The range of phenotypes is large, suggesting that more than one mutation can exist having obesity as part of its phenotype. The results of studies using hyperphagic genetically obese animals suggested that these obese animals either did not send or receive appropriate satiety signals or were not able to respond to them by decreasing their food intake. Likely, the nonresponsivity (that is, an error in the signaling system) is the explanation since parabiotic pairs using genetically lean and obese rats behaved like the force-fed and voluntary feeding pairs. While the genetically obese partner was hyperphagic and obese, the lean partner ceased eating and eventually starved to death.

It is apparent that although there may be controls that influence feeding and body weight, these controls may not fully regulate body fatness. That is, body weight may be set but body fat may change depending on food intake and physical activity. This may explain why aging humans may gain body fat while decreasing food intake to maintain their body weight. As humans age, they decrease their physical activity and their body composition changes; they lose muscle mass and gain body fat. Their body shape changes as well. They may observe an increase in the size of their fat mass in the abdomen and on the thighs and buttocks. Again, epidemiologists have noted the differences in health risks associated with the location of the excess fat stores; the so-called apple and pear shapes. Those persons whose fat stores are distributed equally between storage sites on shoulders, arms, abdomen, hips, and thighs are said to be "apples". Their risk of developing obesity-associated disorders is greater than that in people who have accumulated fat stores at sites below the waist, the "pears". The depots differ in the degree of fatty acid turnover. That is, they differ in how readily they can release their stored fat for use by other tissues. In humans, studies of cells isolated from the femoral, gluteal, and omental (thigh, buttocks, abdomen) depots revealed significant differences in free fatty acid release. On the basis of the rate of free fatty acid release and the size of the depots, the half life of the fat depot in the femoral area was calculated to be 305 days. For the gluteal depot it was 326 days and for the omental depot it was 134 days. Estimates of the half life of the fat in the other depot sites have not been made. An estimate of half life is the estimate of time needed to exhaust one half of the fat store. As the human uses the stored lipid, more lipid is synthesized to replace that which was used. Hence, the term fatty acid turnover means that fatty acids are both used and replaced. If they are used at a greater rate than they are replaced, a net fat loss will occur. As can be seen, however, different depots will shrink at different rates depending on their location. In addition to the aforementioned differences in depot fat use, there are also genetic and sex differences in the extent and location of the fat depots. Women, for example, have larger subcutaneous fat stores than men. Men have larger omental fat depots than women of the same age and weight.

2. Morbidity of Severely Obese People

Health care professionals have observed countless instances of the codevelopment of excess body fat with diabetes mellitus, hypertension, and cardiovascular disease. Epidemiologists have reported that obesity and overweight are risk factors in the development of these diseases. However, there are some inconsistencies with respect to the relationship of obesity to cardiovascular disease and total mortality. Studies by the CDC and those by Sjostrom suggest that weight loss by the obese may not positively affect life span. Long-term studies of mortality by formerly obese people conducted by Williamson et al. of the CDC suggest the reverse. Their preliminary report indicates an increase in mortality in people who have consciously reduced their body fat and remained lean. This report has raised serious questions about the efficacy of weight loss with respect to life span extension.

3. Treatment of Obesity

In almost no other area of medicine have there been so many failures as have occurred in the treatment of obesity. Fully 90% of all those who lose weight regain it. Data from the Chicago Gas and Electric Study suggest that one cycle of loss and regain is a risk factor for death from coronary heart disease independent of body fatness. The gain-loss group when compared to subjects who neither gained nor lost weight had 1.8 times the risk of death from heart disease. This suggests that weight cycling is not a healthy behavior. If weight is to be lost, it must stay lost if health benefits are to be gained. Often this does not occur. Weight cycling consists of intermittent periods of food restriction followed by periods of "normal" eating patterns. These patterns may include periods of gorging or binge eating. One of the major effects of Calorie restriction on metabolism is a reduction in the resting metabolic rate (RMR). This lowers the overall energy requirement and increases energy efficiency, thus allowing a greater percentage of dietary Calories to be partitioned into fat synthesis upon refeeding.

The effects of weight cycling on energy efficiency may be due to the composition of the weight loss during Calorie restriction. One of the consequences of rapid weight loss, especially when induced by very low-Calorie low-carbohydrate diets, is the loss of body protein or lean body mass. This is especially true when the individuals are physically inactive. Maintenance of LBM is an energy-expensive process. Lean body mass is the most metabolically active tissue in the body with respect to energy demands, accounting for the majority of Calories to support the basal energy requirement (i.e., 60 to 70% of daily basal energy requirements for adults). Therefore, the less body protein, the lower the energy requirement. If weight loss consists of significant amounts of body protein, then the formerly overfat person will have a lower basal energetic requirement and an increased energy efficiency in terms of the weight regain as fat.

One of the responses of cycled humans is the tendency to overeat during the initial few days of the refeeding period. This suggests that the regulation of food intake is affected by the weight loss. The regulation of food intake is discussed in the next section. Signals sent to the brain by the starved body seem to set the stage for hyperphagia (increased food intake above normal) once food is no longer restricted. These signals must be fairly enduring because this hyperphagia is of about the same duration as the duration of the restriction period. The origin of these signals is not known but no doubt they exist because food intake is an event regulated by the central nervous system. Studies of starved and refed rats showed that these rats had a preference for dietary fat if given a choice of several energy sources. As a result of this selection, cycled rats regained more body fat than if the food offered was carbohydrate and/or protein. Again, this suggests the involvement of signals from the brain directing the individual to select Calorically rich food. This signal, coupled with the increased efficiency of the body in retaining the ingested energy, helps to explain why the fat regain occurs in people who have restricted their energy intake to lose weight. Food restriction puts into place a metabolic machinery geared to save as much energy as possible and to stimulate the brain to signal the body to consume energy-rich foods.

Thus, even though the patient tries to control eating and food intake, the body seeks to return to its prior overfat state. Constant vigilance is required of the patient to override these biological signals which direct the body to be fat. However, even when the patient carefully monitors food energy intake and consciously decides to regulate it, weight regain may occur due to the body's increased energetic efficiency and its tendency to synthesize and store fat in preference to protein. Here is where a good exercise program might be useful. Exercise, on a regular basis, stimulates muscle protein development as well as increases energy expenditure. Exercise can be a useful adjunct to energy intake restriction because it redirects energy loss from the lean body mass. In the sedentary individual, weight loss occurs at the expense of both fat and protein components of the body. In the exercising food-restricted individual, the weight loss is primarily fat loss. Further, mild to moderate exercise seems to suppress food intake. Thus, food restriction together with exercise are additive in a beneficial way with respect to the loss and regain of body fat.

IV. REGULATION OF FOOD INTAKE

In the preceding section, the health concerns of obesity were discussed as well as a notation that obesity is sometimes characterized by hyperphagia (overeating). In this section food intake and its regulation will be discussed not only from the physiological point of view but also from the sociocultural point of view. It is important for those who study the processes by which humans consume and utilize food to realize how complex the subject is. An individual does not ingest thiamine, vitamin A, protein, and selenium, those nutrients necessary for his well-being; he ingests food, be it sirloin steak, fresh juicy peaches, or chocolate covered ants. He does not choose to eat a green salad because it is nutritionally sound to do so but because of complex conscious and subconscious motivation peculiar to himself. This section is designed to explain the origin of his motivation — its psychological and physiological roots.

A. PSYCHOLOGICAL ASPECTS OF FOOD INTAKE

Humans consume food, not nutrients. Although specific nutrients are necessary for the growth and maintenance of the human organism, it would be shortsighted to attempt to study basic nutritional needs without an appreciation of those factors which influence the intake of a sufficient variety of foods to obtain them. Most animals other than humans eat primarily to satisfy this nutritional need; a human's motivation for eating (or not eating) is frequently to satisfy nonnutritional requirements. Food selection is based on a combination of forces arising from one's culture, family, educational level, economic circumstances, and individual needs and idiosyncrasies.

Culture is the integrated pattern of human behavior which is transmitted to succeeding generations. It dictates the role each person plays in society, as well as his responsibilities to himself, his peer group, and his family. Food habits are largely determined by one's culture. Many habits have existed for centuries and have been maintained as an integral part of a cultural heritage. The Judaic dietary law, based on passages in Leviticus and Deuteronomy in the Old Testament, have very specific regulations about meat consumption. The prohibitions include the flesh of birds and animals of prey, reptiles, creeping insects, animal blood, any animal which does not chew its cud and have a cloven hoof, and any species from the water that does not have fins and scales. This eliminates eagles, ostriches, snakes, lizards, grasshoppers, camels, pigs, rabbits, sharks, oysters, clams, shrimp, and mussels. A large portion of the world's population has its dietary habits controlled by the teachings found in Buddhism, Hinduism, and Jainism (a sect of dissenters from Hinduism). These philosophies support the belief that all life is sacred. This includes killing animals for food. The prohibition against killing animals for food does vary from religion to religion and, even within a religion, varies from cultural group to group. For example, the Hindu reveres the cow and will not kill it for food. However, when a cow or oxen dies, the untouchables (the lowest class in Hindu society) take the animal, skin it for leather, and eat the meat. Since this population ordinarily is the poorest in India, this distribution of calories and protein serves to ensure their survival.

Not only do cultural laws prohibit the eating of certain foods, cultural practices also influence the foods that are eaten. The Jamaican enjoys plantain, ackee (a native food, poisonous when ripe, that looks and tastes like scrambled eggs), eggplant, papaya, mangoes, fish, lobster, naseberries, and otaheite apples. The Otomi Indians of the Mezquital Valley in Mexico make their meals from tortillas and from local plants such as malva, hediondilla, nopal, maguey, garambullo, yucca, purslane, pigweed, sorrel, wild mustard flowers, *lengua de vaca*, sow-thistle, and cactus fruit. They drink an intoxicating beverage, pulque, made from the century plant. A North American raised in a different culture would look askance at this diet, and view it as nutritionally deficient. However, nutritional analyses of the Otomi Indians' diet showed it to be better balanced than that of an urban group from the U.S. Persons from large sections of east and south Asia and tropical Africa refuse to drink milk; other African groups, on the contrary, prize milk as a precious food and serve it only to adult men. The Masai, people from an African nation, not only drink the milk from their cattle but draw blood from the jugular vein and drink that also. Entomophagy, the eating of insects, is accepted in many cultures; the Australian bushmen consume sugar ants and witchetty grubs; inhabitants of Central Africa eat fresh and fried termites; Japanese eat dytiscid beetles (fried and made into a sauce with sugar), grasshoppers, maggots, pupae of the wasp, *Vespula sp.*, and the larvae of silkworms. Several kinds of beetles are used as a confectionary in China.

Within a given culture, the family has a significant influence on food acceptance. This happens not because there is an active effort by elders to teach the children but because the children see the same daily ritual of food preparation. Unconsciously they assimilate it. In primitive societies, meals are important daily social events; females prepare the food and it is distributed on the basis of sex and age. In these societies as well as in our own, important family social events (christenings, weddings, funerals, etc.) are celebrated with food. These family practices become part of the cultural heritage and influence food choice.

Similarly, in progressive, industrial societies, food customs are assimilated by children through the practices of their parents. As technological advances increase the complexity of a society, food as an element in its culture becomes less important. Sociologists who study contemporary society have observed that mealtimes have become less relevant as a time for family social interaction. In the U.S. a large part of the eating is done outside the family environment; convenience foods, sandwiches, fast foods, soft drinks, and many such items are picked up by individuals on a regular basis. Forces outside the family influence food choices. Advertising, peer pressure, lifestyle, and age may well be more important determinants of food choices than family food practices. There has also been a change in the roles of food in festive occasions: whereas 100 years ago a large meal might have been served to celebrate an important life event, such as a wedding or a christening, today these events are more often celebrated with a cocktail party. As in less industrialized societies, children observe these practices and apply them.

The impact that the family has on food choices is often a reflection of the educational level of the one who selects and prepares the food: if this person is limited in education, the diet frequently shows a poor supply of nutrients.

In more recent times in the U.S. a definite correlation has been shown between the education of a homemaker and the nutritional intake of her family. The data for this correlation come from two surveys conducted to examine the extent of malnutrition in the U.S.: (1) the Ten State Survey from 1968 to 1970 mandated by the federal government; and (2) the Health and Nutrition Examination Survey (HANES) conducted by the Center for Disease Control, U.S. Public Health Service. Food intake, clinical tests, physical examinations, anthropometric examinations, medical histories, and educational and financial status were evaluated. The surveys showed that the fewer the years of education the homemaker had, the greater the number of nutritional deficiencies in the diet of the family.

Economic circumstances also exert considerable influence on food choices. The aborigine, living in an arid barren land, is very poor. He hunts for every calorie he consumes. To increase his food supply, his culture has evolved to include a host of insects as part of his daily diet. At the other extreme, in a more affluent society considerable amounts of money are spent on foods of no outstanding nutritional value. Caviar is a prime example. In 1989, Beluga caviar cost just over $400/pound. Caviar is considered a prestigious food by many Americans and Europeans, and they delight in both serving it to guests and eating it themselves. It has no greater nutritional value than cheese, eggs, or hamburger but does impart a certain status to the consumer.

Additionally, there are a host of other factors, which are interrelated, that influence food choices: geography, climate, methods of distribution, and storage facilities. Although the New Zealanders and the Danes live many miles apart, both their diets include an abundance of dairy products. This is a function of, in part, the similarities in their geography and climate. Citrus fruits are easily grown in Egypt. However, the food distribution methods are antiquated. As a result, many people in the country do not enjoy these fruits because they spoil in the process of being shipped. In contrast, in the U.S. because of rapid transportation systems, imported foods such as papaya and plantain are frequently enjoyed and foods produced in one segment of the country are available throughout the nation.

Final among the factors being considered that influence food choices is an individual's physiological and psychological idiosyncrasies. An example of the former is the situation in which an individual lacks the intestinal enzyme, lactase, which is necessary to digest the milk sugar, lactose. When he drinks milk, he experiences abdominal bloating, cramps, and diarrhea. Needless to say, he elects to exclude milk from his diet. Countless other food allergies have been observed: allergies to wheat, corn, chocolate, eggs, strawberries, tomatoes, soy products, to name a few. If an allergy can be identified, frequently a very difficult task, the item is eliminated from one's diet. Sometimes a food item is eliminated instinctively without medical documentation simply because an individual senses a relationship between his food intake and his sense of well-being.

Throughout history there have been individuals who possessed bizarre appetites. During the 19th century lived one Jeremiah Johnson, a mountain man who wandered the unexplored West, living off the land and livers of Crow Indians. Presumably, during the course of his travels, he devoured the livers of 247 Indians. In Hungary in the early 1600s lived the Countess Elisabeth de Bathory, who had a penchant for the blood of young, buxomy virgins, for through their blood she hoped to regain her youth. In her efforts to do so, she is reported to have killed 650 girls, drinking their blood and using it as a fluid in which to bathe.

All in all, a person's reasons for selecting the foods he eats is a very complex issue with apparently little consideration given to his nutritional requirements. The foods one person might consider an elegant repast, another would not deign to touch. Human behavior added to the study of nutrition, makes a difficult subject even more complex.

B. PHYSIOLOGICAL ASPECTS OF FOOD INTAKE

1. Sensory Perception of Food

In addition to the social, cultural, and economic influences on food intake, the selection of foods involves a complex interaction between the special senses: reactions of the eye, ear, nose, mouth, and the sensations of pain and touch are all involved. The appearance, texture, smell, and taste of food, which in many ways are inextricably bound to one's cultural heritage, as well as the sensation of hunger, determine whether the hand will reach out and grasp the food, transport it to the mouth, and consume it. The appearance of the food, its color, its consistency, and its temperature are perceived by the sensory system which includes the eye, the sense of touch, the sense of temperature, and the sense of smell. Temperature, taste, texture, and smell are perceived via sensory receptor systems located in the nose and mouth. Recall that a receptor is a defined organization of molecules within a membrane or cellular organelle which recognizes and binds compounds or elements needed by the cell. A receptor may also serve to translate or transmit or initiate the sending of a message to other parts of the cell or to other parts of the body. For example, the sensory receptors in the oral cavity perceive the attributes of foods such as texture, and taste. The taste/smell/texture translate the stimulus into an electrochemical message which is relayed to the brain. Currently, far more is known about the anatomy of the area in which these events take place than about the physiology of the events themselves.

a. Appearance

Part of the social/cultural force that influences one's acceptance of food is the defined expectation of an acceptable food. In part, this expectation is based on the appearance of that food. Does it have the desired size and shape, and most important, is it the expected color?

Work done on the relationship between food acceptance and color has shown a striking dependence of one on the other. One study showed that when jellies were colored in an atypical manner, the fruit flavors were incorrectly identified. In another study, the flavoring of colorless syrups was incorrectly identified by most of a group of 200 pharmacy students; they were even less able to identify the correct flavor if the solutions were given unusual colors. In a third study, a trained panel of wine tasters showed a dependence on color in their evaluation of wine. Food coloring was added to dry white table wine to simulate the appearance of reisling, sauterne, sherry, rosé, claret, and burgundy. The panel judged the rosé-colored wine to be the most sweet and the claret-colored wine to be the least sweet. Interestingly, subjects who seldom drank wine and participated in the same experiment did not relate color to sweetness.

So important are these visual aspects of food that the USDA food quality grading standards are based on the visual appearance of food. For example, color is an important characteristic for the grading standards of beef and of fruits. Other visual characteristics, such as the presence or absence of blemishes and bruises, are also important.

Food scientists have spent considerable time trying to relate visual characteristics to measurable physical parameters that determine the acceptance or rejection of a given food. Appearance may provide a clue about the juiciness of an apple or the tenderness of a steak; these properties, of course, are also determined in the mouth and perceived there as differences in texture.

b. Texture

The texture of food plays an important role in food acceptance because the sense of touch is highly developed in the mouth. Texture, traditionally defined in terms of how a food "feels" in the mouth, is perceived by four different sets of receptors: the *pain, tactile, pressor,* and *sound* receptors. The pain receptors may be activated if foods are extremely hot or cold or rich in such seasonings as cayenne pepper, for these items chemically burn the surfaces of the mouth and/or tongue. The tactile receptor receives messages about the geometrical characteristics of the food. The size, shape, and frequency of food particles will be ascertained and, if these characteristics are expected, the food will be accepted. If, however, the mashed potatoes are lumpy or the ice cream gritty, the tactile receptors will perceive this and the food may be rejected. These tactile receptors are located in the skin of the tongue, oral cavity, and throat. Not only do they perceive characteristics such as "grittiness" or "lumpiness", they also detect differences in moisture and fat content. These latter characteristics may describe the richness, moistness, or slipperiness of a given food.

Texture is also perceived by pressor receptors located in the muscles, tendons, and joints of the mouth, jaws, and throat. These receptors are elements of the kinesthetic sense. The characteristic resistance to chewing, as in a tough piece of meat, is an example of the perception of texture by the kinesthetic sense. "Hard or tough to chew" means extreme physical resistance to the actions of the teeth and jaws. Strenuous exertion by the voluntary muscles is required; this, in turn, is perceived as changes in the position, movement, and tension of the teeth and jaws. The kinesthetic sense is difficult to study because it is not easily located and identifiable. However, through the use of such drugs as cocaine, which blocks the muscle receptors, it has been learned that the oral kinesthetic sense originates as much from the joints as from the muscles. Four sets of receptors are involved: two in the muscles, one in the tendon, and one in the fascia associated with the muscle. There are free nerve endings (also called pressor receptors) in the muscles which are activated by the chewing of such hard items as nuts, crackers, or bones, and which stimulate a sense of motion.

Some textural characteristics are sensed by sound receptors. The sounds a food makes when chewed contributes to the acceptability of the item. The crunch of crisp celery or the snap of a fresh potato chip contribute to the enjoyment of that food. The stimulation of tactile and kinesthetic receptors and auditory receptors plays important roles in the evaluation of textural characteristics of the food. Individuals will vary in their preferences for smooth, chewy, crisp, hot, cold, or crunchy textures; all of these attributes, however, are based not on taste, smell, or appearance but on mouth "feel" and food sounds. In addition, cultural influences will contribute to the textural expectations of individuals. For example, a soft, smooth, bland textured food may be associated with the food needs of infants or invalids and may not be accepted by the young male with a strong "macho" self-image. Juicy, chewy textures requiring exertion of the jaw muscles may be very acceptable to the young adult but are much less acceptable to the school age child.

c. Smell (Olfaction)

Smell and taste are intimately related. Persons who have lost their sense of smell, as frequently happens with a cold, complain that food is not as tasty as when they are well. This is because part of their appreciation of food has decreased through a temporary impairment of their ability to smell.

Among the special senses, the sense of smell is the most sensitive. The average person can detect one part in a trillion parts of air for some high potency odorants. For example, ethyl mercaptain (ethanethiol) can be detected at 4.0×10^{-11} mg/ml air. However, the perception of a particular aroma quickly diminishes if the aroma persists. This process is called *olfactory adaptation* and begins the first second after an aroma is perceived.

The perception of smell is a subjective phenomenon. Depending upon a person's expectations, an item can have an intrinsically pleasant or unpleasant aroma. One example of such subjectivity is the scent of a gardenia: many people enjoy it but some find the aroma too strong or overpowering. Another is that the Japanese found the body odor of Western man, when first he came to their islands, offensive. This was due to the presence of small amounts of butyric acid in the sweat of their visitor. This butyric acid aroma arises because Americans are heavy meat eaters. Only people who do not eat meat, as the Japanese did not do in any significant quantity during the late 19th century, notice the odor. However, as the Japanese have been exposed to greater numbers of Americans and as the consumption of meat by the Japanese has increased, the difference in body odor has lessened.

Because the perception of smell is so highly subjective, it is difficult to study either qualitatively or quantitatively. Some physiologists contend that whereas taste perception involves the differentiation of four primary tastes, smell involves many primary odors. However, little progress has been made towards identifying and classifying these odors. Although it is difficult to study the phenomenon of smell, the anatomy of the area in which the event occurs has received considerable attention and is fairly well known.

The perception of smell is performed in a specialized area (Figure 18) located in the respiratory tract. The respiratory tract consists of the nose, nasal cavity, pharynx, larynx, trachea, bronchi, and lungs. Within this area, the nasal cavity is divided into two approximately equal and separate chambers known as the nasal fossae or nasal passages. Ambient air enters these chambers, proceeds to the nasopharynx, and exits through rear passageways known as the choanae. In humans, olfaction occurs in an area that occupies 2 to 4 cm² in the superior portion of both nasal passages.

Although the entire nasal cavity is lined by a mucous membrane, that from the olfactory region is distinguished by its yellow to brown color and is known as the *olfactory mucosa* or olfactory membrane. Many small glands of Bowman secrete mucus onto the surface of the olfactory mucosa. The receptor cells for the sense of smell, known as the *olfactory receptor cells* or simply *olfactory cells*, are found in the olfactory mucosa. The olfactory sensory unit is shown in Figure 19. The olfactory cells are long, slender, bipolar, modified nerve cells; they

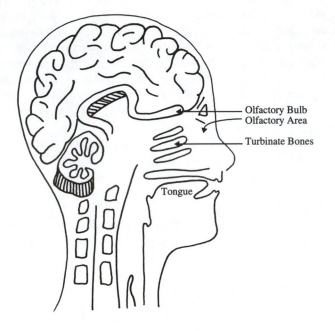

FIGURE 18.   Anatomy of the major components of the olfactory system.

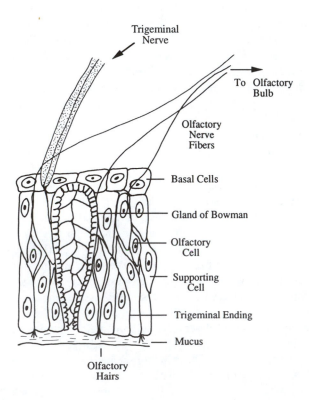

FIGURE 19.   Details of the olfactory sensory unit. The olfactory cells are supplied with both sensory and motor fibers. The sensory fibers proceed in three separate branches to the olfactory bulb.

are interspersed and supported by columnar epithelial cells. Both cells have an underlying layer of *basal cells*. The dendritic end of the olfactory cell has numerous, small (approximately 0.1 micron in diameter and 10 to 200 microns in length) *olfactory hairs* or *cilia* that project into the mucus that coats the olfactory mucosa. The cilia of the olfactory mucosa are distinguishable from the others of the respiratory tract by their motion. Whereas the respiratory tract cilia wave back and forth rhythmically, and by their motion assist in removing impurities from the respiratory tract, the cilia of the olfactory mucosa do not. Their movements appear to be random and uncoordinated. The presence and action of the cilia have been confirmed by electron microscopic examination of mucosal tissue.

From the other end of the olfactory cell extends an axon directly into the central nervous system. Axons from different olfactory cells converge and form the *olfactory nerve*. The olfactory nerve extends through the sievelike openings of the ethmoid bone located behind the bridge of the nose to one of the two *olfactory bulbs* of the forebrain. The two bulbs lie on top of the ethmoid bone beneath the frontal lobes of the brain. Information about different odorants passes directly from the olfactory bulb to the cerebral cortex.

The trigeminal nerve in the cheek is involved in certain responses to odorants. The trigeminal receptors are bare nerve endings found in the nasal passages, mouth, throat, and mucosa around the eyes. They communicate with the brain through the trigeminal nerve. A trigeminally mediated component is part of the odor of such substances as chlorine, peppermint, and menthol. The extent of its involvement is a function of the nature of the odorant and its concentration in the air.

Even though the anatomy involved in olfactory reception is well described, the process by which smells are detected and discriminated is poorly understood. It has been established that the perception of smell involves both a preneural and neural phase. Several features are involved in the preneural phase. A volatile chemical will release molecules into the air. These molecules are inhaled, entering the nasal passages. Under normal conditions, about 2% of the inhaled air will reach the olfactory region and participate in the olfactory event. Sniffing enhances olfaction because inhaled air is forcefully drawn into the upper nostrils, thus increasing the number of odorant molecules to which the olfactory region is exposed. These molecules must then dissolve in the layer of mucus that covers the olfactory. Once they have dissolved in the mucus, they can interact with the receptor site. At one time it was thought that the receptor sites were located only on the cilia. However, it is currently believed that the cilia are not the only possible place; the exact position of other sites has not been established. The nature of the interaction between the odorant molecule and the receptor site is the subject of considerable debate.

This interaction triggers the neural phase; an action potential is initiated in the axon of the receptor cell and transmitted via the olfactory nerve to the olfactory bulb and on to the cerebral cortex. Through this sequence of events, 2000 to 4000 smells can be discriminated.

In attempting to unravel the mystery of the mechanism of smell, the relationship between molecular structure and odor discrimination has been an active area of investigation. Regrettably, an odor cannot be predicted from knowledge of the structure of a molecule because often, but not always, minor alterations in the structure produce marked changes in the smell. The odor of vanillin is a familiar one, drawing to mind visions of fresh-baked cookies. A simple substituent change produces isovanillin, a compound that is practically odorless. Replacing the methoxy group with an ethoxy one makes ethylvanillin, a compound four times more aromatic than vanillin. In contrast, there is no marked change in odor quality if the aldehyde group is replaced with a nitro or cyano group. These structures are shown in Figure 20.

More than 20 theories have been proposed to explain why a specific molecular structure will arouse a specific smell sensation. Most of them deal with the nature of the interaction between the odorant molecule and the receptor site. The "penetrate and puncture" theory of Davies and the stereochemical site theory of Amoore are two such theories.

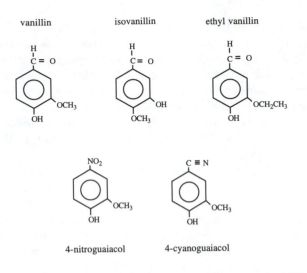

FIGURE 20. Structures of related compounds which vary little but which are perceived differently by the olfactory system.

Davies contends that the odorant molecule is adsorbed by the lipid layer of the membrane wall of the olfactory receptor cell (see Figure 19). This molecule can either desorb from the surface of the cell membrane or penetrate it. If it penetrates, it punctures the membrane and leaves a hole that closes slowly. The outer fluid of the receptor cell has a high sodium ion concentration; the inner fluid has a high concentration of potassium ions. Before the hole closes, ions enter the cell. This stimulates the initiation of an action potential and a signal is sent to the brain.

Amoore proposes an alternative explanation. His stereochemical site theory postulates that the size and shape of a molecule govern the type of odor perceived. An odorous molecule will find a complimentary molecular structure in the receptor cells. Compounds with similar sizes and shapes will fit into the same site on the receptor cell and, thus, elicit the same smell perception. A necessary part of his theory is that primary odors exist, just as do primary tastes, except that there are far more primary odors than primary tastes.

These theories are highly speculative. The study of people with specific anosmias (no smell perception) are providing further insights into the process of olfaction. In albinism, a genetic mutation that results in absence of pigmentation, anosmia is frequently observed. This suggests that there may be a relationship between olfaction and pigment formation analogous to the relationship of visual acuity and visual pigments. However, the presence of a relationship does not imply that olfactory response is dependent on the presence of pigments in the olfactory region. It may mean, instead, that pigmentation and olfaction are dependent variables of a common genetic error in metabolism. If such as this were the case, pigmentation and olfaction would have no relationship to one another; they are manifestations of the same problem.

Other kinds of specific anosmias have also been observed. Some persons are unable to detect the sulfur-containing compound, *n*-butyl mercaptan. Others are insensitive to the "sweet" smell of hydrogen cyanide or to the scent of freesia (a sweet-smelling flower). This suggests that specific chemical structures in both odorants and receptors are needed for odors to be detected. Parosmia (inappropriate odor perception) is probably due to anosmia of a particular substituent in an odorant grouping. Frequently, a loss in olfactory sensitivity is the result of a severe bout of influenza or damage to the trigeminal or fifth cranial nerve. In this latter instance, the error in olfaction resides in the neural phase rather than the preneural phase, as has been the case in the other examples cited. In contrast to all these forms of anosmia, very high sensitivity to odors has been noted in persons with cystic fibrosis (a genetic error in electrolyte exchange characterized by an accumulation of mucous in lungs) or with Addison's disease (deficient adrenal cortical hormone release). In both these diseases, sodium ion loss is excessive; this indicates a need for the movement of sodium in odor perception and acuity. New data are constantly being added to that already accumulated. They may show, in time, that the present theories are inaccurate or incomplete.

d. Taste (Gustation)

The perception of taste, as the perception of smell, is highly subjective. Despite this high level of subjectivity, physiologists have established that humans perceive four primary tastes: sour, salty, sweet, and bitter. Chemicals which can elicit any one of these tastes are called *tastants*. The tastants must be in solution in order to be perceived. Both water-soluble and lipid-soluble compounds can serve as tastants.

Different substances evoke each of the primary tastes. The chemicals which elicit the sour taste are acidic compounds; the hydrogen ion, rather than the associated anion, actually stimulates the receptor. Generally, the sourness is proportional to the concentration of the hydrogen ion. A more acidic compound will trigger a stronger response than a neutral compound. An anion of an inorganic salt produces a salty taste. The halides, chloride, fluoride, bromide, and iodide are usually associated with a salty taste.

A variety of chemicals, mostly organic, trigger the sensation of the sweet taste; sugars, glycols, alcohols, aldehydes, ketones, amides, esters, amino acids, sulfonic acids, halogenated acids, and the inorganic salts of lead and berryllium. The sweetest compound known is the *n*-propyl derivative of 4-alkoxy-e-aminonitrobenzene. Such organic compounds as the glycosides amygdalin (found in almond kernels) and naringin (found in citrus fruit), and the alkaloids caffeine, quinine, strychnine, and nicotine taste bitter. These structures are shown in Figure 21. Inorganic salts of magnesium, ammonium, and calcium also taste bitter.

The average person is more receptive to a bitter taste than to a sour, salty, or sweet taste. For example, a 0.000008 M quinine solution tastes bitter, but it requires a much higher concentration (0.0009 M) of hydrochloric acid to taste sour, and an even higher concentration (0.01 M) of sodium chloride to taste salty or of sucrose to taste sweet.

Additionally, the pleasantness of a given taste relates to the concentration of the tastant. For example, as the concentration of sucrose in a solution is increased, its taste changes from unpleasant to pleasant; the pleasant sensation of sweet arises only at higher concentrations. In contrast, a bitter taste can be pleasant at low concentrations but become unpleasant at high ones. In small quantities, the white membrane of orange or grapefruit sections enhance the flavors of these fruits; however, they are seldom eaten by themselves because of their bitter taste.

Within a given taste modality, some chemicals can be tasted at a lower concentration than others. This can be expressed quantitatively by measuring the detection threshold and, from this, calculating the relative taste indices. Table 10 gives the relative taste indices of several substances. In this table, the intensities of each of the four primary sensations are referred to a reference compound: the acidic substances to hydrochloric acid; the sweet substances to sucrose; the bitter ones to quinine; and the salty ones to sodium chloride. Each of these reference compounds is assigned an index value of 1.

Each of these primary tastes is perceived through the organ of taste, the taste bud. The taste bud is about 1/30 mm in diameter and 1/16 mm in length. It contains two kinds of cells: the receptor cell and the supporting cell. The *gustatory receptor cells,* also called the *taste cells*, are barrel-shaped, modified epithelial cells. From one end of each taste cell protrudes several *microvilli* or *taste hairs*. These microvilli extend through a taste pore within the tongue's surface to contact the fluids of the mouth. For a tastant to be perceived, it must be in solution. The other end of each taste cell is innervated with *gustatory nerve fibers*. One cell may be innervated with several fibers or several fibers may innervate one cell; there is no one-on-one line of communication between the individual taste cell and the central nervous system (CNS).

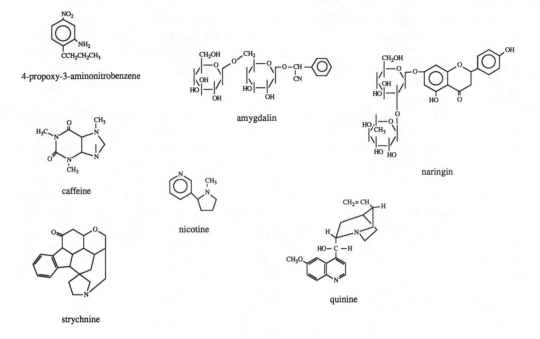

FIGURE 21.   Chemical structures of compounds that elicit a bitter taste.

TABLE 10
Relative Taste Indices of Different Substances

Sour substances	Index	Bitter substances	Index	Sweet substances	Index	Salty substances	Index
Hydrochloric acid	1	Quinine	1	Sucrose	1	NaCl	1
Formic acid	1.1	Strychnine	3.1	4-Propoxy-3-amino-nitrobenzene	5000	NaF	2
Chloracetic acid	0.9	Nicotine	1.3	Saccharin	675	CaCl₂	1
Lactic acid	0.85	Phenylthiourea	0.9	Chloroform	40	NaBr	0.5
Tartaric acid	0.7	Caffeine	0.4	Fructose	1.7	NaI	0.35
Malic acid	0.6	Pilocarpine	0.16	Alanine	1.3	LiCl	0.4
Potassium H tartrate	0.58	Atropine	0.13	Glucose	0.8	NH₄Cl	2.5
Acetic acid	0.55	Cocaine	0.02	Maltose	0.45	KCl	0.6
Citric acid	0.46	Morphine	0.02	Galactose	0.32		
Carbonic acid	0.06			Lactose	0.3		

Adapted from A. C. Guyton, *Textbook of Medical Physiology,* 7th ed., W. B. Saunders, Philadelphia, 1971, p. 639.

The traditional view of taste held that its perception was mediated only by taste buds (Figure 22a) found in the papillae on the surface of the tongue and that there were specific areas where each modality, and only that modality, was perceived (Figure 22b). This is not wholly true. Taste buds are actually found in several places within the oral cavity: on the surface of the tongue, palate, pharynx, and larynx and sometimes on the cheeks.

The surface of the tongue is covered by small structures called papillae. Four distinct kinds of papillae have been described (Figure 22c). Filiform papillae are very small and are scattered over most of the surface of the tongue. Fungiform papillae are raised, pigmented papillae and are intermixed with the filiform papillae on the anterior two thirds of the surface. They are not found beyond the sulcus terminalis, a V-shaped groove near the back of the tongue. Circumvallate papillae are larger and taller and are prevalent on the posterior surface of the tongue.

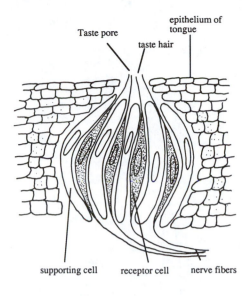

FIGURE 22a. The taste bud.

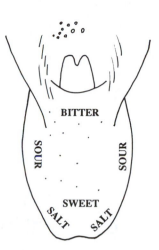

FIGURE 22b. The four taste modalities of the tongue.

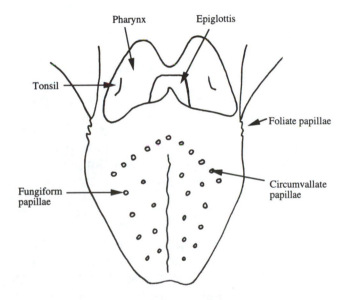

FIGURE 22c. Upper surface of the human tongue.

Foliate papillae are located along the sides near the back of the tongue. The filiform papillae contain no taste buds. Moderate numbers of taste buds are found in the fungiform and foliate papillae, but most of the taste buds are found in the circumvallate papillae. The tongue, although it perceives all four of the taste modalities, is most sensitive to salty and sweet (see Figure 22b). The palate, on the other hand, is more sensitive to the sour and bitter tastes than to the salty and sweet tastes. The pharynx also detects all four tastes but not to the same extent as the tongue and palate (see Figure 23). Scattered over the entire oral cavity of an adult are approximately 10,000 taste buds. The taste cells within the taste buds are epithelial cells, which are short-lived cells with a rapid turnover rate. A human taste cell has an approximate lifetime of 250 hours. The ability to quickly regenerate is in marked contrast to most other elements of the nervous system. As one grows older, the rate at which taste cells are

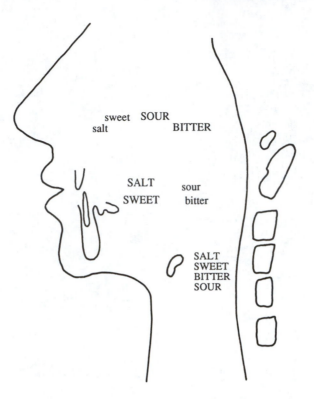

FIGURE 23.   Taste sensing locations of the palate and pharynx.

regenerated is decreased and, as a consequence, there is a concomitant decrease in quantity. With a decrease in number of taste cells, taste acuity declines.

The anatomical features that are involved with gustation have been well studied. So also have the tastants which elicit the sensation. Organic chemists have long known that small structural changes can alter tastes. For instance, the sugars listed in Table 10 are structurally similar. The taste response they elicit, however, varies from very sweet (β-D-fructose) to bitter (β-D-mannose). The most remarkable feature of these compounds is that mutarotation about the anomeric carbon of α-D-mannose to make β-D-mannose changes the taste perceived from sweet to bitter. These structures are shown in Figure 24.

Saccharin is sweet while its *N*-alkylated derivatives are tasteless. The alkali metal salts of cyclamate (cyclohexyl amine sulfate) are sweet while the amine salt is nearly tasteless. It has been found that the dipeptide L-aspartyl-L-phenylalanine methyl ester and certain related compounds are nearly 200 times sweeter than sucrose. Since this compound is composed of natural amino acids and is quite low in calories, it offers intriguing possibilities as a synthetic sweetener. If any other amino acids are substituted for the L-aspartate (even a closely related compound L-glutamate), the resulting product is tasteless. However, sweetness is maintained if phenylalanine is replaced by methionine or tyrosine. The dipeptide-free acid of the methyl ester is not sweet, nor is the ethyl ester as sweet as the methyl ester.

Although much is known about the anatomy of the oral cavity and much is known about the chemistry of the tastants, a thorough understanding of the mechanism of taste has not been assembled. As with smell, the process includes both a preneural and neural phase. The preneural event involves an interaction between the tastant and the receptor cell. It is generally believed that this is a steric interaction between these two sites, possibly involving conformational changes. Then, in some incompletely understood manner, this triggers the neural phase, which is the depolarization of specific taste nerves and the passage of impulses to the brain.

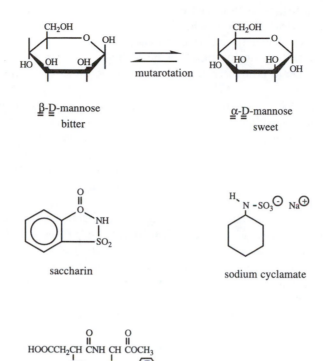

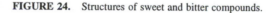

FIGURE 24.   Structures of sweet and bitter compounds.

Electrical signals generated when various tastants have been applied to the tongue have been measured.

For the auditory and visual senses, medical specialties have evolved to diagnose and treat, where possible, deviations from normal. Similar specialties have not been developed to solve problems of taste and smell, nor have great strides been made in the diagnosis and treatment of disorders of these senses. However, abnormalities in taste perception have provided a means for verifying and enlarging the understanding of the mechanism of the taste sensation.

Anatomic abnormalities of both the palate and the tongue have been associated with a decrease in taste sensitivity. Patients with abnormal palate structures have significantly elevated thresholds for sour and bitter tastes but not for sweet and salty ones. An increase in threshold means that a greater concentration of the tastant is required for detection and recognition of that tastant by a subject. However, not all patients with anatomic abnormalities of the hard or soft palate exhibit taste disturbances. For example, those with gross clefts of the back part of the hard palate detect and recognize all four modalities of taste.

People who wear dentures report an increase in the detection and recognition thresholds for sour and bitter tastes, but no change in their response to sweet and salty tastes. Artificial dentures cover and fit close to the palate and hence, cover part of the mouth area containing taste receptors, as a result, there may be an artificial masking of taste receptor sites in these parts of the mouth and taste perception may be affected.

Abnormalities on the surface of the tongue, such as lichen planus and tumors, cause a decrease in taste acuity. Diseases which affect the nerve supply to the tongue (such as postdiphtheritic neuritis, sarcoidosis, and Bell's palsy), severe trauma, and irradiation of the oral cavity as part of treatment for a malignancy will result in a decrease in taste sensitivity. Interestingly enough, congenital underdevelopment or absence of the tongue is not accompanied by a decrease in taste acuity. In all of these abnormal states there is a reduction or omission in the number of taste receptor cells. To this is attributed the cause for the decrease in taste acuity.

Speculation about the specific functions of the taste bud in taste perception have resulted from studies of patients with Type I familial dysautonomia (Riley-Day syndrome). In this syndrome, the tongue's surface is smooth; the sulcus terminalis, taste buds, and fungiform and circumvallate papillae are missing; and the number of unmyelinated free nerve endings is greatly diminished. Patients demonstrate significantly raised detection and recognition thresholds: some cannot consistently distinguish between water and saturated solutions of sodium chloride, sugar, urea, and $0.03 M$ hydrochloric acid. However, when treated with methacholine (an α-adrenergic drug), these patients have normal taste perception while the drug remains in their system. This has led to the suggestion that the taste buds function as a chemical sieve. It is proposed that taste buds have pores of a small, controlled size through which chemical stimuli may reach the nerves. Numerous factors, not yet identified, may control this pore size. In patients with familial dysautonomia, treatment with methacholine causes an increase in membrane permeability, including that of the lingual surface which, in turn, allows a tastant to reach the unmyelinated free nerve endings in the tongue. Thus, the taste threshold is lowered and the patient is more responsive to the tastant.

The divalent cations, particularly copper, zinc, and nickel, have been reported to affect taste sensitivity. When given to patients with hypoguesia, some improvement occurs. Observations of serum and tissue levels of copper in patients with rheumatoid arthritis and Wilson's disease have led to conjectures about copper's role in the regulation of taste acuity. Patients with either of these diseases are often treated with D-penicillamine. With this therapy, patients having Wilson's disease experience no change in their taste acuity; however, patients with rheumatoid arthritis frequently report a decrease in taste acuity. D-Penicillamine therapy is associated with a decrease in serum and tissue copper levels. For the arthritic patients, this does indeed happen. Not so in patients with Wilson's disease; the disease is characterized by abnormally high levels of serum copper. Penicillamine simply reduces this high level to a normal level. The taste acuity of the arthritic patients, if given oral copper sulfate, returns to normal. Thus, copper appears to be directly involved with taste acuity and its depletion leads to hypoguesia.

Recent reports indicate that taste dysfunction may be associated with impaired zinc absorption and decreased saliva levels of zinc. Oral therapy of zinc or nickel returned the taste acuity to normal.

Steroid hormones have also been implicated in the taste mechanism through studies of diseases of the endocrine system. Patients with Addison's disease, decreased adrenal cortical function, or panhypopituitarism have lowered detection thresholds. Patients with Addison's disease are sometimes able to detect concentrations of tastants as low as 0.01 of that perceived by normal subjects. In both cases, the heightened taste sensitivity returns to normal when the missing steroids are given. The mechanism by which the steroids influence taste perception is not known.

A comprehensive, unified theory of taste perception has not yet been realized; but the taste of food, as well as its appearance, texture, and smell are intimately involved in the desire to eat.

C. NEURONAL SIGNALS FOR HUNGER AND SATIETY

Internal cues regulate food intake through a number of signals and responses which ultimately result in the initiation or cessation of feeding. These cues are in addition to those described above which involve the cerebrum. Both short-term and long-term controls are exerted which, over time, serve to regulate the food intake of normal individuals so that they neither gain nor lose weight. Food intake control rests, in part, with the integration of a variety

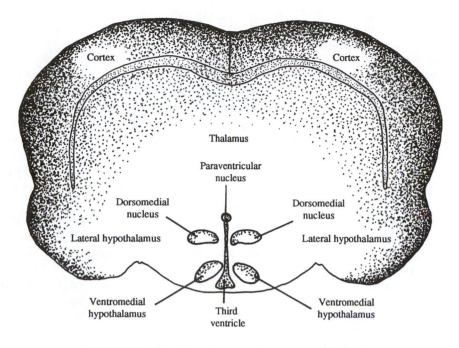

FIGURE 25. Appetite and satiety regulatory areas of the brain.

of hormonal and nonhormonal signals which are generated both peripherally and centrally. The hypothalamus is thought to be the main integrator of these signals. Other discrete areas are also involved. The hypothalamus is located beneath the thalamus, a part of the forebrain, close to the pituitary (Figure 25). The hypothalamus is involved in both the initiation and cessation of both food and water intake. It serves as an endocrine organ which produces the hormones that in turn modulate the release of hormones from the posterior pituitary. It also releases other hormones, called releasing factors or tropins, which control the activity of the anterior pituitary. The area of the brain which includes the thalamus, hypothalamus, and pituitary has been called the center of existence because it controls much of what is known as instinctive behavior. In addition to its regulatory effect on appetite, satiety, and thirst, the hypothalamus serves, through its effect on the pituitary, as the main subcortical control center for the regulation of the parasympathetic and sympathetic systems; for the regulation of heart rate; and for the regulation of vasodilation and vasoconstriction, two important processes for the maintenance of body temperature. If the body temperature rises, vasodilation (increased blood flow through skin capillaries) along with increased respiration and increased sweat loss occurs, increasing body heat loss. Conversely, if body temperature is below normal, vasoconstriction (decreased blood flow) occurs and body heat is conserved. Vasoconstriction, vasodilation, and heart rate are also important to the regulation of blood pressure. Indirectly, the hypothalamus regulates the activity of the gastrointestinal system, the emotions, and spontaneous behavior.

The role of the hypothalamus in the control of eating behavior has been well studied. As early as 1840, extreme obesity in man was reported to occur in patients with hypothalamic tumors. Recognition of the involvement of the ventromedial hypothalamus in the regulation of food intake did not come until it was shown that if the ventromedial hypothalamic area was destroyed or lesioned the animals overate, with a resulting increase in body fat. If the lateral hypothalamus was lesioned, animals became both adipsic (had no thirst response) and aphagic (did not eat). This relationship of feeding behavior to drinking behavior can be understood when the consequences of dehydration due to absence of fluid intake are realized. In adipsic animals, saliva production is significantly reduced; thus, laterally lesioned animals have difficulty, initially, in swallowing dry food. As the lesioned animal recovers or adapts to the lesion, he drinks when he eats dry food but does not eat when water deprived. In addition, the lesioned rat does not drink in response to serum hyperosmolarity (increased levels of solutes in the blood), hyperthermia (increased body temperature), or hypovolemia (decreased blood volume). Animals with lesions in the lateral hypothalamus do not respond to reductions in blood sugar levels (via insulin injections) and will die in severe hypoglycemia rather than eat readily available food. This observation suggests that both the lateral and ventromedial nuclei in the hypothalamus interact via chemical signals to control eating and drinking. Since eating and the cessation of eating is under hypothalamic control, it is reasonable to assume that this behavior is initiated or stopped by a series of signals emitted from and/or received by this tissue. The nature of this signal system is rather complex. As research continued in this area, it was learned that other areas of the brain are involved. The paraventricular nucleus located slightly in front of the dorsomedial nucleus (Figure 25) appears to be involved in the regulation of glucose intake as it relates to the maintenance of glucose homeostasis. The dorsomedial nucleus, found on either side of the third ventricle seems to be involved in the control of body size but not body fat and, because of this involvement, is likely to play a role in food intake. In addition, the area postrema of the brain stem and the caudal medial nucleus have been implicated in food intake regulation. The details of this involvement are not yet in hand.

One school of thought is that eating is a response to variations in the level of circulating glucose. This theory, called the glucostatic theory, proposes that cellular energy requirements determine feeding behavior. In particular, it suggests that brain cells, which use glucose almost exclusively as their metabolic fuel, are exquisitely sensitive to fluctuations in blood glucose levels, and will activate the "feeding center" to initiate feeding when blood glucose levels dip below normal or activate the "satiety center" to stop feeding when blood glucose levels are high. Support for this theory comes from the observation that feeding is initiated by animals injected with insulin and from the observation that gold thioglucose (which destroys the satiety center of the hypothalamus) is ineffective in diabetic animals. In the latter case, eating continues because gold thioglucose does not get into the hypothalamic cells of diabetic animals to destroy the satiety center. This occurs because the penetration of gold thioglucose into the hypothalamic cells is insulin dependent. This is a very simplistic approach to food intake regulation; however, it has provided a framework for the building of a more cohesive explanation of the systems which operate to ensure energy balance.

Another school of thought is that eating behavior is controlled by the fat cell size and number. This is called the lipostatic theory. It speculates that there is a set point for each animal for the number of fat cells and their fat content and that when this set point is reached, the animal ceases to eat. In the absence of eating, these fat stores are mobilized and used until a lower set point is reached and feeding again commences. This theory is supported by observations of animals that had been starved. These animals eat large amounts of food when realimented after starvation until they regain their prestarvation weight; then, they resume their prestarvation eating behavior. In other words, they overate to fill their fat depots, then ate only enough to maintain these depots. Modulation of food intake by signals arising in adipose tissue has been an important component of many theories of energy balance.

It is possible that the theories described above (as well as some others) may be integrated into one to more readily allow for the understanding of the signals needed to initiate, maintain, and stop feeding. Both the brain and the GI tract release a variety of hormones which regulate quite specific components of the food intake/utilization system. Most of these hormonal signals have short-term effects on feeding, but do not affect the overall long-term food consumption. These signals may truly be hunger or satiety signals, however, one must not confuse a satiety signal with a food intake inhibition signal or confuse a hunger signal with a food intake initiation signal. The initiation may occur but not be sustained sufficiently to result in significant food consumption. Similarly, inhibition may occur but may not significantly alter overall food intake. One needs to examine, therefore, not only the stop and start

TABLE 11
Factors That Affect Food Intake

Enhances	Suppresses	
Insulin	Insulin cachectin (Tumor necrosis factor)	Anorectin
Testosterone	Estrogen	Corticotropin-releasing hormone
Glucocorticoids	Phenylethylamines[a]	Neurotensin
Thyroxine	Mazindol	Bombesin
Low serotonin levels	Substance P	Cyclo-his-pro
Dynorphin	Glucagon	High protein diets
β-Endorphin	"Satietin" (a blood-borne factor)	High blood glucose
Neuropeptide Y	High fat diet	Enterostatin
Galanin	Serotonin	Calcitonin
Opioid peptides	Fluoxetine	Thyrotropin releasing factor
Growth hormone-releasing hormone	Pain	Somatostatin
Desacetyl-melanocyte stimulating hormone	Histidine (precursor of histamine)	
	Amino acid imbalance in diet	
	Tryptophane (precursor of serotonin)	
Antidepressants[b]	Cholecystokinin (CCK)	

[a] These are drugs and, except for the drug phenylpropanolamine, are controlled substances. Many have serious side effects. They are structurally related to the catecholamines. Most are active as short-term appetite suppressants and act through their effects on the central nervous system, particularly through the β adrenergic and/or dopaminergic receptors. This group includes amphetamine, methamphetamine, phenmetrazine, phentermine, diethylpropion, fenfluramine, and phenylpropanolamine. Phenylpropanolamine-induced anorexia is not reversed by the dopamine antagonist, haloperidol.

[b] All of these drugs are controlled substances and their use must be carefully monitored. This groups includes amitriptyline, buspirone, chlordiazepoxide, chlorpromazine, cisplatin, clozapine, ergotamine, fluphenazine, impramine, iprindole, and others that block 5-HT receptors.

signals, but also the overall control of food intake that has a long-term effect on energy balance. Sustaining feeding or food abstinence may involve not only the factors listed in Table 11 but other factors as well. Initiation of feeding may be hormonally induced yet sustained because the food is found to be pleasing as per the discussion on the hedonistic qualities of food — its taste, smell, texture, etc. Similarly, cessation of feeding even though hormones have signalled initiation, may occur if the food is not palatable or acceptable.

A number of hormones, diet ingredients, metabolites, and drugs have been shown to influence food intake and feeding behavior. Some of the more important ones are shown in Table 12. Hormones that can enhance food intake at one level can suppress it at another level. Insulin is a prime example. Thyroxine is another. Normal individuals given a low dose of insulin will experience hunger. However, large doses of insulin can provoke a serious hypoglycemia that will have the opposite effect. Campfield and Smith have studied the signals for feeding that occur in the rat. They have shown that feeding is initiated when the brain perceives a small fall in blood glucose. Transient declines within the normal range of blood glucose levels were found to precede meal initiation. This feeding response could be attenuated if blood glucose levels were elevated via an intravenous infusion of glucose. Preceding the transient fall in blood glucose was a transient insulin spike which probably was responsible for the transient fall in glucose. Individuals soon after a high glucose meal will feel satiated; their blood and brain glucose levels have risen as has blood insulin, and their appetite is suppressed. Other hormones are involved as well. In hypothyroidism, hunger signals are poorly perceived. The patient, although not anorexic, does not have a strong drive to eat. In contrast, hyperthyroidism is characterized by strong, almost unremitting hunger.

Within this framework are a number of afferent and efferent systems which influence food intake by providing information to the brain and relaying instructions via neuronal signals from the brain to the rest of the body. Bray has recently reviewed the actions of peptides that

TABLE 12
Some Drugs That Affect Nutrient Intakes and Use

Drug	Effect
Phenylethylamine and related compounds	Anorexia
Amphetamine	Anorexia
Ethanol	Inhibits intestinal absorption of folate, B_{12}, increases need for niacin, riboflavin, thiamin, and pyridoxine
Diphenylhydantoin (Dilantin)	Impairs use of folate
Oral contraceptives	Increased folate turnover
Azulfidine	Decreases folate absorption, B_{12}, and fat-soluble vitamins
Neomycin	Decreases lipid absorption
p-Aminosalicylic acid	Promotes diarrhea and results in decreased absorption of almost all nutrients
Colchicine	Promotes diarrhea and results in decreased absorption of almost all nutrients
Biguanides (penformin, metformin)	Decreased absorption of B_{12}
Bile salt sequestrants	Decreased fat and fat-soluble vitamin absorption

affect the intake of specific nutrients and the sympathetic nervous system. Food intake can be increased or decreased with reciprocal effects on the central nervous system when these peptides are administered. Galanin, neuropeptide Y, opioid peptides, growth hormone releasing hormone, and desacetyl-melanocyte stimulating hormone increase food intake, whereas insulin excess, glucagon, cholecystokinen, anorectin, corticotropin-releasing hormone, neurotensin, bombesin, cyclo-his-pro, and thyrotropin-releasing hormone reduce food intake. Several of these hormones or peptides have specific actions with respect to the intake of specific food components. For example, increases in neuropeptide Y result in increased carbohydrate intake while increases in the level of galanin and opioid peptides increase fat intake. Fat intake is suppressed when the blood level of enterostatin rises. Rising blood levels of glucagon suppresses protein intake. All of the above are short-term signals that appear to regulate food selection as well as the amount of food consumed. Although most of these studies have been done in carefully prepared experimental animals (usually rats), there is sufficient indirect evidence to suggest that short-term food intake is similarly regulated in humans. In humans, serotoninergic agents are being developed for use as treatments for obesity and eating disorders. These agents are successful because they either block the binding of serotonin (5-hydroxytryptamine, 5-HT) to its receptor, or upregulate the receptors' binding affinity. 5-HT receptors are widespread throughout the cerebral cortex, the limbic system, the striatum, the brain stem, the choroid plexus, and almost every other region of the central nervous system. Because serotonin suppresses feeding if the receptor is blocked, feeding is enhanced. Thus, drugs that block these receptors are useful in treating anorexia (decreased desire to eat), especially the anorexia that accompanies anxiety, depression, obsessive-compulsive disorders, panic disorders, migraine, and chemotherapy emesis. In contrast, drugs that potentiate the binding of 5-HT to its receptor will result in a suppression of appetite and may be useful in treating the hyperphagia of Prader Willi syndrome and that associated with genetic obesity.

Drugs, particularly those used in cancer chemotherapy, frequently have as a side effect, appetite suppression. In part, this reduction in food intake may be due to disease and/or drug induced changes in taste and aroma perception and in part due to the effects of the disease and/or drugs on the central nervous system, particularly the adrenergic and serotonergic receptors. Several of the drugs listed in Table 12 are appetite suppressants and are chemically related to the catecholamines. As indicated, some of these drugs can be addictive and are therefore controlled substances. It appears that none of the drugs listed in Table 12 are free of side effects.

Some steroids affect food intake. Adrenalectomized animals or humans with Addison's disease, both glucocorticoid-deficient states, do not perceive normal hunger signals. If without food for extended periods of time, these individuals are difficult to realiment. However, once eating commences, a normal feeding pattern will be maintained. In excess, glucocorticoid stimulates feeding and patients with Cushing's disease (excess glucocorticoid production) or patients who are receiving long-term glucocorticoid treatment will report increased hunger and food intake. Patients with Cushing's disease are often characterized by large fat depots across the shoulders and in the abdomen. In addition, obese patients are frequently characterized by excess blood levels of both glucocorticoids and insulin. As noted above, these hormones stimulate the appetite and feeding.

Within the normal range, doses of testosterone and estrogen, although also steroids, have opposite effects with respect to food intake. In experimental animals, day-to-day variations in food intake by females will follow the same pattern as their day-to-day variation in estrogen level. When estrogen is high, food intake is suppressed and vice versa. Women who are anestrus due to ovariectomy or who are postmenopausal frequently lose their day-to-day estrogen-mediated food intake pattern. With this loss is a more even (and somewhat increased) food intake and subsequent body fat gain. This has been found as well in castrated female rats.

The gain in body weight as fat is explained by the loss in food intake control exerted by the estrogens rather than by an estrogen inhibiting effect on lipogenesis. Testosterone increases food intake marginally, but it also stimulates protein synthesis and spontaneous physical activity. As a result, body fat does not increase. As testosterone levels in males decline with age, protein synthesis declines and the body tends to sustain its fat synthetic activity. This results in a change in body composition with an increase in body fat stores. The age-related decline in testosterone production may not be accompanied by a decline in food intake.

Although food intake can vary from day-to-day in response to minor day-to-day variations in food supply, activity, and hormonal status, body weight is relatively constant. The mechanisms that control body weight are very complex and the fine details of this regulation are far from clear. However, suffice it to say that major long-term deviations in either food intake or physiological state can affect body weight or energy balance. If food intake (energy intake) is curtailed for days to months, body weight will fall; similarly, if food intake is dramatically increased, body weight will increase. This relationship assumes no change in body energy demand. As described in the section on trauma, the energy requirement can be increased up to tenfold by major illness despite the fact that the patient may be recumbent and perhaps sedated. Similarly, an individual who has markedly changed his or her activity level will affect his or her energy balance. If strenuous exercise is added without an increase in food intake, this exercise will increase energy expenditure and negative energy balance or weight loss will occur. In most individuals, therefore, long-term changes in energy balance, either through changes in intake or expenditure, will result in a body weight change.

D. ANOREXIA NERVOSA

That food intake can be consciously controlled is evident in the condition known as *anorexia nervosa*. This condition is frequently observed in adolescent females and is related to their inaccurate perception of their body fatness. They become obsessed with the desire to be thin and either refuse to eat and adequately nourish their bodies, or they eat but after eating force themselves to regurgitate food. Self-induced vomiting is called *bulimia*. Additional behavior related to an obsession with body image includes the regular use of laxatives and diuretics and the extensive participation in exercise designed to increase energy expenditure. Although the patients may be eating some food, these patients are not consuming enough food to meet their macro- and micronutrient requirements. Because of this, they are in negative energy and protein balance. These patients are characterized by little body fat. Because ovulation requires a minimal amount of fat in the body, ovulation ceases. Amenorrhea, hypothermia, and hypotension also develop and, if untreated, anorexics will starve to death. In many respects, these patients' physiological/biochemical features are similar to those patients described in the section on starvation. Their catabolic hormone levels are high and their body energy stores are being raided as a result. Insulin resistance due to the catabolic hormones is observed. Liver and muscle glycogen levels are low. Fat stores are minimal. As the weight loss proceeds further, these individuals have a reduced bone mass, a decreased metabolic rate, decreased heart rate, hypoglycemia, hypothyroidism, electrolyte imbalance, elevated free fatty acid and cholesterol levels, peripheral edema, and lastly, cardiac and renal failure. When their fat stores fall below 2% of total body weight, they will die. This 2% represents the lipids essential to the structure and function of membranes as well as those complex lipids that comprise the central nervous system.

With this scenario in mind, then, the clinician faces the challenge of reversing the condition. Just as it is difficult to reverse starvation-induced changes in the metabolism of unintentionally starving humans (see sections on starvation, protein-calorie malnutrition, and trauma), reversing the weight loss of anorexic patients presents some special challenges. The energy requirements for weight regain in anorexic patients are highly variable and depend largely on the physiological status of the patient at the time of treatment initiation and on the pre-anorexia body weight. Those patients who had been obese prior to their self-induced anorexia regained their lost weight faster than patients who had been of normal body weight. Pharmaceutical agents to stimulate appetite and reverse depression (if present) can be used. If the person is clinically depressed, frequently, treatment of the depression will have a positive effect on food intake. This is not always true, however. In contrast, treatment of the anorexia with appetite stimulating drugs, nutritional support, and counseling can reverse the condition of weight loss and secondarily, positively affect the depression. Again, this is not always true. The outcome of the treatment depends on the time at which it is instituted. If anorexia nervosa is recognized early in the sequence of hormonal and metabolic change, then the chances of success are much greater than if treatment is initiated after irreversible tissue changes have occurred. While controversy exists as to the success of treatment as well as the accuracy of diagnosis, it is generally agreed that aggressive treatment can achieve reversal in 50% of the cases. Mortality is estimated at 6% of cases. This leaves an estimate of approximately 44% who recover spontaneously without medical intervention. Treatment success also depends on the degree of self-prescribed food intake restriction. Total food abstinence is far more threatening than mild abstinence. Included in the mortality figure of 6% are those who commit suicide. This implies a relationship between the development of depression and anorexia — two self destructive behaviors that represent abnormalities in the CNS system.

Restoring the weight loss of the anorexic patient follows a slightly different pattern from the weight regain by traumatized individuals and formerly obese individuals. In the latter groups the fat regain precedes the protein regain. In fact, in the genetically obese individual fat regain takes precedence over protein regain. In the recovering anorexic who was not genetically obese prior to anorexia, protein regain keeps pace with fat regain. As both synthetic processes utilize micronutrients these must be provided at levels similar to those prescribed for growing children. Recovering anorexics are "growing" new tissue to replace that which was raided during the energy deficit period. They must consume sufficient nutrients to support this regrowth.

Bulimic and nonbulimic anorexics differ in their weight recovery. Those who were bulimic recover their lost weight more rapidly than those who were anorexic only. This is probably due to the difference in rate of weight loss. Those anorexics who were also bulimic were more severely starved and lost weight faster than nonbulimic anorexics. Because of this they are more likely to be diagnosed and treated sooner than nonbulimic anorexics. In anorexics, as with prolonged starvation, gut absorptive capacity is compromised due to a loss of cells lining the gastrointestinal tract. In the early phase of treatment, malabsorption is likely to occur. Because of the development of malabsorption, the recovering anorexic requires more food than the recovering bulimic anorexic. The recovering anorexic has lost more absorptive cells than the bulimic anorexic. Of interest is the report that even after weight regain, the recovered anorexic has a higher than normal energy requirement and, if not met, will begin to lose weight once again. This suggests that not all of the anorexia nervosa is self inflicted. It may begin with a conscious effort to consume less food but then may continue because of a change in the signals for food intake initiation and cessation and a change in the efficiency with which the body uses the food consumed.

E. ABNORMAL APPETITE

Humans, as well as some lower animals, will sometimes or habitually consume items of no nutritional value. In some cases, the item in question will have a deleterious effect on the person's health. The habit is called *pica*, after the Latin word for magpie. The magpie is a bird which will consume all manner of food and nonfood items. Pica has been observed for centuries and was described by Aetius of Amida in 1542. Many different items are consumed; however, the most common are clay (geophagia), laundry starch (amylophagia), or ice (pagophagia). A number of studies on the prevalence of pica have shown that up to 70% of some population groups may have this habit. Pregnant women as well as children are the most frequently affected and black women were 3 to 4 times more affected than white women of the same socioeconomic group. The most common cravings were for laundry starch (as much as 8 oz. a day) and clay. When both men and women were studied, few men exhibited the practice and it has been suggested that men use liquor or tobacco to meet their nonfood oral needs.

The question of why pica exists has not been satisfactorily answered. From the various epidemiological studies, age, sex, social status, and race appear to be important factors in the development of the habit. Several studies have noted that pica was associated with anemia. For example, it has been reported that frequent nosebleeds and other spontaneous losses of blood accompanied or preceded an increased craving for certain food and nonfood items. Clay, rice, French fries, ice, green vegetables, bread, hot tea, and grapefruit were mentioned as being consumed in large quantities by these patients. The patients were treated for their anemias by iron supplements and were tested for their iron-binding capacity. Some of the patients had low uptakes of iron while others were normal. Those with poor iron-binding capacities were usually the clay eaters; those with normal iron-binding capacities were ice cream eaters. Clay, even the small amount residing in the gastrointestinal tract of patients having no access to clay while hospitalized, could have adsorbed the oral iron supplements. Thus, it seems unlikely that an innate lowered iron-binding capacity was responsible for either the anemia or the pica. However, pica does appear to *follow* the development of anemia rather than precede it.

In addition to anemia, other conditions have been observed in pica patients. Muscular weakness and low serum potassium levels have been reported in geophagic patients. Both these conditions could be attributed to the binding of potassium in the intestine by the clay. This may also be true in patients consuming large quantities of laundry starch.

A more serious aspect of pica is the consumption of paint chips (plumbism) by young children. If the paint contains lead oxide as the pigment, lead intoxication can develop. This is characterized by anemia, low serum iron and copper values, growth depression, ataxia, kidney damage, coma, convulsions, and death. The ataxia, stupor, coma, and convulsions reflect the effect of lead on the central nervous system. This can be understood as the effect of lead on hemoglobin synthesis. Both copper and iron utilization is impaired and the anemia typical of lead intoxication is microcytic and hypochromic in character. In addition, lead may replace either copper, iron, or calcium in a number of tissues and, because it is metabolically inert, inhibit the functionality of that tissue. In the case of hemoglobin synthesis, it becomes obvious that the oxygen carrying capacity of the red blood cells is decreased. Those tissues with a high oxygen requirement, i.e., the neural tissue, will be the most affected. Thus, one can understand the neuromuscular response to chronic lead ingestion. If neuronal tissue suffers from prolonged oxygen deprivation it will die and this damage is irreversible. Subjects with lead poisoning can be treated with compounds such as EDTA, which will bind the circulating lead and allow the body to excrete the EDTA-lead complex. It is not possible, however, to rid the body of all of its accumulated lead nor to protect the patients from future ill effects of their lead-induced pathology. Lead will remain in its storage sites like bone and, when mobilized, will have untoward effects.

In the U.S. today, the majority of lead intoxication cases are young children ages 1 to 6, with pica. Adults who work in lead-related industries or consume lead-contaminated illicit beverages are also affected. Increasing the levels of lead exposure generally increases the blood and tissue lead levels, yet individual variation due to age, sex, and nutritional status occurs. The factors which determine the fractions of the body where lead is deposited have not been determined. It is known that well-nourished individuals are more resistant to the deleterious effects of lead than are poorly nourished individuals.

SUPPLEMENTAL READINGS

ARTICLES

Alpert, S. (1990) Growth, thermogenesis and hyperphagia, *Am. J. Clin. Nutr.*, 52:782–792.

Aw, T. Y. and Jones, D. P. (1989) Nutrient supply and mitochondrial function, *Ann. Rev. Nutr.*, 9:229–251.

Booth, D. A. (1992) Integration of internal and external signals in intake control, *Proc. Nutr. Soc.*, 51:21–28.

Bouchard, C. (1989) Genetic factors in obesity, *Med. Clin. N. Am.*, 73:67–81.

Bouchard, C., Savard, R., and Despres, J. P. (1985) Body composition in adopted and biological siblings, *Human Biol.*, 57:61–75.

Bray, G. (1992) Drug treatment of obesity, *Am. J. Clin. Nutr.*, 55:5385–5445.

Champigny, O. and Recquier, D. (1990) Effects of fasting and refeeding on the level of uncoupling protein mRNA in brown adipose tissue. Evidence for diet induced and cold induced responses, *J. Nutr.*, 120:1730–1736.

Crenshaw, L. I. (1980) Temperature regulation in vertebrates, *Ann. Rev. Physiol.*, 42:473–491.

de Quiroga, G. B. (1992) Brown fat thermogenesis and exercise. Two examples of physiological oxidative stress?, *Free Radical Biol. Med.*, 13:325–340.

Frisch, R. (1991) Body weight, body fat and ovulation, *Trends Endocrinol. Metab.*, 2:191–197.

Geloen, A., Collet, A. J., Guay, G., and Bukowiecki, L. J. (1990) In vivo differentiation of brown adipocytes in adult mice. An electron microscopic study, *Am. J. Anat.*, 188:366–372.

Geloen, A. and Trayhurn, P. (1990) Regulation of the level of uncoupling protein in brown adipose tissue by insulin requires mediation of the sympathetic nervous system, *FEBS Lett.*, 267:265–267.

Giles, R. E., Blanc, H., Cann, H. M., and Wallace, D. C. (1980) Maternal inheritance of human mitochondrial DNA, *Proc. Natl. Acad. Sci. U.S.A.*, 77:6715–6719.

Hamm, P., Shakelle, R. B., and Stamler, J. (1989) Large fluctuations in body weight during young adulthood and twenty-five year risk of coronary death in men, *Am. J. Epidemiol.*, 129:312–318.

Harris, R. B. S. (1990) Role of set point theory in regulation of body weight, *FASEB J.*, 4:3310–3318.

Hatefi, Y. (1985) The mitochondrial electron transport and oxidative phosphorylation system, *Ann. Rev. Biochem.*, 54:1015–1069.

Hervey, G. R. and Tobin, G. (1982) The part played by variation of energy expenditure in the regulation of energy balance, *Proc. Nutr. Soc.*, 41:137–153.

Heusner, A. A. (1982) Energy metabolism and body size I. Is the 0.75 mass exponent of Kleibers equation a statistical artifact, *Respiration Physiol.*, 48:1–12.

Himms-Hagen, J. (1989) Brown fat thermogenesis and obesity, *Prog. Lipid Res.*, 28:67–115.

Ide, T. and Sugano, M. (1988) Effects of dietary fat types on the thermogenesis of brown adipocytes isolated from rat, *Agric. Biol. Chem.*, 52:511–518.

Issartel, J. P., Dupuis, A., Garin, J., Lunardi, J., Michel, L., and Vignais, P. V. (1992) The ATP synthase (F_0F_1) complex in oxidative phosphorylation, *Experientia*, 48:351–362.

Jakobsen, K. and Thorbek, G. (1993) The respiratory quotient in relation to fat deposition in fattening-growing pigs, *Br. J. Nutr.*, 69:333–343.

Jeanrenaud, J. (1985) An hypothesis on the aetiology of obesity: dysfunction of the central nervous system, *Diabetologia*, 28:502–513.

Kaul, R., Heldmaier, G., and Schmidt, I. (1990) Defective thermoregulatory thermogenesis does not cause onset of obesity in Zucker rats, *Am. J. Physiol.*, 259:E11–E18.

Martin, R. J., White, D. B., and Hulsey, M. G. (1991) The regulation of body weight, *Am. Sci.,* 79:528–541.

Ricquier, D., Casteilla, L., and Bouillaud, F. (1991) Molecular studies of the uncoupling protein, *FASEB J.,* 5:2237–2242.

Roberts, S. B., Fuss, P., Evans, W. J., Heyman, M. B., and Young, V. R. (1993) Energy expenditure, aging and body composition, *J. Nutr.,* 123:474–482.

Sjostrom, L. V. (1992) Morbidity of severely obese subjects, *Am. J. Clin. Nutr.,* 55:508S–515S.

Stunkard, A. J., Harris, J. R., Pedersen, N. L., and McClearn, G. E. (1990) The body mass index of twins who have been reared apart, *N. Engl. J. Med.,* 322:1483–1487.

Stunkard, A. J., Sorensen, T. I. A., Harris, C., Teasdale, T. W., Chakraborty, R., Schull, W. J., and Schulsinger, F. (1986) An adoption study of human obesity, *N. Engl. J. Med.,* 314:193–198.

Trayhurn, P. and Jennings, G. (1986) Evidence that fasting can induce a selective loss of uncoupling protein from brown adipose tissue mitochondria of mice, *Biosci. Rep.,* 6:805–810.

Wallace, D. C. (1992) Diseases of the mitochondrial DNA, *Ann. Rev. Biochem.,* 61:1175–1212.

Webster, A. J. F. (1993) Energy partitioning, tissue growth and appetite control, *Proc. Nutr. Soc.,* 52:69–76.

Welch, G. R. (1991) Thermodynamics and living systems: problems and paradigms, *J. Nutr.,* 121:1902–1906.

Welle, S. L., Amatruda, J. M., Forbes, G. B., and Lockwood, D. H. (1984) Resting metabolic rates of obese women after rapid weight loss, *J. Clin. Endocrinol. Metab.,* 59:41–44.

Westerteys, K. R. (1993) Food quotient, respiratory quotient and energy balance, *Am. J. Clin. Nutr.,* 57:759S–765S.

BOOKS

Bjorntorp, P. and Brodoff, B. N., Eds. (1992) *Obesity,* J. B. Lippincott, Philadelphia, 805 pps.

Mitchell, P. (1986) *Chemiosmotic Coupling and Energy Transduction,* Glynn Research, Bodmin, U.K.

Trayhurn, P. and Nicholls, D. G., Eds. (1986) *Brown Adipose Tissue,* Edward Arnold, London, 299–338.

Unit 4

PROTEINS

TABLE OF CONTENTS

I. OVERVIEW

After the energy need is met, protein is the next most important macronutrient need. The proteins provide the amino acids which are needed to synthesize the body protein. Protein, in its many forms, is an essential and universal constituent of all living cells. As much as one half of the dry weight of the cell is protein. The human body on the average is 18% protein. Besides being plentiful, proteins serve a variety of functions. They serve as structural components, as biocatalysts (in the form of enzymes), as antibodies, as lubricants, as messengers (in the form of hormones), and as carriers. Proteins are composed of amino acids which must be provided in food. On the average, Americans consume about 100 g protein per day. After digestion, the amino acids which comprise the food proteins are absorbed and used to synthesize body proteins. In this unit, the chemistry and physiology of the proteins are discussed.

II. AMINO ACIDS

A. CHEMISTRY

Amino acids consist of carbon, hydrogen, oxygen, nitrogen, and occasionally sulfur. All amino acids with the exception of proline have a terminal carboxyl group,

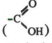

and an unsubstituted amino (-NH$_2$) group attached to the α carbon. Proline has a substituted amino group and a carboxyl group. Also attached to the α carbon is a functional group identified as R; R differs for each amino acid (Table 1). The general structure of amino acids can be represented as

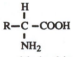

While it is convenient to represent amino acids in this manner, in reality the amino acids exist as the dipolar ion in the range of pH values (5.0 to 8.0) found within the body.

TABLE 1
Structures and Abbreviations of the Amino Acids

Name	Abbreviation	Structure
Glycine	Gly	$\begin{array}{c} H \\ | \\ H-C-COOH \\ | \\ NH_2 \end{array}$
Alanine	Ala	$\begin{array}{c} CH_3-CH-COOH \\ | \\ NH_2 \end{array}$
Valine	Val	$\begin{array}{c} CH_3 \\ \diagdown \\ CH-CH-COOH \\ \diagup \quad | \\ H_3C \quad NH_2 \end{array}$
Leucine	Leu	$\begin{array}{c} CH_3 \\ \diagdown \\ CH-CH_2-CH-COOH \\ \diagup \qquad | \\ H_3C \qquad NH_2 \end{array}$
Isoleucine	Ile	$\begin{array}{c} CH_3 \\ \diagdown \\ CH_2 \\ \diagdown \\ CH-CH-COOH \\ \diagup \quad | \\ H_3C \quad NH_2 \end{array}$
Serine	Ser	$\begin{array}{c} CH_2-CH-COOH \\ | \qquad | \\ OH \quad NH_2 \end{array}$
Threonine	Thr	$\begin{array}{c} CH_3-CH-CH-COOH \\ | \qquad | \\ OH \quad NH_2 \end{array}$
Cysteine (Cystein)	Cys	$\begin{array}{c} CH_2-CH-COOH \\ | \qquad | \\ SH \quad NH_2 \end{array}$
Methionine	Met	$\begin{array}{c} CH_2-CH_2-CH-COOH \\ | \qquad\qquad | \\ S-CH_3 \qquad NH_2 \end{array}$
Aspartic Acid	Asp	$\begin{array}{c} HOOC-CH_2-CH-COOH \\ | \\ NH_2 \end{array}$

TABLE 1 (continued)
Structures and Abbreviations of the Amino Acids

Name	Abbreviation	Structure
Asparagine	Asn	$H_2N-\overset{\overset{\displaystyle}{\|}}{\underset{O}{C}}-CH_2-\overset{\overset{\displaystyle}{\|}}{\underset{NH_2}{CH}}-COOH$
Glutamic Acid	Glu	$HOOC-CH_2-CH_2-\overset{\overset{\displaystyle}{\|}}{\underset{NH_2}{CH}}-COOH$
Glutamine	Gln	$H_2N-\overset{\overset{\displaystyle}{\|}}{\underset{O}{C}}-CH_2-CH_2-\overset{\overset{\displaystyle}{\|}}{\underset{NH_2}{CH}}-COOH$
Arginine	Arg	$H_2N-\overset{\overset{\displaystyle}{\|}}{\underset{NH}{C}}-\overset{\overset{\displaystyle}{\|}}{\underset{H}{N}}-CH_2-CH_2-CH_2-\overset{\overset{\displaystyle}{\|}}{\underset{NH_2}{CH}}-COOH$
Lysine	Lys	$\overset{\overset{\displaystyle}{\|}}{\underset{NH_2}{CH_2}}-CH_2-CH_2-CH_2-\overset{\overset{\displaystyle}{\|}}{\underset{NH_2}{CH}}-COOH$
Hydroxylysine	Hyl	$\overset{\overset{\displaystyle}{\|}}{\underset{NH_2}{CH_2}}-\overset{\overset{\displaystyle}{\|}}{\underset{OH}{CH}}-CH_2-CH_2-\overset{\overset{\displaystyle}{\|}}{\underset{NH_2}{CH}}-COOH$
Histidine	His	$CH_2-\overset{\overset{\displaystyle}{\|}}{\underset{NH_2}{CH}}-COOH$ (imidazole ring, HN, N)
Phenylalanine	Phe	$C_6H_5-CH_2-\overset{\overset{\displaystyle}{\|}}{\underset{NH_2}{CH}}-COOH$
Tyrosine	Tyr	$HO-C_6H_4-CH_2-\overset{\overset{\displaystyle}{\|}}{\underset{NH_2}{CH}}-COOH$
Tryptophan	Trp	indole ring $-CH_2-\overset{\overset{\displaystyle}{\|}}{\underset{NH_2}{CH}}-COOH$
Proline	Pro	pyrrolidine ring $-COOH$

TABLE 1 (continued)
Structures and Abbreviations of the Amino Acids

Name	Abbreviation	Structure
Hydroxyproline	Hyp	(structure of hydroxyproline)

The student will find it useful to remember the basic structure of alanine and then remember that all of the rest of the amino acids have R groups that replace the terminal methyl group in alanine. For example, in valine, the methyl group is replaced with an isopropyl group; in phenylalanine it is replaced with a phenyl group.

$$R-\underset{\underset{NH_3^+}{|}}{\overset{\overset{H}{|}}{C}}-COO-$$

There are several ways to classify the amino acids. Protein chemists use the polarity of the R group as the basis for their classification of the amino acids. This classification system divides the amino acids into four groups: (1) nonpolar; (2) polar but not charged; (3) positively charged at pH 6.0 to 7.0; and (4) negatively charged at pH 6.0 to 7.0. The distribution of the amino acids into these groups is shown in Table 2. This classification system is considered more useful than others because it relates to the functions of the amino acids in protein structures. Another classification that is frequently useful is based on the chemical nature of the amino acids. This grouping is listed in Table 3.

Nutritionists, while interested in the physical and chemical characteristics of the individual amino acids, classify the amino acids on the basis of whether the body can synthesize them in sufficient quantities to meet the body's need or whether the diet must provide them. For these purposes, then, amino acids are classified as essential or nonessential. The definition of essentiality rests with the species of animal in question and its physiological need. In the adult human, for example, histidine need not be in the diet. While essential, it is stored in muscle as carnosine and can be mobilized in times of need. However, during periods of high rates of protein synthesis, growth for example, not enough histidine can be synthesized. Additional supplies must then be provided in the diet. Table 4 lists the essential and nonessential amino acids for adults.

Occasionally, through a mutation in one or more genes which code for enzymes needed for amino acid interconversion, or through a specific illness, certain of the nonessential amino acids cannot be synthesized. In these instances, the amino acid in question then becomes essential and must be provided in the diet. An example of the former is the mutation in the gene for phenylalanine hydroxylase which results in phenylketonuria (PKU). This mutation is clinically characterized by severe mental retardation. Phenylalanine hydroxylase catalyzes the conversion of phenylalanine to tyrosine. In the patient with phenylketonuria, tyrosine cannot be synthesized and thus becomes an essential amino acid. Phenylalanine metabolites other than tyrosine are made and accumulated, and it is this accumulation of neurotoxic compounds that destroy cells in the brain, which in turn results in the characteristic symptom of phenylketonuria, mental retardation. Another example is renal disease. In this condition, the kidney, which is a major site (in addition to the liver) for arginine synthesis, may be destroyed by the disease process. Because of damage to the kidney, the body may not be able to synthesize sufficient arginine to meet its requirement. Thus, arginine becomes an essential amino acid. In uremia, histidine may also become an essential amino acid for the same reason given for arginine. Care must be taken in each of the above instances to provide the needed

TABLE 2
Classification of Amino Acids Based on
Polarity of the Functional Groups

Nonpolar R Groups

Alanine	Phenylalanine	Methionine
Valine	Tryptophan	Proline
	Leucine	Isoleucine

Polar Uncharged R Groups

Serine	Asparagine	Cysteine	Glycine
Threonine	Glutamine	Hydroxyproline	Tyrosine

Positively Charged R Groups

Lysine	Hydroxylysine
Arginine	Histidine

Negatively Charged R Groups

Aspartic acid
Glutamic acid

TABLE 3
Amino Acids Classified According to Chemical Nature

Monoamino monocarboxylic: glycine, alanine, valine, leucine, isoleucine
Diamino monocarboxylic (basic): arginine, lysine
Monoamino dicarboxylic (acidic): glutamic acid, aspartic acid
Sulfur containing: cystine (and cysteine), methionine
Aromatic: tyrosine, phenylalanine
Heterocyclic: proline, hydroxyproline, histidine, tryptophan

TABLE 4
Essential and Nonessential Amino
Acids for Adult Mammals

Essential	Nonessential
Valine	Hydroxyproline
Leucine	Cysteine
Isoleucine	Glycine
Threonine	Alanine
Phenylalanine	Serine
Methionine	Proline
Tryptophan	
Lysine	Glutamic Acid
Histidine	Aspartic Acid
[a]Arginine	

[a]   Not essential for maintenance of most adult mammals.

amino acids in the diet in sufficient quantities to maintain tissue protein synthesis without exceeding the body's capacity to utilize these amino acids. If too much of the amino acid is provided, unusual amounts of some metabolites of these amino acids may be formed and these metabolites may be toxic and destructive.

1. Stereochemistry

Amino acids, like the simple sugars, exist as stereoisomers. Their absolute configuration, similarly, is related to the configuration of glyceraldehyde. The Fischer projection of D-glyceraldehyde shows the hydroxyl function on the α carbon to the right. At a similar point in a D-amino acid, the amino function is to the right.

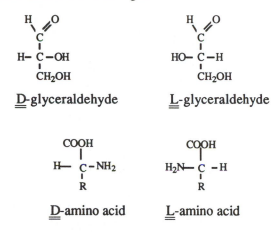

All of the amino acids except glycine (which has no asymmetric carbon atom) possess optical activity. The amino acids of nutritional importance are all L-amino acids whereas the nutritionally important sugars are of the D-series. Species differences exist in the utilization of L vs. D amino acids. There are a number of D amino acids that are of use to single-cell organisms and, further, some D amino acids combine to form potent antibiotics. Gramicidin D and actinomycin D for example, contain D-amino acids. Their utility as antibiotics rests with the fact that mammalian cells cannot absorb them as readily as microorganisms. Pathogenic organisms incorporate them into their intracellular material and these materials then become antimetabolites, successfully terminating the metabolic activity of the pathogen in question.

2. Acid-Base Properties

Because amino acids possess acidic carboxyl and basic amino groups, they can function as either hydrogen acceptors or donors. At low pH, amino acids can exist in the fully protonated form:

$$
\begin{array}{c}
H \\
| \\
R\!-\!C\!-\!COOH \\
| \\
NH_3^+
\end{array}
$$

At higher pH levels, H^+ from the carboxyl function will be released and the amino acid exists as the dipolar ion,

$$
\begin{array}{c}
H \\
| \\
R\!-\!C\!-\!COO^- \\
| \\
NH_3
\end{array}
$$

At even higher pH values, the amino function dissociates and the amino acid exists in the negatively charged form

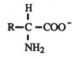

If the amino acid has more than one amino or carboxyl group, further dissociation can occur and the range in pH over which this occurs is much broader. For example, aspartic acid exists

"at pH 1 as:"
$$\begin{array}{l} COOH \\ | \\ CH_2 \\ | \\ CH\text{-}NH_3{}^+ \\ | \\ COOH \end{array}$$

"at pH 3 as:"
$$\begin{array}{l} COOH \\ | \\ CH_2 \\ | \\ CH\text{-}NH_3{}^+ \\ | \\ COO^- \end{array}$$

"at pH 6 to 8 as:"
$$\begin{array}{l} COO^- \\ | \\ CH_2 \\ | \\ CH\text{-}NH_3{}^+ \\ | \\ COO^- \end{array}$$

"and at PH 11 as:"
$$\begin{array}{l} COO^- \\ | \\ CH_2 \\ | \\ CH\text{-}NH_2 \\ | \\ COO^- \end{array}$$

With each change in the form of the amino acid that occurs, from the lowest to the highest pH, a hydrogen ion is released. The capacity to accept or release hydrogen ions is characteristic of all amino acids; however, only a few (glutamate, aspartate, histidine, and, perhaps, arginine) serve as buffers with respect to the regulation of hydrogen ion concentration in the body. Glutamine is especially important as a buffer in the kidney. However, because free amino acids are in low concentrations relative to the other buffering systems in the body, their buffering power is much less important than that of the carbonate and phosphate buffering system. Even these amino acids are not as potent buffers as are some of the other compounds in the body.

3. Reactions

The amino acids undergo characteristic chemical reactions at the α-carboxyl group, at the α-amino group, and at the functional groups of the side chains. Such characteristic reactions are particularly useful to the biochemist, for they assist in the quantitative determination of the amino acid composition and sequence in a given protein. These reactions are summarized in Table 5.

Among the reactions that the functional groups on the side chains of the amino acids undergo, those that involve the thiol or sulfhydryl group of cysteine are important. This group is weakly acidic and quite reactive. It is very susceptible to oxidation by either oxygen in the presence of iron salts or by other oxidizing agents. When oxidized, cysteine is converted to cystine. In this conversion, two cysteine residues are joined together by a disulfide (-S-S-) bridge. Within the extracellular proteins, sulfhydryl groups react with one another to form disulfide bridges. These bridges stabilize the internal structure of the protein. Sulfhydryl groups also react with heavy metals to form mercaptides. This reaction is of great interest to the nutritionist since protein-mineral interactions, or more truly, mineral-sulfhydryl reactions, are important not only for an understanding of how minerals serve as cofactors in enzymatic reactions and for mineral transport into and out of cells, but also to an understanding of the mechanisms involved in heavy metal intoxication. Figure 1 illustrates these reactions.

No discussion of the chemical reactions of the amino acids would be complete without discussing the formation of the peptide bond (Figure 2). Without question, this is the most important reaction of these compounds. The formation of the peptide bond involves the removal of one molecule of water with the resultant linkage between the carbon of one amino

TABLE 5
Characteristic Chemical Reactions of Amino Acids

Reaction Name	Reagent	Use
Ninhydrin reaction	Ninhydrin	To estimate amino acids quantitatively in small amounts
Sanger reaction	1-Fluoro-2,4-dinitrobenzene	To identify the amino terminal group of a peptide
Dansyl chloride reaction	1-dimethylamino-naphthalene (also called dansylchloride)	To measure very small amounts of amino acids quantitatively
Edmann degradation	Phenylisothiocyanate	To identify the terminal NH_2 group in a protein
Schiff base	Aldehydes	Labile intermediate in some enzymatic reactions involving α-amino acid substrates

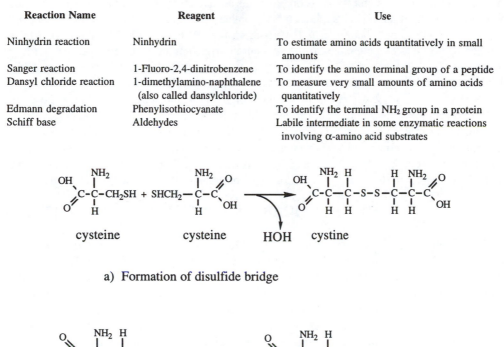

cysteine   cysteine   HOH   cystine

a) Formation of disulfide bridge

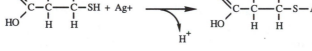

cysteine   cysteine silver mercaptide

b) Formation of a mercaptide

FIGURE 1. Examples of sulfhydryl group reactions; (a) formation of disulfide bridge; (b) formation of a mercaptide.

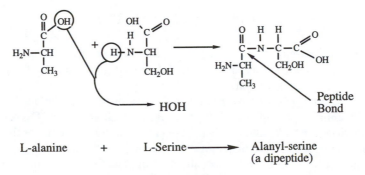

L-alanine   +   L-Serine ⟶ Alanyl-serine (a dipeptide)

FIGURE 2. The formation of a peptide bond.

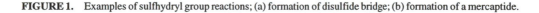

acid to the α-amino group of a second amino acid. The water is formed when the hydroxyl ion of the carboxyl group of one amino acid combines with a hydrogen atom from the amino group of a second amino group. Peptide bonding is the basis for the formation of peptides, polypeptides, and proteins and is the linkage used in the primary structure of any sequence of amino acids.

The number of possible combinations of the 20 amino acids commonly found in proteins to make different protein molecules is almost limitless. In a dipeptide which contains two different amino acids (A and B), two combinations are available: A-B and B-A. In a tripeptide with three different amino acids, six combinations are available if all three amino acids are used and each used only one time: A-B-C; B-A-C; A-C-B; B-C-A; C-A-B; and C-B-A. The number of possible combinations of the sequential arrangement of different amino acids is determined by the expression $n!$ (n factorial), where n is the number of different amino acids. If 20 amino acids are present in a protein, the number of possible combinations would be $20 \times 19 \times 18 \times 17 \ldots \times 1 = 2 \times 10^{18}$. The molecular weight of this molecule is about 2400 (average molecular weight of an amino acid × number of amino acids = 120×20), a relatively small protein. If the molecule were larger, and if the amino acids were used more than once, the number of possible combinations is increased even more. That nature can consistently reproduce the same protein, when there are so many choices of amino acids and sequences, is due to its dependence on the codes for each of these proteins in the genetic material, DNA.

III. PEPTIDES AND PROTEINS

Two amino acids joined together form a dipeptide, three form a tripeptide, and so on. Each amino acid in a chain is referred to as an amino acid residue. A chain of up to 100 amino acids joined together is called a polypeptide. If more than 100 amino acids are involved, then the compound is called a protein. Proteins have been identified which have as many as 300,000 amino acids residues and molecular weights in excess of 4×10^7.

The sequence of the amino acids which comprise a given protein is represented by a sequential arrangement of abbreviations for each. For example, the polypeptide bradykinin is represented in the following manner: Arg-Pro-Pro-Gly-Phe-Ser-Pro-Phe-Arg. The right-hand side of the chain represents the carboxyl terminal while the left-hand side represents the amino terminal. The systematic name for bradykinin is arginyldiprolylglycylphenylalanyl-serylprolylphenylalanylarginine. This systematic name is seldom used except when one wishes to give the amino acid sequence of this protein. The amino acid sequence of a given protein can vary and its variation is controlled genetically. Some of the proteins of importance in nutrition have been sequenced, but these are few in number compared to the vast array of proteins in nature. Even if the proteins were sequenced, their systematic names would not be used because such a name would be very cumbersome.

IV. PROTEIN STRUCTURE

Proteins are complex molecules having characteristic primary, secondary, tertiary, and quaternary structures. The primary structure is determined genetically as the particular sequence of amino acids in a given protein.

The genetic material, DNA (deoxyribonucleic acid), in the cell nucleus holds the code that dictates the amino acid sequence of the protein. A small amount of DNA is also found in the mitochondria (mtDNA). Should there be a change in the sequence of the nucleotides which comprise the code, the sequence of amino acids will be different. A change in the normal sequence of bases in the DNA is called a mutation. It can be either a spontaneous mutation or one induced by drugs or a virus or any one of a number of external variants that target the genetic material of the cell. Whether the substitution of one or more amino acids for another has an adverse effect on the activity of the protein being synthesized depends wholly on the amino acids in question. If these amino acids have functional groups in their R side chain that modify the three-dimensional structure and the function of the protein, then its activity will be abnormal. Throughout this text examples of genetic mutations and their consequences are given to illustrate the importance of heredity in determining nutrient needs and tolerances.

Under normal pH and temperature conditions a protein is characterized not only by its amino acid sequence but also by its three-dimensional structure; that is, how the chain of amino acids twists and turns and what shape this long chain of amino acids assumes. This three-dimensional shape, unique to each protein's particular amino acid sequence, is known as the native conformation of the protein. This assumption of shape may be spontaneous or may be catalyzed by enzymes, and reflects the lowest energy state of the protein in its native environment. Protein conformation is usually divided into two categories: secondary and tertiary. The secondary and tertiary structures of a protein result from interactions between the reactive groups on the amino acids in the protein.

Secondary structure is the *local* conformation of the protein molecule. It is due to the formation of hydrogen bonds, disulfide bridges, and ionic bonds (in the case of the polar amino acids) between adjacent or nearby amino acids in an amino acid chain. As a result of these bonds, there is a regular recurring arrangement in space of the amino acids within the chain which can extend over the entire chain or only in small segments of it. Two kinds of periodic structures are found in proteins: the helix and the pleated sheet. In the helix, the amino acid chain can be viewed as wrapping itself around a long cylinder. The most common helical arrays are the α-helix and triple helix. The other periodic shape is the pleated sheet. It is essentially a linear array of the amino acid chain. These structures are shown in Figure 3. All of these structures are stabilized by hydrogen bonding and sulfide bridges.

Tertiary structure is the *regional* conformation a protein molecule possesses; it develops after the secondary structure is established. Tertiary structure refers to how the amino acid chain bends or folds in three dimensions to form a compact or tightly folded protein. Tertiary structure results from hydrogen bonding, disulfide cross-linkages, ionic bonds between polar amino acids, and interactions between hydrophobic R groups. This last feature tends to locate the hydrophobic R groups internally in the protein structure, away from the aqueous environment. A protein which clearly demonstrates tertiary structure is hemoglobin. Some parts of the amino acid chains in this molecule can form helices; others cannot. This gives the molecule the fluidity to assume different three-dimensional shapes along the chain: it will bend back upon itself to accomplish the maximum number of hydrogen bonds and disulfide bridges.

As a result of the various bonds that can form within a protein molecule, essentially two kinds of proteins exist: fibrous protein and globular protein. Fibrous proteins resemble long ribbons or hairs. They tend to be insoluble in most solvents and include such tough, resilient protein structures as collagen and elastin. Fibrous protein can have either the helical or pleated sheet structure. Collagen is an example of the triple helix; silk, a pleated sheet structure. Whereas the fibrous proteins appear to have a long "stringy" shape, globular proteins are roughly spherical or elliptical. Many enzymes and antibodies have a globular structure.

The quaternary structure refers to how groups of individual amino acid chains are arranged in relation to each other within a given protein. It is the structure which results when two or more polypeptide chains combine. The chains (subunits) may be different or identical, yet each subunit still possesses its own primary, secondary, and tertiary structure. The number of subunits in a protein may vary; some proteins have only two subunits while others have as many as 2130 subunits. The protein hemoglobin, for example, consists of four subunits and is one of the few proteins whose primary, secondary, tertiary, and quaternary structures are known. It contains four separate peptide chains: two α chains which contain 141 amino acid residues and two β chains which contain 146 amino acid residues. To each of these is bound a heme (iron) residue in a noncovalent linkage.

A. PROTEIN DENATURATION

One of the most striking characteristics of proteins is the response to heat, alcohol, and other treatments which affect their quaternary, tertiary, and secondary structures. This characteristic response is called *denaturation*. Denaturation results in the unfolding of a protein molecule, thus breaking its hydrogen bonds and the associations between functional groups;

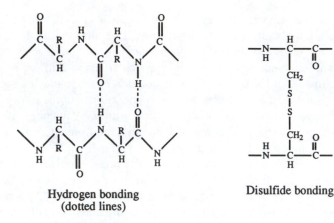

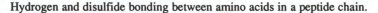

Hydrogen bonding
(dotted lines)

Disulfide bonding

Hydrogen and disulfide bonding between amino acids in a peptide chain.

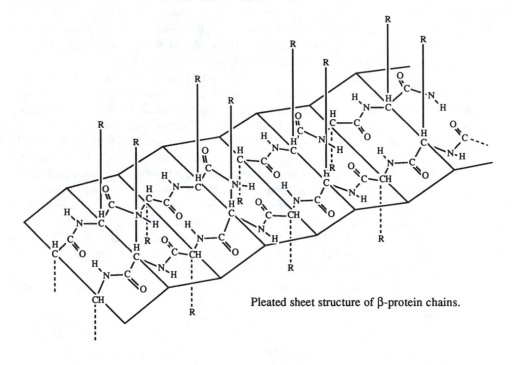

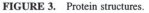

Pleated sheet structure of β-protein chains.

FIGURE 3.   Protein structures.

as a result, the three-dimensional structure is lost. Denaturation affects many of the properties of the protein molecule. Its physical shape is changed, its solubility in water is decreased, and its reactivity with other proteins may be lost. When denatured, the protein loses its biological activity. Most proteins are denatured at temperatures greater than 50 to 60°C; some are denatured at temperatures less than 15°C. A very good example of protein denaturation is the coagulation of egg white when heated. Heat denaturation, unless extreme, does not affect the amino acid composition of protein and, indeed, may make these amino acids more available to the body because heating provokes the unfolding or uncoiling of the protein and exposes more of the amino acid chain to the action of the proteolytic digestive enzymes. For this reason, many cooked proteins are of higher biological value than those same proteins if consumed without heat treatment. If only mild denaturation occurs, it can be reversed. This process is called *renaturation*. If a protein is renatured, it will resume its original shape and biological activity.

V. CLASSIFICATION OF PROTEINS

A. CLASSIFICATION BY SOLUBILITY AND PROSTHETIC GROUPS

In addition to the conformational classification of proteins as described above, proteins have been classified on the basis of their solubility characteristics. As more and more information has been acquired about proteins, this classification system has become outmoded. However, because the vocabulary from this system has become so firmly entrenched in discussions of protein, it is necessary to become familiar with it. In this system, proteins are classed as simple or conjugated proteins. Simple proteins are those which contain only L-amino acids or their derivatives and no prosthetic group. Examples of simple proteins and their characteristics are given in Table 6.

Conjugated proteins contain some nonprotein substances linked by a bond other than an ionic bond. Since most proteins occur in cells in combination with prosthetic groups, conjugated proteins are the ones most nutritionists will recognize. Table 7 and the text below describe representative conjugated proteins.

1. Glycoproteins

A majority of the naturally occurring conjugated proteins are glycoproteins. Sugar molecules are covalently bound to proteins, especially those proteins that are secreted from cells (mucin, for example) and those that comprise the mucin which is found in outer surface of the plasma membrane. Different types of covalent linkages have been found. The most common are the N-glycosidic linkages formed between asparagine amide group and a sugar. Another common linkage is the O-glycosidic linkage between either the serine or threonine hydroxyl group and a sugar. Glycoproteins include the mucin in saliva as well as the conjugated proteins of plasma, collagen, ovalbumin (the major protein of egg white), and plant agglutinins. The glycoproteins range in size from a molecular weight of 15,000 to more than 1 million; the carbohydrate component of these proteins varies from 1 to 85%. Glycoproteins having more than 80% of their molecules as carbohydrates are called *proteoglycans*.

Only 8 of the 100 or so carbohydrates that are known to occur in nature are found in glycoproteins (Table 8). These carbohydrates occur in chains containing no more than 15 saccharide units. Of the 20 amino acids in these proteins only four (Table 8) actually bind to the carbohydrate moiety. The carbohydrates are linked to these amino acids by a nitrogen-oxygen glucosidic bond or through an oxygen bond. Some proteins contain small amounts of carbohydrate in loose association rather than as integral and characteristic parts of their structure. An example of this association is the glycosylated hemoglobin found in the blood of poorly controlled diabetics. In diabetes, blood glucose levels may fluctuate and exceed the normal range of 80 to 120 mg/dl. Some of this excess of glucose may be picked up by the hemoglobin and form glycosylated hemoglobin. Levels of glycosylated hemoglobin are used as indicators of the degree of control of the diabetic state.

The function of the carbohydrate moiety of glycoproteins is not well defined. Some of the glycoproteins, those located on the exterior aspect of the plasma membrane, are part of the cell recognition system. Others are essential to the immune mechanism as a component of γ-globulin. Glycoproteins are essential components of membrane transport systems and are components of many receptors.

2. Lipoproteins

Lipoproteins are multicomponent complexes of lipids and protein that form distinct molecular aggregates with approximate stoichiometry between each of the components. They contain polar and neutral lipids, cholesterol, or cholesterol esters in addition to protein. The proteins and lipids are held together by noncovalent forces. The protein component (apolipoprotein) is located on the outer surface of the micellular lipid structure, where it serves a hydrophilic function. Lipids, primarily hydrophobic molecules, are not easily transported through an aqueous environment such as blood. However, when they combine with proteins the resulting

TABLE 6
Simple Proteins

Name	Characteristics	Example
Albumins	Soluble in water, coagulated by heat, precipitated by saturated salt solutions	Lactalbumin Serum albumin
Globulins	Soluble in salt solutions; insoluble in water; coagulated by heat	Serum globulin Ovoglobulin
Glutelins	Soluble in dilute acids and bases; insoluble in neutral solvents, coagulated by heat	Glutenin from wheat
Prolamins	Soluble in 70–80% alcohol; insoluble in absolute alcohol, water and other neutral solvents	Zein from corn Gliadin from wheat
Scleroproteins	Insoluble in all neutral solvents and in dilute acids and bases	Keratin Collagen
Histones	Soluble in water and very dilute acids; insoluble in very dilute NH_4OH; not coagulated by heat; basic amino acids predominate	Nucleoproteins
Protamines	Basic polypeptides, soluble in water or in NH_4OH; not coagulated by heat; basic amino acids predominate	Eggs

TABLE 7
Some Conjugated Proteins

Name	Prosthetic group	Example
Glycoproteins and mucoproteins	Nucleic acid carbohydrates which hydrolyze to amino acid sugars; mucoproteins contain 4% hexosamines and glycoproteins contain less	Serum alpha, beta, and gamma globulins; Mucin
Lipoproteins	Neutral fats, phospholipids, cholesterol	Cell membranes Blood lipid carrying proteins
Nucleoproteins	Nucleic acid	Chromosomes
Phosphoproteins	Phosphate joined in ester linkage	Milk casein
Hemoproteins	Iron	Catalase, Hemoglobin, Cytochromes
Flavoproteins	Flavin adenine nucleotide (FAD)	FAD linked-succinate dehydrogenase
Metalloproteins	Metals (not part of a nonprotein prosthetic	Ferritin

compound becomes hydrophilic and can be transported in the blood to tissue which can use or store these lipids. The importance of these lipoproteins as carriers is discussed later in Unit 6. Membrane lipoproteins, like the glycoproteins, are essential components of membrane transport systems and, as such, are important in the overall regulation of cellular activity.

3. Nucleoproteins

Nucleoproteins are combinations of nucleic acids and simple proteins. The protein usually consists of a large number of the basic amino acids. Nucleoproteins are ubiquitous molecules that tend to have very complex structures and numerous functional activities. All living cells contain nucleoproteins. Some cells, such as viruses, seem to be entirely composed of nucleo-protein.

4. Other Conjugated Proteins

The phosphoproteins and the metalloproteins are associations of proteins with phosphate groups or such ions as zinc, copper, and iron. The association may be fairly loose as with the phosphate carrying protein or tight as with the phosphate in casein and the iron in ferritin.

Hemoproteins sometimes are grouped with the metalloproteins because of the iron which they contain. Flavoproteins are primarily enzymes and have as their prosthetic group a

TABLE 8
Components of Glycoproteins

Sugars found in glycoproteins	Amino acids which bind to the carbohydrates in glycoproteins
Glucose	Asparagine
Acetylgalactosamine	Serine
Galactose	Threonine
Arabinose	Hydroxylysine
Mannose	
Xylose	
Fucase (6-deoxy galactose)	
Acetylglucosamine	

phosphate-containing adenine nucleotide which functions as an acceptor or donor of reducing equivalents.

B. CLASSIFICATION BY FUNCTION

In addition to the system described above for the classification of proteins, the biochemist classifies these compounds on the basis of their function. Thus, proteins are classified as enzymes, storage proteins such as casein or ferritin, transport proteins such as hemoglobin, contractile proteins such as myosin, immune proteins such as antibodies, toxin proteins such as the *Clostrodium botulinum* toxin, hormones such as insulin, receptor proteins such as the insulin receptor, and structural proteins such as elastin and collagen. The functions of body proteins are discussed in Section VII. The nutritionist might not use this system for classifying food proteins, yet will want to understand these functions as part of his/her knowledge about the protein nutrient class.

C. CLASSIFICATION BY NUTRITIVE VALUE

In nutrition, we are interested in food proteins as sources of needed amino acids. Those proteins which contain the essential amino acids in the proportions needed by the body are referred to as *complete* proteins. They are primarily of animal origin. Eggs, milk, meat, and fish are sources of complete protein. Proteins lacking in one or more essential amino acids or which have a poor balance of amino acids relative to the body's need are *incomplete* or *imbalanced* proteins. These proteins are usually of plant origin, although some animal proteins are incomplete. The connective tissue protein called collagen, from which gelatin is isolated, lacks tryptophan; zein, the protein in corn, is low in lysine as well as tryptophan. Table 9 gives the protein and Table 10 gives amino acid content of several food proteins. When food selection is limited by the availability of protein-rich foods, incomplete proteins can be combined so that all of the essential amino acids are provided. For example, corn or wheat and soy or peanut proteins can be combined in the same meal so that all of the essential amino acids are provided. When these proteins are combined they will provide sufficient amounts of the needed amino acids. The combination of incomplete proteins needed to provide all the needed amino acids must be consumed within a relatively short time interval (less than 4 hours) to obtain the appropriate and needed amounts of amino acids. Maximum benefit is obtained when the combination is consumed at the same time. Supplementation of incomplete proteins with missing amino acids has been suggested for populations consuming diets having a single dietary item as its main protein source. This supplementation is not very practical over a long period of time due to the cost of the pure amino acid supplement. Such populations are also likely to develop other nutritional disorders when their food supply is so limited. With judicious use of a variety of foods available to these populations, amino acid deficiencies or imbalances can be overcome.

TABLE 9
Protein Content of Representative
Foods in the Human Diet

Food	Protein, g
Milk 244 g (8 oz)	8
Cheddar cheese, 84 g (3 oz)	21.3
Egg, 50 g, (1 large)	6.1
Apple, 212 g (1–3 1/4" diameter)	0.4
Banana, 74 g (1–8 3/4" long)	1.2
Potato, cooked, 136 g (1 potato)	2.5
Bread, white, slice, 25 g	2.1
Fish, cod, poached, 100 g (3 1/2 oz)	20.9
Oysters, 100 g (3 1/2 oz)	13.5
Beef, pot roast, 85 g (3 oz)	22
Liver, pan fried, 85 g (3 oz)	23
Pork chop, bone in, 87 g (3.1 oz)	23.9
Ham, boiled, 2 pieces, 114 g	20
Peanut butter, 16 g (1 tablespoon)	4.6
Pecans, 28 g (1 oz)	2.2
Snap beans, 125 g (1 cup)	2.4
Carrots, sliced, 78 g (1/2 cup)	0.8

From Handbook #8, USDA, Composition of Foods.
U.S. Government Printing Office, Washington, D.C.

In addition to the amino acid content, protein quality, or rather the quality of the food containing the protein, is classed according to its total protein content. Potatoes, for example, contain a very good distribution of essential and nonessential amino acids, yet, because the potato contains so little protein (1.7%), it is not considered a good protein source. One would have to consume a lot of potatoes (3.18 kg or ~7 lb) to meet one's daily amino acid and total nitrogen requirements. Total protein content can be determined rather easily, but analysis of a food to establish the individual amino acid content can be tedious and difficult.

1. Protein Analysis

Total protein content is estimated from the total nitrogen content of the food as determined by the classical Kjeldahl method. This method also determines nonprotein nitrogen as well; however, the amount of error in the method due to the inclusion of these compounds is very small. Most proteins contain 16% nitrogen. To convert the nitrogen content to protein, one uses the following formula:

$$P_G = N_G \times \frac{100}{16} = N_G \times 6.25$$

where P_G = grams of protein in 100 g of food and N_G = grams of nitrogen in 100 g of food.

This conversion factor is an average factor. If one wishes more exact figures, established conversion factors for each food category are available. For example, cereals generally have less protein nitrogen and more nonprotein nitrogen, thus, the conversion factor of 5.7 is used for cereal foods. On the other hand, milk has more protein nitrogen and the factor of 6.4 may be used. Generally speaking, because humans usually consume a mixed diet, the lower and higher factors tend to average out and the value of 6.25 is correct to use when the protein intake of a day's food intake is chemically determined.

The amino acid determination of a protein has two phases: qualitative identification and quantitative estimation of the residues. The peptide bond that connects the residues is cleaved

TABLE 10
Average Amino Acid Content of Selected Foods (mg/100 g)

	Tryptophan	Threonine	Isoleucine	Leucine	Lysine	Methionine	Cystine	Phenylalanine	Tyrosine	Valine	Arginine	Histidine	Alanine	Aspartic acid	Glutamic acid	Glycine	Proline	Serine
Milk	90	294	407	626	496	156	57	309	325	438	233	168	220	465	1491	126	709	376
Cheddar Cheese	87	237	430	622	468	166	36	342	305	458	233	208	179	372	1745	98	731	384
Whole Egg	103	311	415	550	400	196	146	361	269	464	410	150	0	438	773	221	265	525
Beef	73	276	327	512	546	155	79	257	212	347	403	217	361	583	946	387	308	262
Lamb	81	286	324	484	506	150	82	254	217	308	407	174	349	576	948	365	289	250
Bacon	65	210	274	500	403	97	73	298	161	298	427	169	0	589	702	589	331	242
Chicken	76	266	330	452	549	163	84	246	220	307	395	180	0	614	1004	418	0	0
Fish	62	271	317	472	548	182	84	232	169	333	352	0	0	551	796	345	381	193
Baked Beans	61	295	314	524	381	64	19	359	179	336	270	20	0	0	0	0	0	0
Pecans	78	219	312	436	245	86	122	318	178	296	668	154	0	0	0	0	0	0
White Bread	61	189	288	448	151	95	134	312	163	292	228	129	180	286	1980	202	675	0
Corn Meal	38	249	289	810	180	116	81	284	382	319	220	129	622	776	1103	212	522	353
Rice	64	233	279	513	235	107	81	299	272	416	343	100	0	281	815	407	288	302
Banana	95	0	0	0	289	55	0	0	162	0	0	0	0	0	0	0	0	0
Oranges	39	0	0	0	221	33	0	0	0	0	0	0	0	0	0	0	0	0
Peas	52	229	287	390	295	50	68	240	152	256	555	102	183	596	442	202	0	0
Brussels Sprouts	63	218	264	276	280	66	0	210	0	274	396	150	0	0	0	0	0	0
Potatoes	67	246	274	311	333	78	60	276	112	334	308	90	292	0	625	0	208	250

From Handbook #8, Amino Acid Composition of Foods, USDA, U.S. Government Printing Office, Washington, D.C.

by acid, base, or enzyme-catalyzed hydrolysis to give a mixture of separated amino acids. The free amino acids are separated from one another and identified using chromatographic and/or electrophoretic techniques. Once separated and identified, each amino acid present can be determined quantitatively. Several of the reactions given in Table 5 can be used. These assays do not establish the sequence of the amino acids, nor the protein's primary structure, but merely tell how much of each amino acid is present. The sequence of amino acids can be determined by cleaving the amino acids in the chain one by one, and following this cleavage with an analysis of the individual amino acids. Usually, high performance liquid chromatography (HPLC) is used for this aspect of sequence analysis.

2. Biological Value of Dietary Protein

Although the total protein (nitrogen) content can be readily determined, and although the amino acid content of the food can also be determined, albeit with greater difficulty, the determination of the *biological value* of a given protein within a food is even more difficult. By biological value, one means how well the food is digested and absorbed and how well the component amino acids meet the amino acid needs of the consumer. The biological value of a food protein depends not only on amino acid content, but also on the needs of the consumer. Growth carries with it a demand for particular amino acids as part of the total nitrogen requirement, whereas maintenance (as in the adult, nongrowing animal) has a total nitrogen requirement with less stringent demands for specific amino acids.

There is also a species dependence to biological value. Chickens, because they grow feathers, need more sulfur-containing amino acids in their diets than humans. Thus, proteins having a higher proportion of sulfur-containing amino acids will have relatively higher biological values for chickens than for other species. Rats, the usual test animal in nutrition studies, grow fur which contains a lot of arginine. This means that proteins rich in arginine will have a higher biological value for rats than for humans. A number of methods of assessing biological values have been used. Each has its advantages and disadvantages.

Using an *holistic* approach to assessing protein quality, H. H. Mitchell devised the nitrogen balance technique in 1924. This technique was based on Folin's definitions of endogenous and exogenous nitrogen excretion. By definition, the endogenous nitrogen comes from the nitrogen-containing excretory products synthesized in the body and not recycled. Exogenous nitrogen was defined as those nitrogen-containing products that are excreted in direct proportion to the amount of nitrogen consumed in the food. These are arbitrary definitions and there is some crossover between categories. However, they are useful in the context of evaluating the biological usefulness of dietary protein. *Endogenous* nitrogen comes from the breakdown of body tissue and represents nitrogenous compounds produced as a result of one-way reactions. For example, when muscles contract, creatine phosphate breaks down to creatine and phosphate. The contraction uses the energy released by this compound as it breaks down. While the phosphate can be recycled, creatine is converted to creatinine and excreted in the urine. Its excretion is relatively constant, presuming that the individual is a normal healthy adult who follows a fairly regular daily routine. Other nitrogenous compounds considered to be in the endogenous category are uric acid, allantoin, 3-methyl histidine, and ammonia. Regardless of the dietary protein intake, the excretion of these compounds by normal individuals is relatively constant.

In contrast, *exogenous* nitrogen fluctuates in response to the dietary protein intake. The main compound providing this nitrogen is urea. Urea results when excess amino acids are deaminated. The body converts the -NH_3 to urea via the urea cycle and excretes the urea in the urine. Exogenous nitrogen is also found in the feces and represents undigested food protein. Fecal nitrogen also represents the nitrogen of intestinal flora, desquamated intestinal cells, and intestinal enzymes. Figure 4 illustrates the principle of nitrogen balance.

These definitions, developed initially by Folin, were used by Thomas and Mitchell when they devised the nitrogen balance technique for evaluating protein quality. The method

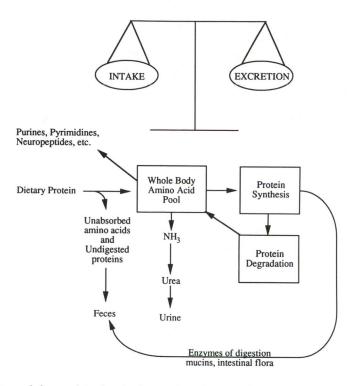

FIGURE 4. Nitrogen balance exists when the diet contains sufficient high-quality protein to provide amino acids for the synthesis of proteins lost through degradation.

assumes that a given protein, when fed at maintenance levels, will completely replace the protein being catabolized during the normal course of metabolic events in the body. It also assumes that all nitrogen gain and loss can be measured. Thus, for good-quality proteins, nitrogen balance (intake vs. excretion) should be zero for an adult individual, and for poor-quality proteins, nitrogen balance will be negative. For growing individuals, good-quality proteins result in high nitrogen retentions while poor-quality proteins result in low nitrogen retention. The amount of protein retained can be determined by analyzing the total nitrogen content of the food, the feces, and the urine.

The biological value (BV) was conceived as a ratio of the nitrogen retained to that absorbed multiplied by 100. In the original method, animals were fed a nitrogen-free diet for 7 to 10 days, then fed a diet containing the test protein at a level commensurate with their protein maintenance requirements for the same time interval. During each of these periods, the urine and feces were collected and analyzed for total nitrogen. Knowing the nitrogen intake and the nitrogen excretion during both the nitrogen-free and test periods, the biological value was calculated as follows:

$$BV = 100 \times \frac{\text{N retained}}{\text{N absorbed}} = 100 \times \frac{N_I - (N_{FT} - N_{FF}) - (N_{UT} - N_{UF})}{N_I - (N_{FT} - N_{FF})}$$

where BV $\;=\;$ biological value
$N_I \;\;=\;$ nitrogen intake
$N_{FT} =$ fecal nitrogen during test period
$N_{FF} =$ fecal nitrogen during nitrogen-free period
$N_{UT} =$ urinary nitrogen during test period
$N_{UF} =$ urinary nitrogen during nitrogen-free period

This method is noninvasive and very useful for work with humans. However, nitrogen can be lost via routes other than urine and feces. In hot climates or in physically active subjects, significant nitrogen losses can occur through the sweat. On an adequate protein intake, it has been estimated that up to 1 g N/dL can be lost. On an inadequate or low protein diet, sweat losses can amount to 0.5 g N/dL. Hair, nail, and menstrual losses can also contribute error to the nitrogen balance technique. Usually sweat, hair, skin, and nail losses are ignored since they are minor in comparison to the urine and fecal losses. Other errors in the method include the possibility of daily cumulative errors in the collection and analysis of the food, urine, and feces, and the effects of poor nutritional status on the responses of the subject to this procedure. Good subject cooperation is essential to insure quantitative ingestion of the food and the quantitative collection of the urine and feces.

The main disadvantage of this method is theoretical in character. The basic assumption of "replaceability" of body protein by a food protein is valid only when comparing good-quality proteins. When poor proteins such as zein, gelatin, or gluten are evaluated, unrealistically high values result. This overestimation results from the failure of the method to account for the mobilization of body protein to meet particular amino acid needs. If there is a deficiency of one or more of the essential amino acids in the test protein, the animal will catabolize body proteins in an effort to provide the missing amino acid so as to support the synthesis of vital or needed proteins. There appears to be a hierarchy of body proteins: those which are most essential to the survival of the animal are synthesized in preference to those, such as muscle protein, which are not as essential. In any event, when the body proteins are mobilized, the needed amino acids they contain are utilized and the remaining ones are deaminated and used for energy. The amino group is then converted to urea and excreted, contributing to the urinary nitrogen level. The Mitchell nitrogen balance technique does not differentiate the source of the nitrogen in the excreta and, because of this, is not as valid as a technique to evaluate incomplete proteins. In efforts to circumvent the problem of overestimating the biological values of incomplete or imbalanced proteins, other methods, some of which are variations of the original nitrogen balance technique, have been proposed and used.

The nitrogen balance index (NBI) of Allison and co-workers relates the absorbed nitrogen to the nitrogen excretion of a separate but concurrent group of individuals fed a nitrogen-free diet. This technique requires less time than the Thomas-Mitchell method but is subject to many of the same kind of errors. Both methods suffer from the inaccuracies contributed by the methodological measure of the so-called endogenous nitrogen loss. Both methods assume that this loss is represented by the nitrogen excreted by the animal during the nitrogen-free period.

One must consider the dynamic state of the body proteins, that is, the constant need to synthesize proteins having a short half-life. This synthesis must be accommodated by the catabolism of tissue protein; a catabolic process unlikely to occur extensively if good-quality proteins are consumed. Because this overestimation of endogenous loss is more serious with proteins of poor quality, inconsistent biological values are obtained. This is particularly true when unrefined proteins or food mixtures are evaluated. The relationship of the nitrogen balance technique to the nitrogen balance index can best be seen in Figure 5.

A more accurate method for the evaluation of protein quality is one which actually measures the retention of nitrogen in the carcass from the ingested protein nitrogen. This is called the NPU-BV or NPU method. Using the methods which calculate biological value from the change in carcass protein, groups of animals, usually rats, are fed diets containing graded amounts of the test protein or a nitrogen-free diet. After a period of 7 to 10 days, the animals are killed and the nitrogen content of the carcasses determined. Obviously, proteins of high quality will evoke a greater retention of nitrogen in the carcass than proteins of poor quality. Using this technique, biological value can be calculated as follows:

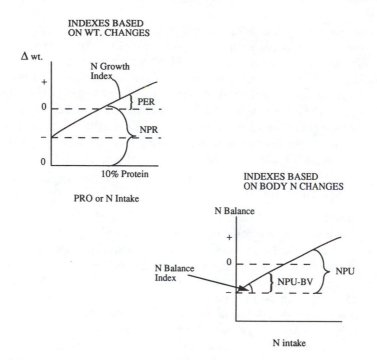

FIGURE 5. Illustrations of the indexes of protein quality. Those that are based on weight changes are shown in the upper panel, while those that are based on changes in body nitrogen are shown in the lower panel.

$$NPU \text{-} BV = \frac{B_f - B_k + I_k}{I_f} \times 100$$

where B_f = carcass nitrogen of animals fed test protein diet
B_k = carcass nitrogen of animals fed nitrogen-free diet
I_k = absorbed nitrogen of animals fed nitrogen-free diet
I_f = absorbed nitrogen of animals fed test protein diet

While this method has the obvious advantage of actually measuring nitrogen retention, its disadvantages are also obvious. This method is inappropriate for large animals because of the technical difficulties associated with the determination of body composition and because of the excessive cost. Obviously, too, human studies would not be possible. However, conceptually, the method has merit and several investigators have devised variations which are useful in a variety of species.

One variation that is useful in humans is to measure the changes in body composition indirectly. Using a stable isotope of nitrogen, ^{15}N, one can study the rates of total body protein synthesis and breakdown as a response to variation in amounts of dietary protein. Constant infusions of ^{15}N-glycine allows one to assess the value of given proteins in the homeostatic situation where there is constant protein synthesis and breakdown. While a very useful technique, it is also very expensive and requires sophisticated techniques and equipment to make the appropriate measurements.

Another variation of the carcass retention method which uses a radioactive isotope, measures the change in ^{40}K concentration in the body as a result of consuming a given protein for a period of 7 to 10 days. This method is based on the constancy of potassium as an intracellular ion. The concentration of potassium in the body can be directly related to the number of cells in the body and indirectly related to the protein in the body. Since a set percentage of this potassium exists as the naturally occurring radioactive isotope ^{40}K, measuring ^{40}K levels is a direct measure of body cell number and an indirect measure of body protein. Again, while this method has the advantage of its applicability to the human, its disadvantage is one of cost and availability of the whole-body counters needed to determine the presence of the isotope.

By far, the easiest variation of the carcass retention methods is the protein efficiency ratio (PER). In this method, carcass composition is not determined. It makes the assumption that the gain in body weight of a given animal is related to the quality of the protein fed. Thus, young growing animals are fed test protein-containing diets for a period of 28 days. The weight gain is computed and divided by the total protein intake. The formula, $PER = \dfrac{\text{weight gain in grams}}{\text{protein intake in grams}}$ is easy to use and the method requires no specialized expensive equipment. This is the method used for protein quality evaluation by most food companies and has been adopted by the regulatory agencies of the U.S. and Canada as their method of choice in evaluating the nutritional quality of foods. The ease and simplicity of the method, however, should not lull the reader into thinking that it is a "choice" method. PER can vary from species to species, and within a given species from strain to strain. Examples of within-species variation in the PER of a given protein is given in Table 11. Variation can be introduced if levels of protein intake higher or lower than 10% by weight are used. In addition, the methods make no allowance for the maintenance requirement of the animal. Values obtained from a variety of food proteins are nonlinear. That is, a protein having a PER of 2 may not have twice the nutritional value of a protein having a PER of 1. Examples of the PER for a variety of food proteins is shown in Table 12.

A modification of the PER is the net protein ratio. This method attempts to account for the maintenance needs of the animals. In this method, two groups of animals are used. One is fed a nitrogen-free diet, the other the test diet. This modification is accompanied by all the pitfalls of using the nitrogen-free diets that have been discussed.

A variety of methods employing the assay of enzymes concerned with protein metabolism have also been devised. The determination of the activity of transaminase, xanthine dehydrogenase, renal arginase, and others have been reported as indicators of protein quality. Unfortunately, these methods have not been rigorously tested and compared to the presently available whole-body methods.

The holistic approach, while valuable and useful, is nonetheless time consuming and expensive. The approaches discussed above do have the advantage that digestibility and amino acid availability are given due consideration.

Attempts to circumvent the time and expense of whole-animal work have resulted in a number of useful techniques. One method, the amino acid score or chemical score, is a nonbiological method and requires the amino acid analysis of the test protein. The amount of the most limiting amino acid (only the essential amino acids are considered) is related to the content of that same amino acid in a reference protein. In most cases, this reference is egg protein, however, a theoretical protein based on the amino acid requirements of the species in question could also be used. Thus

$$\text{Chemical Score} = \frac{\text{mg of limiting amino acid/g test protein}}{\text{mg of amino acid/g ideal protein}} \times 100$$

While this method is quick and does not use animals, it does not make any allowance for digestibility or availability of the constituent amino acids. This is a rather important aspect of protein nutrition. Some amino acids form sugar-amino acid complexes which render the amino acids less available to the body. This occurs with the browning of baked goods such as bread; while bread is not considered a prime protein source, evaluation of its protein quality using the amino acid score would be in error due to the browning reaction.

TABLE 11
The PER of a Test Protein as Calculated Using the
Weight Gain of Rats from Seven Different Strains

Rat strain	PER			
	Week 1	Week 2	Week 3	Week 4
Holtzman	4.14	3.94	3.61	3.50
Charles River	4.29	3.64	3.54	3.60
ARS-Sprague Dawley	4.31	3.76	3.32	3.36
Osborne-Mendel	4.20	3.52	3.24	3.39
Wistar	4.47	3.59	3.33	3.37
Wistar Lewis	3.69	3.64	3.37	3.28
SSB/PL (NIH)	3.80	3.37	2.96	2.47

TABLE 12
PER of Various Foods

Eggs	3.9–4.0
Fish	3.5
Milk	3.0–3.1
Beef	2.3
Soybeans	2.3
Beans	1.4–1.9
Nuts	1.8
Peanuts	1.7
Gluten	1.0
Rice	2.0
Corn	1.2

A variation on this chemical method tries to account for digestibility. In this method, test proteins are first digested *in vitro* using conditions resembling those in the gastrointestinal tract. The amino acid score is then determined on the products of this digestion. This is a relatively new but promising approach to evaluating protein quality. It will require considerably more work to validate it, but at present it represents an innovative approach to the problems associated with assessing protein quality.

VI.   PROTEIN USE

A. DIGESTION
The daily protein intake of about 100 g plus that protein that appears in the gut as enzymes, sloughed epithelial gut cells, and mucins is almost completely digested and absorbed. This is a very efficient process that ensures a continuous supply of amino acids to the whole-body amino acid pool (see Figure 4). Less than 1% of the total protein that passes through the gastrointestinal tract appears in the feces. If the food contributes between 70 and 100 g of protein and the endogenous protein contributes another 100 g (range: 35 to 200 g) then one might expect to see about 1 to 2 g of nitrogen in the feces. This is equivalent to 6 to 12 g protein. Of the dietary protein, the fecal protein might include the hard to chew/digest tough fibrous connective tissue of meat, or nitrogen-containing indigestible kernel coats of grains, or particles of nuts that are not attacked by the digestive enzymes. For example, peanuts that are eaten whole, have a structure that is difficult to broach by the digestive enzymes. Unless chewed very finely, much of the nutritive value of this food may be lost. Peanut butter, on the other hand, is very well digested because the preparation of the peanut butter ensures that its particle size is very small and is thus quite digestible.

The purpose of protein digestion is to liberate the amino acids which comprise the consumed proteins. Except for the period shortly after birth, the enterocyte cannot absorb protein intact. It must be hydrolyzed to its component amino acids. This is accomplished through a series of enzymes which have specific target linkages as their point of action. These enzymes are summarized in Table 13. The protein hydrolases, called peptidases, fall into two categories. Those that attack internal peptide bonds and liberate large peptide fragments for subsequent attack by other enzymes are called the endopeptidases. Those that attack the terminal peptide bonds and liberate single amino acids from the protein structure are called exopeptidases. The exopeptidases are further subdivided according to whether they attack at the carboxy end of the amino acid chain (carboxypeptidases) or the amino end of the chain (aminopeptidases). The initial attack on an intact protein is catalyzed by endopeptidases while the final digestive action is catalyzed by the exopeptidases. The final products of digestion are free amino acids and some di- and tripeptides that are absorbed by the intestinal epithelial cells.

In contrast to carbohydrate and lipid digestion which is initiated in the mouth with the salivary amylase and the lingual lipase, protein digestion does not begin until the protein reaches the stomach and the food is acidified with the gastric hydrochloric acid. The HCl serves several functions. It acidifies the ingested food, killing potential pathogenic organisms. Unfortunately, not all pathogens are killed. Some are acid resistant or are so plentiful in the food that the amount of gastric acidification is insufficient to kill all of the pathogens.

Hydrochloric acid also serves to denature the food proteins, thus making them more vulnerable to attack by pepsin, an endopeptidase. Actually, pepsin is not a single enzyme. It consists of pepsin A which attacks peptide bonds involving phenylalanine or tyrosine and several other enzymes which have specific attack points. The pepsins are released into the gastric cavity as pepsinogen. When the food entering the stomach stimulates HCl release and the pH of the gastric contents fall below 2, the pepsinogen loses a 44-amino acid sequence. The activation of the pepsins from pepsinogen occurs by one of two processes. The first, called *autoactivation*, occurs when the pH drops below 5. At low pH the bond between the 44th and 45th amino acid residue falls apart and the 44-amino acid residue (from the amino terminus) is liberated. The liberated residue acts as an inhibitor of pepsin by binding to the catalytic site until pH 2 is achieved. The inhibition is relieved when this fragment is degraded, as happens at pH 2 or below or when it is attacked by pepsin. Since the fragment binds at the catalytic site of pepsin, this can happen. The other process is called *autocatalysis* and occurs when already active pepsin attacks the precursor pepsinogen. This is a self-repeating process and serves to ensure ongoing catalysis of the resident protein.

The cleavage of the 44-amino acid residue, in addition to providing activated pepsin, has another purpose. That is, it serves as a signal peptide for cholecystokinin release in the duodenum. This, then, sets the stage for the subsequent pancreatic phase of protein digestion. As described in the units on lipids and carbohydrates, (Units 6 and 5, respectively), cholecystokinin stimulates both the exocrine pancreas and the intestinal mucosal epithelial cell to release its digestive enzymes. The intestinal cell releases an enzyme, enteropeptidase or enterokinase, which serves to activate the protease, trypsin, released as trypsinogen by the exocrine pancreas. This trypsin not only acts on food proteins, it also acts on other preproteases released by the exocrine pancreas, activating them. Thus, trypsin acts as an endoprotease on chymotrypsinogen by releasing chymotrypsin, on proelastase by releasing elastase, and on procarboxypeptidase by releasing carboxypeptidase. Trypsin, chymotrypsin, and elastase are all endoproteases, each having specificity for particular peptide bonds, as detailed in Table 13. Each of these three proteases have serine as part of their catalytic site so any compound that ties up the serine will inhibit the activity of these proteases. Such inhibitors as diisopropylphosphofluoridate react with this serine and in so doing bring a halt to protein digestion.

Through the action of pepsin, trypsin, chymotrypsin, and elastase, numerous oligopeptides are produced which then are attacked by the amino and carboxypeptidases of the pancreatic

TABLE 13
Digestive Enzymes and Their Target Linkages

Enzyme	Location	Target
Pepsin	Stomach	Peptide bonds involving the aromatic amino acids
Trypsin	Small intestine	Peptide bonds involving arginine and lysine
Chymotrypsin	Small intestine	Peptide bonds involving tyrosine, tryptophan, phenylalanine, methionine, and leucine
Elastase	Small intestine	Peptide bonds involving alanine, serine and glycine
Carboxypeptidase A	Small intestine	Peptide bonds involving valine, leucine, isoleucine, alanine
Carboxypeptidase B	Small intestine	Peptide bonds involving lysine and arginine
Endopeptidase, aminopeptidase, dipeptidase	Cells of brush border	Di- and tripeptides that enter the brush border of the absorptive cells

juice and those on the brush border of the absorptive cells. One by one, the amino acids are liberated from these chains, and one by one they are absorbed and appear in the portal blood.

B. ABSORPTION

Although single amino acids are liberated in the intestinal contents, there is insufficient power in the enzymes of the pancreatic juice to render all of the amino acids singly for absorption. The brush border of the absorptive cell, therefore, not only absorbs the single amino acid but also the di- and tripeptides. In the process of absorbing these small peptides it hydrolyzes them to their amino acid constituents. There are specific transport systems for each group of functionally similar amino acids and for peptides. Most of the biologically important L-amino acids are transported by an active carrier system against a concentration gradient (see Figure 6). In several instances, the carrier is a shared carrier. That is, the carrier will transport more than one amino acid. Such is the case with the neutral amino acids and those with short or polar side chains (serine, threonine, and alanine). Other shared carriers are listed in Table 14. The mechanism whereby these carriers participate in amino acid absorption is similar to that described for glucose uptake (see Unit 5). This mechanism is illustrated in Figure 6.

C. METABOLISM

The amino acids leaving the absorptive cell enter a whole-body amino acid pool from which all cells withdraw amino acids for use in the synthesis of biologically important proteins, peptides, and amino acid derivatives. The peptides may be hormones or one of the many signal peptides that comprise the various signal transduction systems found in the body. Amino acids not used for peptide or protein synthesis can be deaminated and the carbon unit used for energy or for the synthesis of glucose or fatty acids. Amino acids can also be carboxylated to form amines. Amines are quite potent compounds that act as intracellular effectors such as the neurotransmitters, or as high-energy compounds such as creatin phosphate.

1. Hormones: Regulators of Protein Metabolism

Hormones serve as internal messengers regulating the ebb and flow of a variety of cellular functions. As internal signals, hormones regulate such processes as heartbeat, vascular contraction, salt conservation, glucose uptake and utilization, glucose production, and oxygen consumption. Hormones can be viewed as system regulators. They are substances that are released into the bloodstream by a tissue or organ and have an action distal to that tissue. Not all hormones are proteins. Some are dipeptides, some are steroids, some are small polypeptides. All, however, serve as coordinators of activity in specific tissues. Their actions are mediated by specific interactions with specific proteins in the membrane or cytosol or certain of the organelles within the cell. These proteins are called receptors. In turn, the hormones themselves are released via

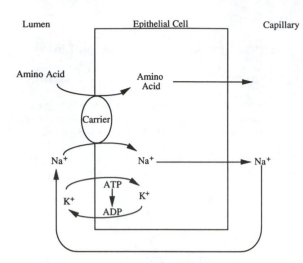

FIGURE 6. Carrier-mediated sodium-dependent amino acid transport. The amino acid leaves the absorptive cell with sodium. The sodium is recirculated back to the lumen for reuse. As sodium enters the cell, potassium is pumped out via a Na⁺K⁺ ATPase system. As sodium leaves the cell, potassium flows back in and the electrolyte balance is maintained.

TABLE 14
Carriers for Amino Acids

Carrier	Amino acids carried
1	Serine, threonine, alanine
2[a]	Phenylalanine, tyrosine, methionine, valine, leucine, isoleucine
3	Proline, hydroxyproline
4	Taurine, β-alanine
5	Lysine, arginine, cysteine-cysteine
6	Aspartic and glutamic acids

[a] When a mutation in the gene that codes for this carrier occurs, the individual is unable to absorb these amino acids from the gut contents or reabsorb these amino acids through the renal tubule. Patients with this disorder will manifest symptoms of protein malnutrition. These people can absorb these amino acids as partners in a dipeptide or tripeptide, however, because of the defect in the renal tubule cannot conserve their supply. This genetic disease is called Hartnup's disease or neutral amino aciduria.

a cascade of sequential reactions that usually begin in the central nervous system, followed by signals generated in the hypothalamus, then the pituitary, and finally by the endocrine cell itself. This cascaded signaling system is a means to amplify a specific signal. The stimulus may originate from the environment of which nutrients are a part. As discussed in Unit 3, food intake elicits a variety of signals from both the CNS and the gut. Specific electrical and/or chemical signals are generated which stimulate the hypothalamus, which then either directly or indirectly (via releasing hormones) stimulates the anterior pituitary which, in turn, directly or indirectly signals the target endocrine cell to synthesize and/or release its hormone, which finally has the needed effect on metabolism. This cascade of signals is illustrated in Figure 7. Not all hormone release mechanisms use all the steps in this cascade. Sometimes short loops are used which bypass some of the initial steps in the cascade. In addition, there is some negative feedback involved which tells the target endocrine cell that enough hormone has been released.

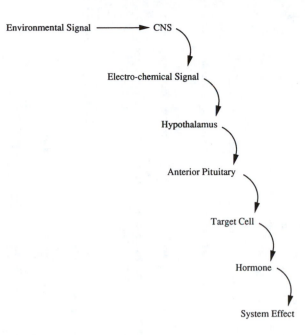

FIGURE 7. Signaling cascade that begins with an initial signal originating in the environment and ends with a whole-body systemic response.

Some of the peptide and protein hormones in the body are listed in Table 15. In general, these hormones function through one of several mechanisms:

1. They induce enzyme synthesis by stimulating mRNA transcription. An increase in mRNA synthesis leads to an increase in enzyme protein synthesis. Hormones acting in this way are thought to be functioning as modifiers of gene expression.
2. Hormones stimulate enzyme synthesis through enhancing the translation of messenger RNA. Growth hormone, a small protein, appears to act in this fashion.
3. Hormones directly activate enzymes by either changing the phosphorylation state of the cell or one of its compartments or by changing the flux of ions as cofactors in the reactions.
4. Hormones activate membrane transport systems which have G proteins as part of their structures.

In the cascade system illustrated in Figure 7, hormones or signals must emanate from one level of the cascade to the next in order for the system to work. The precision of the signaling system depends largely on the specificity of the signal for its target and the specificity of the target for its signal. Some hormones are more specific than others. In general, the protein and peptide hormones are more specific than the steroid hormones. The polypeptide hormones bind to their cognate receptors lodged in the plasma membrane. These receptors generally penetrate the membrane and have a tyrosine-rich tail protruding into the cytosol. Part of the hormone-receptor binding and subsequent cellular events involve G proteins. The G protein is a protein which has a high affinity for GTP (guanine triphosphate). It serves as the signal transducer for the hormone. The G proteins have several subunits which interact and then react with enzymes such as adenyl cyclase or phospholipase C. This process is illustrated in Figure 8. These enzymes may be either activated or inhibited, depending on the hormone in question. Both adenyl cyclase and phospholipase C are components of the intracellular signaling system, the former is a component of the cyclic AMP or protein kinase system and the latter, a component of the phosphatidylinositol (PIP) system. The former leads to a cellular

TABLE 15
Some Protein and Peptide Hormones and Their Function

Hormone	Source	Type	Function
Thyroid, thyroxine, triiodothyionine	Thyroid gland	Dipeptide of tyrosine	Regulates oxygen consumption by tissues
Thyroid stimulating hormone (TSH)	Pituitary	Polypeptide	Stimulates synthesis and release of thyroid hormone by thyroid gland
Thyroid releasing factor	Hypothalamus	Tripeptide	Stimulates pituitary to release thyroid stimulating hormone
Calcitonin	Thyroid gland	Polypeptide	Stimulates bone uptake of calcium
Parathyroid hormone	Parathyroid glands	Polypeptide	Raises serum clacium levels, lowers serum phosphorus levels; increases urinary phosphorus excretion, decreases urinary calcium excretion; activates vitamin D in renal tissue
Insulin	β Cells of islets of Langerhans (pancreas)	Protein	Regulates glucose utilization; stimulates glucose uptake; influences lipid and protein synthesis
Glucagon	α Cells of islets of Langerhans (pancreas)	Polypeptide	Rapid mobilization of hepatic glucose from glycogen; mobilizes fatty acids from adipose tissue stores; enhances hapatic glucose production from amino acids and glycerol
Somatostatin	D Cells of islets of Langerhans (pancreas)	Polypeptide	Inhibits food passage along gastrointestinal system, decreases glall bladder release of bile, slows uptake of nutrients from intestinal lumen; inhibit growth hormone release
Epinephrine	Adrenal medulla	Tyrosine derivative	Stimulates lipolysis, stimulates glycogen breakdown; increases vasodilation of arterioles of skeletal muscles, vasoconstriction of arterioles in skin and viscera
Norepinephrine	Adrenal medulla	Tyrosine derivative	Exerts an overall vasoconstriction effect on vascular system
ACTH	Pituitary	Polypeptide	Stimulates production and release of adrenal corticoid hormones
Antidiuretic hormone (ADH) (Vasopressin)	Pituitary	Polypeptide	Promotes water conservation; controls water resorption by kidney; raises blood pressure
Follicle stimulating hormone (FSH)	Anterior pituitary	Peptide	Controls testicular function; spermatogenesis; stimulates ovum production; enhances release of estrogen
Luteotropic hormone (LH) (Prolactin)	Anterior pituitary	Small protein	Controls testicular function and spermatogenesis; stimulates ovum production; enhances release of estrogen
Growth hormone	Anterior pituitary	Small protein	Stimulates growth of long bones and muscles; stimulates production of somatomedin
Gastrin	Gastric glands	Polypeptide	Stimulates acid and pepsin secretion; stimulates growth of gastric mucosa
Cholecystokinin	Intestine, pancreas	Polypeptide	Stimulates gall bladder contraction; stimulates pancreatic enzyme release
Secretin	Intestine, pancreas	Polypeptide	Stimulates pancreatic secretion; augments action of cholecystokinin

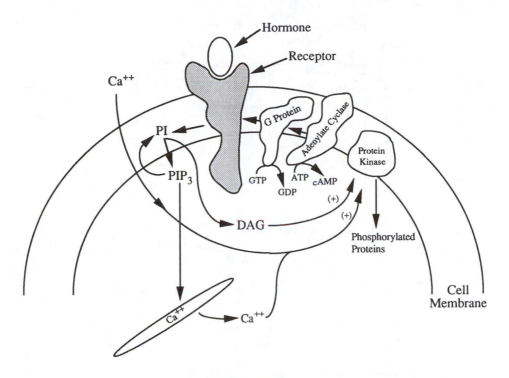

FIGURE 8.   Hormone-receptor reaction that involves the G proteins, adenylate cyclase, proteins, the PIP cycle, and cAMP. When the hormone binds to the receptor, the G protein moves over to the receptor protein and binds GTP. Adenylate cyclase moves over and binds to the G protein and ATP is converted to cAMP.

effect such as the release of cortisol when ACTH binds to the receptor on the membrane of the adrenocortical cell while the latter leads to the release of calcium from intracellular stores. The calcium ion, in turn, plays a role in exocytosis or may be active in the exchange of metabolites across intracellular membranes.

While the details of the synthesis of all of these peptide and protein hormones have yet to be elucidated, some pathways are well known. The synthesis of thyroxine from tyrosine by the thyroid gland (Figure 9) and the synthesis of dopamine, epinephrine, and norepinephrine, also from tyrosine, by the adrenal medulla and CNS are established. Note in Figure 9 that a cascade of signals are needed for the release of these hormones. The synthesis of the pancreatic hormones and the synthesis of the more complicated protein hormones are not clear. The enzymes needed for some of these synthetic pathways have not been fully described nor have the control points in the synthetic pathways been fully elucidated. This is a very active area for research in endocrinology as is the study of the signal transduction systems that explain the actions of each of these hormones.

One of the more interesting observations is that many of the peptide hormones are encoded together in a single gene and that many copies of the same message can exist in this gene. For example, one gene has been found to encode ACTH (adrenocorticotropin hormone), β-lipotropin, γ-lipotropin, α-MSH (melanocyte stimulating hormone), β-MSH, CLIP (corticotropin-like peptide), β-endorphin, and some of the enkephalins. This gene encodes for proopiomelanocortin as illustrated in Figure 10, which in turn can generate the above eight hormones. Not all are generated by the same tissue or cell type but occur separately, generated by specific signals for specific cells. In the above example, one of the gene products, ACTH, is produced and released by the anterior pituitary under the control of the corticotropin releasing hormone. Enzymes are present in the corticotrophic cell that cleave the amino acid sequence of proopiomelanocortin at specific sites, releasing ACTH and β-lipotropin into the circulation. These products can be cleaved further by cells of the pars intermedia to produce

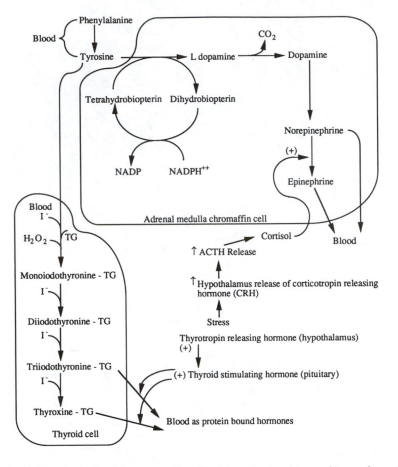

FIGURE 9. Amino acids in the blood flow to specific cells of the endocrine system and are used to make thyroid hormone and catecholamines. These hormones are released into the circulation and are carried to their target cells where they have their effects. Thyroxine synthesis occurs as a sequential iodination of tyrosine residues contained by the protein thyroglobulin (TG).

and release γ-MSH, CLIP, γ-lipotropin, and β-endorphin. CLIP is an abbreviation for corticotropin-like intermediary peptide. α-Lipotropin and β-endorphin can be split further to produce β-MSH and met-enkephalin. The reason why all these gene products arise from the same initial compound has to do with the unique location in the different cell types of specific proteases which act on specific linkages and thus release these smaller peptides into the circulation. Only a few cell types possess these specific proteases.

Many polypeptide hormones are encoded together. Just as ACTH and β-lipotropin are components of the proopiomelanocortin, so too are other hormones split off of prohormone molecules. Vasopressin and neurophysin II arise from the same molecule. Oxytocin and neurophysin I also have the same parent peptide. Although the above examples are all peptide hormones, no doubt we will find that nonhormone peptides can arise in similar fashion. Amino acids in the circulation enter a vast array of cell types and each cell type has many uses for the amino acids brought to it by the circulation. As mentioned, small, medium, and large molecules can be made. The largest of these molecules are the proteins.

2.   Protein Synthesis
Protein synthesis is dependent upon the simultaneous presence of all the amino acids necessary for the protein being synthesized and upon the provision of energy. If there is an insufficient supply of either, protein biosynthesis will not proceed at its normal pace. Chemically, the polymerization

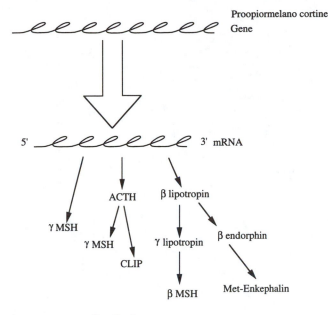

Gene Products

FIGURE 10. One gene encodes several signal peptides, depending on the cell type and signals generated to synthesize one or more of these products. ACTH and β-lipotropin gene products are under the control of the corticotropin releasing hormone (CRH), whereas αMSH, CLIP, γ-lipotropin, and β-endorphin gene products in the pituitary are under control of dopamine. MSH = melanocyte stimulating hormone; CLIP = corticotropin-like intermediary peptide.

of amino acids into protein is a dehydration reaction between two amino acids (see Section IV, this chapter).

The process whereby proteins are synthesized provides the basis for understanding genetic differences. It is also the basis for understanding how the unique properties of each cell type are maintained since the properties that make cells unique are usually conferred by the proteins within them. Some of these proteins are the structural elements of the cell. Others are enzymes that catalyze specific reactions and processes that characterize the cell in question. Still other proteins confer a particular biochemical function on the cell. The amino acid sequence of a particular protein is genetically controlled. This control is exerted through the polynucleotide, deoxyribonucleic acid (DNA).

DNA is composed of four bases: adenine, guanine, thymine, and cytosine. These bases are condensed to form the DNA chain in a process analogous to the condensation of amino acids which comprise the primary structure of a protein. Species vary in the percent distribution of these bases in their DNA. In mammals the adenine-thymidine content varies from 45 to 53%. Small amounts of the base 5-methyl-cytosine as well as methylated derivatives of the other bases can be found.

The sequence of amino acids in each protein synthesized by the body is determined from a subunit of the DNA molecule known as the gene. The gene, through the sequence of bases that are found in its constituent nucleotides, codes for a polypeptide. The DNA in the nucleus is very stable with respect to the base sequence and content. It can be damaged by certain chemicals, free radicals, X-rays, and other agents. However, it also can repair this damage to some extent. If a change in the base sequence does occur and is not repaired, a mutation is said to have occurred. This mutation will then become part of the genetic information transmitted to the next generation.

The chain of nucleotides which comprise DNA is formed by joining these bases through phosphodiester bonds. A typical segment of the chain is illustrated in Figure 11. The hydrophobic properties of the bases plus the strong charges of the polar groups within each

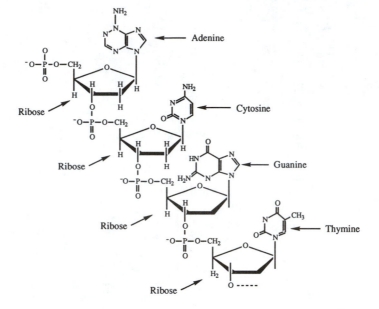

FIGURE 11. The bases which comprise the DNA polynucleotide chain are joined together by phosphodiester bonds using ribose as the common link between the bases.

of the component units are responsible for the helical conformation of the DNA chain. The bases themselves interact such that two chains are intertwined. Hence, the term double helix applies to the nuclear DNA. Hydrogen bonding between the bases stabilizes this conformation as shown in Figure 12. Other factors as well serve to stabilize the structure of the DNA. Unwinding of the DNA, a necessary step in the initiation of protein synthesis, occurs when these stabilizing factors are perturbed. Unwinding exposes a small segment of the DNA, allowing its base sequence to be available for complementary base pairing as happens when messenger RNA is synthesized. The coding segments of most genes contain from 600 to 1800 nucleotides; these nucleotides can code for 200 to 600 amino acids in a polypeptide chain. The nucleotides which code for a specific protein may not be adjacent to each other on the DNA strand but may be located nearby as the DNA exists in a doubly coiled chain of bases, the double helix.

The DNA base sequence is unique for every protein that is synthesized in the body. While only a few bases are used for the DNA, the combinations and sequences of the combinations provide a specific code for each and every protein and peptide. The Human Genome Project sponsored by the National Institutes of Health has as its goal the determination of the complete sequence and the mapping of subsequences. By mapping we mean the identification, within the double helix, of each segment and the protein it encodes. Thus, the function of DNA is to determine the properties of the cell through the provision of a code that directs protein synthesis. It also functions to transmit genetic information from one generation to the next in a given species. Thus, DNA has a broad spectrum of function — it ensures the identity of both specific cell types and specific species. Not all DNA is located in the nucleus. Some is found in the mitochondria. In this organelle, it exists in a circular form rather than as a double-stranded coil (helix) as is found in the nucleus.

In the nucleus, the DNA is found in the chromosomal chromatin. Chromatin contains very long double strands of DNA and a nearly equal mass of histone and nonhistone proteins. Histones are highly basic proteins varying in molecular weight from ~11,000 to ~21,000. As a result of their high content of basic amino acids, histones serve to interact with the polyanionic phosphate backbone of the DNA so as to produce uncharged nucleoproteins. The histones also serve to keep the DNA in a very compact form. The nuclear DNA, as soon as its replication is completed, becomes highly condensed into distinct chromosomes of characteristic shapes.

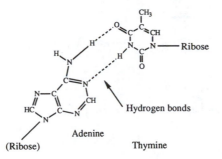

FIGURE 12. Hydrogen bonds form between complementary bases: adenine complements thymine; guanine complements cytosine.

These chromosomes exist as pairs and are numbered. There are 46 chromosomes in the human. Included in this number are the sex chromosomes, the X and Y chromosomes. If the individual has one X and one Y he is a male; if two Xs are present, she is a female. The chromosomes are the result of a mixing of the nuclear DNA of the egg and sperm. Approximately half of each pair comes from each parent. If identical codes for a given protein are inherited from each parent, the resultant progeny will be a homozygote for that protein. If nonidentical codes are inherited, the progeny will be a heterozygote. Within the heterozygote population there may be certain codes which are dominant such as eye color or hair color, for example. These are dominant traits and are expressed despite the fact that the individual has inherited two different codes for this trait. A mutation in a code that is not expressed is a recessive trait. If by chance two identical mutated genes are present that encode a certain protein, the expression of this mutated code will be observed. This is the basis for genetic diseases of the autosomal recessive or dominant type. Autosomal means a mutation in any of the chromosomal DNA except that which is in the X or Y chromosome. A mutation of the DNA in this chromosome is called a sex-linked mutation. If it results in a disease, it is called sex-linked genetic disease.

Having the codes in the nucleus for the synthesis of protein in the cytoplasm implies a communication between the cytoplasm and the nucleus and between the nucleus and the cytoplasm. Signals are sent to the nucleus which "informs" this organelle of the need to synthesize certain proteins. We do not know what all these signals are. Some are substrates for the needed proteins, some are hormones, and some are signaling compounds that have yet to be identified. The communication between the nucleus and the cytoplasm is carried out by messenger RNA (mRNA).

Messenger RNA is used to carry genetic information from the DNA of the chromosomes to the surface of the ribosomes. It is synthesized in the nucleus by a process known as transcription. Chemically, RNA is similar to DNA. It is an unbranched linear polymer in which the monomeric subunits are the ribonucleoside-5'-monophosphates. The bases are the purines adenine and guanine, and the pyrmidines uracil and cytosine. Note that thymine is not used in RNA and that uracil is not present in DNA. RNA is single stranded rather than double stranded. It is held together by molecular base pairing and will contract if in a solution of high ionic strength. RNA, particularly the mRNA, is a much smaller molecule than DNA and is far less stable.

The synthesis of mRNA transcription has been elucidated for many of the important proteins. All known transcription reactions follow the same pattern in that the RNA is made through the use of a DNA template. The synthesis makes use of the RNA polymerase enzymes. Actually, transcription is divided into three parts. The first part is initiation. Initiation refers to the recognition of an active gene starting point by RNA polymerase and the beginning of the bond formation process. The second part is elongation. This is the synthesis or joining together of the nucleotides. The third and last part is the termination of the chain. This is illustrated in Figure 13. The RNA polymerases all synthesize the mRNA in the 5' to 3' direction using the DNA template. Following transcription is translation. This refers to the

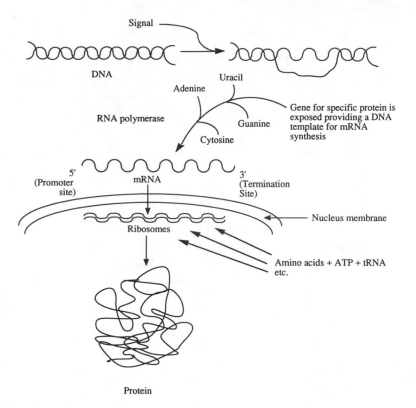

FIGURE 13. Protein synthesis. Signals are transmitted to the nucleus that stimulate the exposure of a gene for a specific protein. A specific messenger RNA is synthesized. The mRNA moves out into the cytosol and attaches to the ribosome, whereupon tRNAs attached to amino acids dock at appropriate complementary bases and the amino acids are joined together to make protein.

synthesis of the protein using the order of the assemblage of constituent amino acids as dictated by the mRNA. As described, this mRNA code is dictated by DNA. There are a number of instances in the nutritional biochemistry literature where a specific nutrient serves to stimulate the transcription of a specific mRNA. Glucose, for example, binds at a specific site on the nuclear DNA which codes for the enzyme glucokinase and has a putative effect on glucokinase mRNA transcription. As the individual consumes a high glucose diet, the glucose in the diet serves as one of the signals which activate the *de novo* synthesis of glucokinase by the pancreatic β cell and the liver cell. The DNA in these cell types has a glucose-sensitive promoter region just preceding the sequence which codes for the glucokinase. Other cell types may not have this promoter region exposed for glucose activation and glucokinase may not be found in these cells. Similar instances of nutrients acting on promoters of mRNA transcription have been described (see *Nutrition and Gene Expression*, in the Supplemental Reading Section).

Ribosomal RNA makes up a large fraction of total cellular RNA. It serves as the "docking" point for the activated amino acids bound to the transfer RNA and the mRNA which dictates the amino acid polymerization sequence. Transfer RNA (tRNA) is used to bring an amino acid to the polysome (ribosome), the site of protein synthesis. Each amino acid has a specific tRNA. Each tRNA molecule is thought to have a cloverleaf arrangement of nucleotides. With this arrangement of nucleotides, there is the opportunity for the maximum number of hydrogen bonds to form between base pairs. A molecule which has many hydrogen bonds is very stable. Transfer RNA also contains a triplet of bases known, in this instance, as the anticodon. The amino acid carried by tRNA is identified by the codon of mRNA through its anticodon; the amino acid itself is not involved in this identification.

The actual site of protein assembly is on the ribosomes; some ribosomes are located on the membrane of the endoplasmic reticulum and some are free in the cell matrix. Ribosomes consist almost entirely of ribosomal RNA and ribosomal protein. RNA is synthesized in the cell nucleus as a large molecule; there, this molecule is cleaved and leaves the nucleus as two subunits, a large one and a small one. The ribosome is reformed in the cytoplasm by the reassociation of the two subunits; the subunits, however, are not necessarily derived from the same precursor.

A few general statements can be made about the distribution of ribosomes in cells which have different capacities for the synthesis of proteins:

1. Cells which synthesize large numbers of protein have numerous ribosomes; conversely, cells which synthesize small numbers of proteins contain few.
2. Of the proteins synthesized by a cell to be secreted from that cell for use elsewhere, most of the ribosomes are attached to the endoplasmic reticulum.
3. Those cells which synthesize protein primarily for intracellular use have relatively few ribosomes attached to the membrane.

Small groups of ribosomes called polysomes are involved in protein synthesis; under physiologic conditions polysomes are bound to the endoplasmic reticulum. The ribosome is bound to the membrane through its large subunit; the small subunit is involved in the binding of mRNA to the ribosome. The ribosomes have two binding sites used in protein synthesis: the amino-acyl site and the peptidyl site. These two sites have specific functions in protein synthesis.

The synthesis of a protein takes place in four stages. Each stage requires specific cofactors and enzymes. In the first stage, which occurs in the cytosol, the amino acids are activated by esterifying each one to its specific tRNA. This requires a molecule of ATP. In addition to a specific tRNA, each amino acid requires a specific enzyme for this reaction.

During the second stage, the initiation of the synthesis of the polypeptide chain occurs. An initiation complex is formed by the binding of mRNA and the first activated amino acid-tRNA complex to the small ribosomal subunit. The large ribosomal unit then attaches, thus forming a functional ribosome. Three specific protein initiation factors are involved in this initiation step.

In the third stage of protein synthesis, the peptide chain is elongated by the sequential addition of amino acids from the tRNA complexes. The amino acid is recognized by base pairing of the codon of mRNA to the bases found in the anticodon of tRNA and a peptide bond is formed between the peptide chain and the newly arrived amino acid. The ribosome then moves along the mRNA; this brings the next codon in the proper position for attachment of the next activated amino acyl-tRNA complex. The mRNA and nascent polypeptide appear to "track" through a groove in the ribosomal subunits. This protects them from attack by enzymes in the surrounding environment.

The final stage of protein synthesis is the termination of the chain. The termination is signaled by one of three special codons (stop codons) in the mRNA. After the carboxy terminal amino acid is attached to the peptide chain, it is still covalently attached to tRNA which, in turn, is bonded to the ribosome. A protein release factor promotes the hydrolysis of the ester link between the tRNA and the amino acid. Once the polypeptide chain is generated and free of the ribosome, it assumes its characteristic three-dimensional structure.

If, during the course of synthesis, there is any interference in the continuity of assembly for lack of a supply of the proper amino acid, synthesis is stopped. Here lies the basis for the time factor of protein synthesis, a feature that nutritionists have recognized for several decades. It was established on the basis of animal feeding experiments that protein synthesis would not occur if all the amino acids were not provided at the proper time. In addition, since protein biosynthesis is very costly in terms of its energy requirement, synthesis is severely inhibited by starvation or caloric restriction. In experimental animals, it has been shown that starvation inhibits the polymerization of mRNA units, thus significantly reducing the activity of the transcription process. Other studies have shown that animals starved and then refed "overcompensate" for this period of reduced mRNA synthesis by markedly increasing mRNA synthesis above normal during the period of realimentation after the starvation period. This starved-refed induced increase in mRNA is manifested as an increase in the synthesis of enzymes necessary for the metabolism of the various ingredients in the diet used for realimentation. The signal(s) for the release of the starvation-induced inhibition of mRNA and enzyme synthesis include the macronutrients in the diet as well as the hormones glucocorticoid, thyroxine, insulin, and others.

If there is a mutation in the sequence of bases that comprise the genetic code for a given protein, the amino acid sequence generated in a protein will be incorrect. Whether this substitution of one amino acid for another in the protein being generated affects the functionality of the protein being generated depends entirely on the amino acid in question. Some amino acids can be replaced without affecting the secondary, tertiary, or quaternary structures of the protein (and hence, its chemical and physical properties) whereas others cannot. In addition, genetic errors in amino acid sequence may pose no threat to the individual if the protein in question is of little importance in the maintenance of health and well-being, or it can have large effects on health if the protein is a critical one. In the synthesis of the important protein, hemoglobin, if the genetic code calls for the use of valine instead of the usual glutamic acid in the synthesis of the β chain in the hemoglobin molecule, the resulting protein is less able to carry oxygen. This amino acid substitution not only affects the oxygen-carrying capacity of the red blood cell but also affects the solubility of the hemoglobin in the red blood cell sap. This, in turn, affects the shape of the red blood cell, changing it from a "dumbbell"-shaped donut to a shape resembling a sickle, hence the name sickle cell anemia. The decreased solubility of the hemoglobin can be understood if one remembers the relative polarity of the glutamic acid and valine molecules. The glutamic acid side chain is more ionic and thus contributes more to the solubility of the protein than the nonpolar side chain of the valine. This change in pH decreases its solubility in water and, of course, a change in solubility leads to an increased viscosity of the blood as the red cells rupture spilling their contents into the blood stream.

The amino acid sequence within a given species for a given protein is usually similar. However, some individual variation does occur. Because of these differences, individuals are able to "recognize" foreign proteins and, through the immune system, reject them. Again, this recognition depends wholly on the amino acid substitutions made and whether the amino acids in question contribute reactive groups that participate in the functional characteristics of the protein or are exposed sufficiently to be "recognized" as a foreign protein. An example of an "acceptable" amino acid substitution would be some of the ones that account for the species differences in the hormone insulin. As a hormone, it serves a variety of important functions in the regulation of carbohydrate, lipid, and protein metabolism. Yet, even though there are species differences in the amino acid sequence of this protein, insulin from one species can be given to another species and be functionally active. Obviously, the species differences in the amino acid sequence of this protein are not at locations in the chains which determine its biological function in promoting glucose use.

3. Protein Turnover

Protein turnover consists of two processes: synthesis and degradation. Synthesis is described in the preceding section. The proteins synthesized by the body have a finite existence. They are subject to a variety of insults and modifications. Some of these modifications have been touched upon as metabolic control processes have been discussed; a prohormone is converted to an active hormone, an enzyme is activated or inactivated with the addition or removal of a substituent, and so forth. Thus it is that a dynamic state within the body exists with respect to its full complement of peptides and proteins. Some proteins have very short lifetimes and very rapid turnover times; other proteins are quite stable and long lived — their turnover time is quite long. The estimate of the life of a protein, that is, how long it will exist in the body, is its half-life. A half-life is that time interval that occurs when half of the amount of a compound synthesized at time X will have been degraded. Given the dynamic state of metabolism, some of these time estimates will be very short. Half-lives of biologically active compounds are very difficult to estimate, yet the concept is handy when one is trying to understand and quantitate the turnover of body protein. Hormones are examples of short-lived proteins. They may be released, serve their function, and be degraded within a very short period (seconds to minutes to hours) of time. The protein of the lens is an example of a long-lived protein; once synthesized, the lens protein is not degraded nor recycled.

4. Protein Degradation

Protein degradation ultimately results in amino acids which are usually recycled (Figure 4). There are some exceptions to this general rule; histidine in the muscle protein is methylated and excreted as such. Most of the liberated amino acids join the body amino acid pool from which the synthetic processes withdraw their needed supply. The process of degradation first reduces the protein to peptides and then reduces these peptides to their constituent amino acids. If these amino acids are not reused for protein synthesis, they are degraded. Figure 14 illustrates the degradative pathway for proteins in general.

Although the proteases of digestion are important to the degradation of dietary protein, they have no role in the intracellular protein degradation. This degradation is primarily the responsibility of the lysosomes. Proteins in the extracellular environment are brought into the cell by endocytosis. This is a process similar to pinocytosis, where the cell membrane engulfs and encapsulates the extracellular material. Endocytosis occurs at indentations in the plasma membrane that are internally coated with a protein called *clathin*. As in pinocytosis, the extracellular protein is surrounded by the plasma membrane to form an intracellular vesicle which, in turn, fuses with a lysosome. Degradation then occurs via calcium-dependent proteases called calpains or cathepsin. Both the Golgi and the endoplasmic reticulum are involved in providing proteases that degrade peptide fragments that arise during the maturation of proteins in the secretory pathway.

Protein degradation (Figure 14) requires energy from ATP and the highly conserved 76-amino acid protein called ubiquitin. Ubiquitin seems to serve as a marker of proteins targeted for degradation. Since proteolysis is not an energy-dependent process, the need for ATP is puzzling except that ATP is needed for the bonding of ubiquitin to the target protein. The rate of degradation varies from protein to protein and this rate is determined by the amino acid at the amino end of the protein amino acid chain. A protein having methionine at its amino end, for example, is less readily degraded than one having lysine or aspartic acid or tryptophan. Proteins that are degraded slowly, therefore, have slower turnover times and longer half lives.

5. Amino Acid Catabolism

Those amino acids in the body's amino acid pool that are not used for peptide or protein synthesis and that are not used to synthesize metabolically important intermediates are deaminated, and the carbon skeletons are either oxidized or used for the synthesis of glucose or fatty acids. There are three general reactions for the removal of NH_3 from the amino acids:

1. They can be transaminated with the amino group transferred to another carbon chain as shown in Figure 15.
2. They can be oxidatively deaminated to yield NH_3 (see Figure 15).
3. They can be deaminated through the activity of an amino acid oxidase (Figure 15).

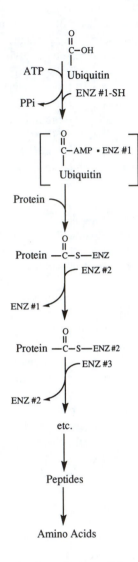

FIGURE 14. General pathway for intracellular protein degradation.

Transamination and deamination are important metabolic reactions. The importance of the alanine cycle in maintaining glucose homeostasis (Unit 5), the contribution of aspartate and glutamate to the shuttling of reducing equivalents between cytosolic and mitochondrial compartments (Unit 3), the use of methionine to make carnitine (Unit 6), and the use of tyrosine for the synthesis of the catecholamines and thyroxine is described in this unit.

The amino acids can be loosely grouped in terms of their catabolism. Valine, leucine, and isoleucine, the branched chain amino acids, are similar in that each has a methyl group on its carbon chain. They can be transaminated with α-ketoglutarate to form branch chain keto acids. These acids are considered homologs of pyruvate and are oxidized by a series of enzymes which are similar to those that catalyze the oxidation of α-ketoglutarate and pyruvate. The degradative steps are shown in Figures 15 and 16. Valine ultimately is converted to propionyl CoA, whereas isoleucine ends up as either acetyl CoA or propionyl CoA and leucine catabolism results in HMG CoA (β-hydroxy-β-methylglutaryl coenzyme CoA). HMG CoA is split

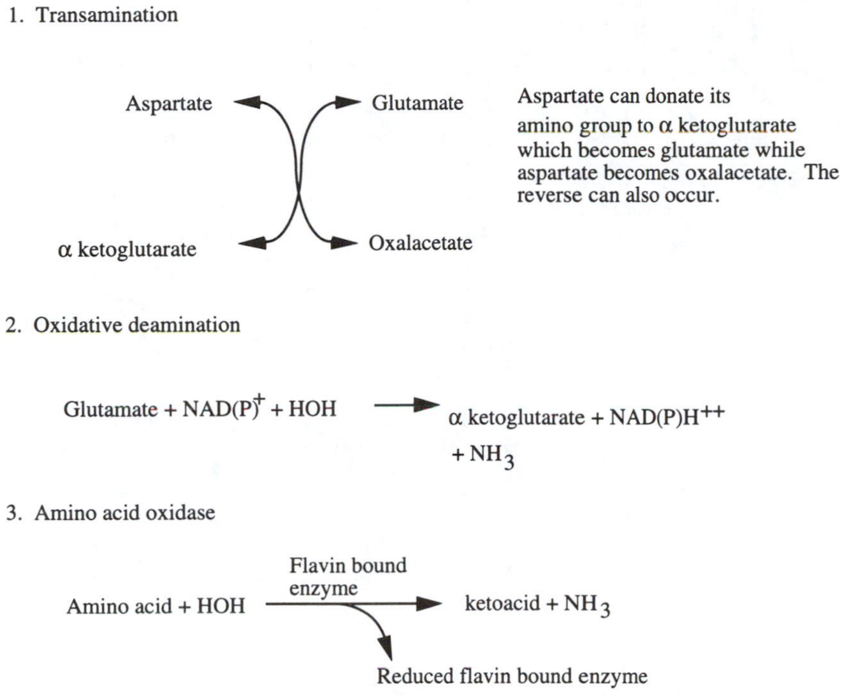

1. Transamination

Aspartate ⟷ Glutamate

α ketoglutarate ⟷ Oxalacetate

Aspartate can donate its amino group to α ketoglutarate which becomes glutamate while aspartate becomes oxalacetate. The reverse can also occur.

2. Oxidative deamination

$$Glutamate + NAD(P)^+ + HOH \longrightarrow \text{α ketoglutarate} + NAD(P)H^{++} + NH_3$$

3. Amino acid oxidase

$$Amino\ acid + HOH \xrightarrow{\text{Flavin bound enzyme}} ketoacid + NH_3$$

Reduced flavin bound enzyme

FIGURE 15. Amino acid reactions that result in the removal of the amino group.

to acetyl CoA and acetoacetate. Propionate is also the result of methionine catabolism. Should there be a defect in propionyl CoA carboxylase, propionate will accumulate.

Accumulations of propionate is characteristic of vitamin B_{12} deficiency. Propionate can serve as the substrate for long-chain odd-numbered fatty acids which are incorporated into myelin, the fatty covering of nerves. For some unknown reason, this myelin is abnormal in its function and fails to protect the peripheral nerve endings, which then die. This may explain the peripheral paresthesia that characterizes B_{12} deficiency. The HMG CoA produced in the catabolism of leucine is not used for cholesterol synthesis because it is produced in the mitochondria and does not travel to the cytosol where cholesterol is synthesized. Instead, HMG CoA is further metabolized to acetoacetate and acetyl CoA. Serine, threonine, and glycine are hydroxyamino acids. All three are gluconeogenic precursors (see Unit 5). Serine can be transaminated to provide pyruvate or dehydrated to form glycine and a methyl group useful in the one carbon metabolism which involves the vitamin folacin. Threonine can be degraded to pyruvate or carboxylated after deamination to form propionyl CoA. The catabolism of threonine is shown in Figure 17. Glutamate is converted to and formed from proline, ornithine, and arginine, the latter two are essential components of the urea cycle (Figure 18). The urea cycle functions to reduce the potentially toxic amounts of ammonia that arise when the ammonia group is removed from amino acids. Energetically speaking, this is a very expensive process. While urea cycle activity can be high when protein-rich diets are consumed and low when low protein diets are consumed, the cycle never shuts down completely. The cycle, shown in Figure 18, is fine tuned by the first reaction, the synthesis of carbamoyl phosphate. This reaction, which occurs in the mitochondria, is catalyzed by the enzyme carbamoyl phosphate synthetase. The enzyme is inactive in the absence of its allosteric activator, N-acetylglutamate, a compound synthesized from acetyl CoA and glutamate in the liver. As arginine levels increase in the liver, N-acetylglutamate synthetase is activated which

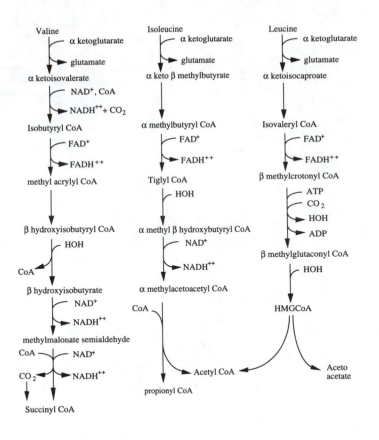

FIGURE 16. Catabolism of branched chain amino acids showing their use in the production of metabolites that are either lipid precursors or metabolites that can be oxidized via the Krebs cycle.

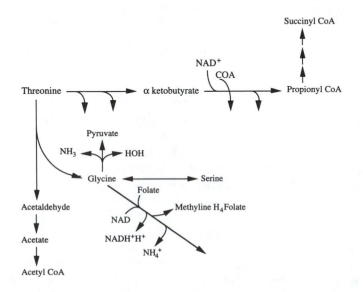

FIGURE 17. Catabolism of threonine showing its relationship to that of serine and glycine.

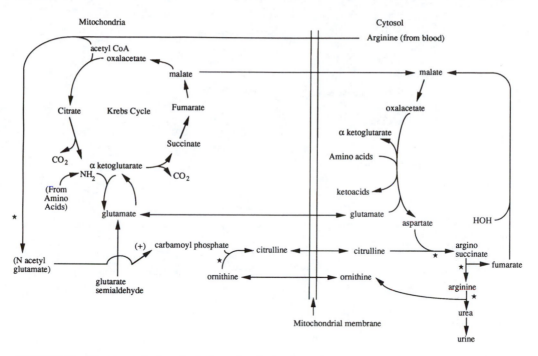

FIGURE 18. The urea cycle. Locations of mutations in the urea cycle enzymes are indicated with a star. Persons with these mutations have very short lives with evidence of mental retardation, seizures, coma, and early death due to the toxic effects of ammonia accumulation.

results in an increase in N-acetylglutamate. One of the more interesting aspects of the urea cycle is that it is initiated in the hepatic mitochondria but finished in the cytosol when urea is liberated via arginase. The urea is transported to the kidney and excreted in the urine. The ornithine returns to the liver to be recycled into citrulline with the addition of carbamoyl phosphate. Rising levels of arginine in the blood turn on N-acetylglutamate synthetase which provides the N-acetylglutamate which, in turn, activates carbamoyl phosphate synthetase and the cycle goes on.

Phenylalanine is the precursor of tyrosine and the use of tyrosine as a hormone precursor has been described (see Figure 7). Phenylalanine is converted to tyrosine via a hydroxylase reaction. Tyrosine, if not used to make one of several hormones, is then deaminated and, through a series of reactions, ends up as fumaryl acetate which is split to provide acetoacetate and fumarate. Tryptophan catabolism shows no similarity to the catabolic pathways of any of the other amino acids. The pathway used by phenylalanine and tyrosine is outlined in Figure 19 and the pathway for tryptophan is shown in Figure 20. Tryptophan is the precursor of serotonin, an important neurotransmitter that serves a variety of functions in the regulation of smooth muscle tone, especially those smooth muscles of the vascular tree. In so doing, it plays an especially important role in the maintenance of blood pressure and the control of the blood supply to the brain and vital organs. Several important drugs that address the problem of clinical depression alter the synthesis of serotonin from tryptophan or alter the action of serotonin once formed. Some of these drugs alter food intake as well (see Unit 3).

Histidine, an amino acid especially important for muscle protein biosynthesis, is also of great importance in one-carbon metabolism. The principle pathway of histidine catabolism leads to glutamate formation and as shown in Figure 21 (as well as in other figures where glutamate and α-ketoglutarate act in transamination) glutamate is an important component of the urea cycle (Figure 18). The decarboxylation of histidine yields histamine. This amine serves to stimulate gastric hydrochloric acid production and to stimulate vasoconstriction. A number of cold remedies and sinus remedies contain substances known as antihistamines,

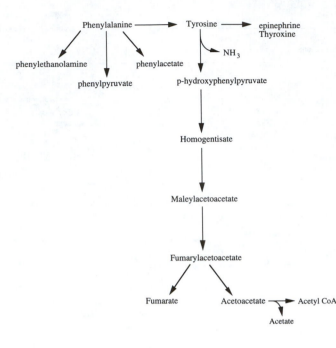

FIGURE 19.   Phenylalanine and tyrosine catabolism. This pathway has a number of mutations resulting in a variety of genetic diseases (see Table 18).

which interfere with the vasoconstrictor action of histamine. Histidine in muscle can be methylated and the end product, 3-methyl-histidine, can be measured in the urine and used as a measure of muscle protein turnover.

Lysine is one of the two essential amino acids whose amino group does not contribute to the total body amino acid pool; the other is threonine. Although lysine can donate its amino group to other carbon chains, the reverse does not occur. Lysine is catabolized to acetoacetyl CoA which then enters the Krebs cycle as acetyl CoA.

Methionine, cysteine, and cystine are important sulfur group donors. The importance of disulfide bridges in the structure of proteins has been described in Sections IV.D and IV.F. Methionine, as discussed in Unit 6, is important for carnitine synthesis. The pathway for methionine and cysteine is shown in Figure 22. Just as mutations in the metabolism of carbohydrate and lipid can occur with sometimes serious life-threatening effects, so too are there mutations in the metabolism of amino acids. Some of these are shown in Table 16.

6. Amino Acid Derivatives
a. *Creatine Phosphate*
The energy needed to drive the energy-dependent reactions of the body is provided by the high-energy bonds of the adenine nucleotides, the guanine nucleotides, and the uridylnucleotides. The concentrations of these nucleotides are carefully regulated and their energy is metered out as needed. Short, quick bursts of energy from these nucleotides are not possible. However, Mother Nature has devised another compound, creatine phosphate, that can do just this. Creatine is formed from glycine, arginine, methionine, and ATP in a three-step reaction sequence as shown in Figure 23. Creatine phosphate has the same free energy of hydrolysis as ATP but creatine cannot be recycled due to the reactivity of the phosphoguanidine group in which the carboxyl group displaces the phosphate. The resultant cyclic compound is creatinine which is then excreted in the urine. Creatine phosphate is found almost exclusively in the muscle and provides the quick burst of energy needed each time a muscle contracts.

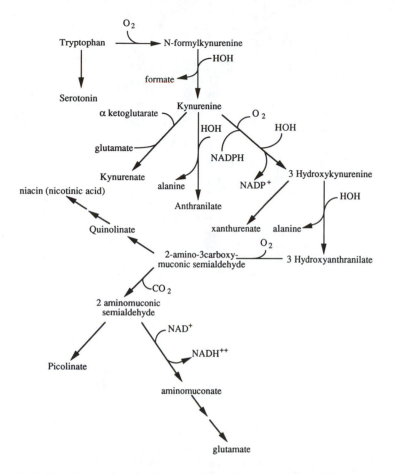

FIGURE 20. Catabolism of tryptophan showing conversion to the vitamin, niacin. This conversion is not very efficient, taking approximately 60 molecules of tryptophan to produce 1 molecule of niacin. Tryptophan catabolism also results in picolinate, which is believed by some to play a role in trace mineral conservation.

Since the muscle activity produces the end product, creatinine, measuring creatinine allows for the estimation of the muscle mass (see Unit 2). Because creatinine excretion is reasonably constant from day to day, researchers use the amount of creatinine in the 24-hour urine collection as an assurance of the completeness of the urine sample. Variations can occur if the usually sedentary subject has an unusually active day. A dramatic increase in muscle use will result in an increase in creatine phosphate breakdown and an increase in creatinine excretion.

b. Choline

Choline is a highly methylated compound synthesized from serine. Choline is an essential component of the neurotransmitter, acetylcholine, as well as an essential ingredient of the phospholipid, phosphatidylcholine.

c. Polyamines

Certain amino acids can be decarboxylated to form the polyamines. Some polyamines are very short-lived compounds that are neurotransmitters. They are quickly broken down so as to limit their effects. The catecholamines fall into this category of polyamines. Other polyamines, putrescine and spermine, bind nucleic acids and other polyanions. They are thus thought to have a role in cell division. However, the mechanism of their action has yet to be elucidated.

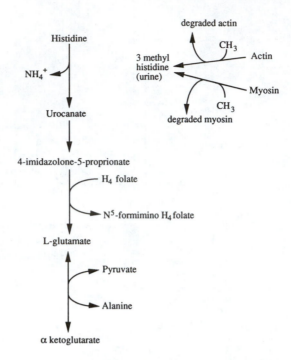

FIGURE 21. Catabolism of histidine. Note that 3-methyl-histadine is not part of the pathway. This metabolite is formed in the muscle when the contractile proteins, actin and myosin, are methylated.

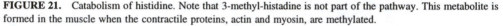

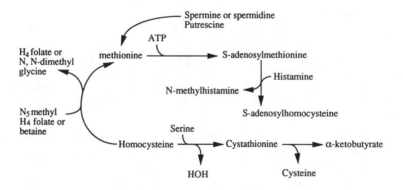

FIGURE 22. Conservation of the SH group via methionine-cysteine interconversion.

VII. FUNCTIONS OF PROTEINS

A variety of proteins are found in the body. Each of the various proteins serves a specific function in the maintenance of life. Any loss in body protein, in effect, means a loss in cellular function. In contrast to lipids and carbohydrates, which have a body reserve to be used in times of need, the functioning body has no true protein reserve. Humans, when they are deprived of or insufficiently supplied with protein, will compensate for this dietary deficiency by catabolizing some, but not all, of their tissue protein with a consequent loss in tissue functionality. Cells, tissues, organs, and whole systems cannot exist without the proteins serving their various functions.

TABLE 16
Genetic Mutations in Enzymes of Amino Acid Metabolism

Disease	Mutation	Characteristics
Maple syrup urine disease	Branched chain keto acid dehydrogenase (several variants)	Elevated levels of α ketoacids and their metabolites in blood and urine; mental retardation, ketoacidosis, early death
Methylmalonuria	Methylmalonyl CoA mutase (several variants). Inability to use vitamin B_{12}	High blood levels of methylmalonate; pernicious anemia, early death
Nonketotic hyperglycinemia	Glycine cleavage enzyme	Severe mental retardation, early death, high blood glycine levels
Hypermethioninemia	Methionine adenosyltransferase (↑ Km not deficiency per se)	Accumulation of methionine in blood (condition is benign)
Homocysteinemia	Cystathionine synthase	Elevated blood levels of methionine, homocysteine; abnormal collagen (no cross linking); dislocated lenses and other ocular malformations; osteoporosis; mental retardation, thromboembolism and vascular occlusions; short life span
Cystathioninuria	Cystathionase	Elevated levels of cystathionine in urine (condition is benign)
Phenylketonuria	Phenylalanine hydroxylase (several variants)	Increased levels of phenylalanine and deaminated metabolites in blood and urine; mental retardation; decreased neurotransmitter synthesis; shortened life span
Tyrosinemia	Tyrosine transaminase	Eye and skin lesions, mental retardation
	Fumarylacetoacetate hydrolase	Liver failure, renal failure
	p-Hydroxylphenylpyruvate oxidase	Increased need for ascorbic acid
Albinism	Tyrosinase	Lack of melanin (skin pigment) formation; increased sensitivity to sunlight; lack of eye pigment
Alcaptonuria	Homogentisate oxidase	Elevated urine levels of homogentisate; slow deposits of homogentisate in bones, connective tissue and internal organs resulting in gradual darkening of these structures. Increased susceptibility to arthritis
Parkinson's disease	Enzyme not identified	Decreased dopamine production by certain brain areas resulting in muscle tremors
Histidenemia	Histidase	Elevated levels of histidine in blood and urine. Can give false positive result in test for phenylketonuria. Elevated urocanase levels in sweat. Decreased histamine formation

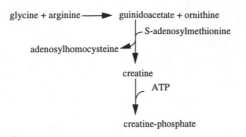

FIGURE 23. Formation of creatine phosphate.

A. PROTEINS AS ENZYMES

From conception to death, living cells use oxygen and metabolize fuel. Cells synthesize new products, degrade others, and generally are in a state of metabolic flux. For these processes to occur, catalysts are needed to enhance each of the many thousands of reactions occurring in the cell. These catalysts, called enzymes, are proteins. Enzymes make up the largest and most specialized class of proteins. Each enzyme is unique and catalyzes a specific kind of reaction. In the cell, enzymes are found in all the cellular compartments (cytoplasm, nucleus, mitochondria, etc.) as well as the membranes within and around the cell. The membrane-associated enzymes are part of the protein component of the cell wall. The location of an enzyme is one of its characteristics and dictates, in part, its role in metabolism.

Enzymes consist of specific sequences of amino acids. Should the sequence deviate, alterations in enzyme activity can be anticipated unless, of course, the change in amino acid does not affect the active site of the enzyme or its molecular shape. The importance of the amino acid sequence is obvious and is related to the availability of R groups (on the amino acids) which will complement reactive groups on the substrates, the molecule on which the enzyme exerts its catalytic action. The catalytic function of the enzyme is intimately related to its amino acid sequence. Enzymes must possess a shape which will complement the molecular shape of the substrate in much the same way as a key fits into a lock. This shape, of course, is a function of the enzyme protein's primary, secondary, tertiary, and quaternary structure. Just as enzymes must have a specific shape, substrates must also have specific shapes in order to be catalyzed by their respective enzymes. This is the reason why only D-sugars or only L-amino acids can be metabolized by mammalian cells. These stereoisomers conform to the shape required by the enzyme which serves as its catalyst. While enzymes show absolute specificity, the specificity generally applies to only a portion of the substrate molecule. If the substrate is a small compound, this specificity applies to the entire molecule. If, however, the substrate is large and complex, the structural requirements are less stringent in that only that part of the substrate involved in the enzyme-substrate complex must have the appropriate molecular arrangement. The portion of the substrate not involved in the reaction (i.e., the nature of the R group) need not be the appropriate conformation. How does this specificity work? Many substrate-enzyme complexes form with a three-point attachment which leaves a fourth atom or R group free. If the attachment site can be approached from only one direction and only complementary atoms can attach, the substrate molecule can bind in only one way.

Some enzymes are specific for only one substrate; others may catalyze several related reactions. While some are specific for a particular substrate, others are specific for certain bonds. This is called *group specificity*. For example, glycosidases act on glycosides (any glycoside), pepsin and trypsin act on peptide bonds, and esterases act on ester linkages. Within these groups, certain enzymes exhibit greater specificity. Chymotrypsin preferentially acts on peptide bonds in which the carboxyl group is a part of the aromatic amino acids (phenylalanine, tyrosine, or tryptophan). Enzymes such as carboxypeptidase or aminopeptidase catalyze the hydrolysis of the carboxy-terminal or amino-terminal amino acid of a polypeptide chain. This bond specificity, rather than molecular specificity, is useful to the animal in that it reduces the number of enzymes needed within the organism. Incidentally, the above enzymes are very useful to the protein chemist in his/her determination of the amino acid sequence of a given protein.

Cells synthesize enzymes in much the same fashion as they synthesize other proteins; yet enzymes are relatively short-lived. Cells must continually synthesize their enzymes if they are to survive. A variety of signals serve as stimulants or inhibitors of this synthesis. One of these signals is the substrate. An excess of substrate will not only activate any preexisting enzyme in the cell but will also serve to stimulate enzyme synthesis. The substrate may act at the level of mRNA transcription or at the level of translation or protein assembly. Hormones such as insulin, thyroid hormone, and cortisol may also serve in this way to stimulate enzyme synthesis and/or activation. Hormonal inhibition of enzyme synthesis also occurs and serves as an internal regulator of the synthetic process.

B. PROTEINS AS CARRIERS

A large variety of compounds are carried in the blood between tissues and organs of the body. Some of the compounds require a specific protein for their transport. Not only is this protein necessary for the transport of compounds insoluble in blood, but it is also necessary to protect these compounds from further reactions during the transport process. Some of the membrane proteins are carriers and some are both carriers and enzymes. Both intracellular and extracellular carriers have been identified; however, the plasma proteins as carriers of lipid have been studied the most due to their possible involvement in the pathophysiology of cardiovascular disease. These are discussed in Unit 6.

The plasma proteins which can have a carrier function are the albumin and the α- and β-globulins. Perhaps the best-studied of the plasma carriers are those associated with the transport of lipid, since these lipoproteins (carriers plus lipids), when levels are elevated, appear to be related to the development of a variety of diseases. These lipoproteins comprise about 3% of the plasma proteins. They are loose associations of such lipids as phospholipids, triacylglycerols, and cholesterols, and represent an example of how proteins function as carriers. The lipids they carry are either from the diet or are synthesized *de novo* in tissues such as the liver. The β-globulin proteins carry these lipids to such sites as muscle or adipose tissue where they are either used or stored. The release of the lipid from the protein carrier is a complicated process. In adipose tissue the lipoprotein is attached to a membrane receptor site; an enzyme, lipoprotein lipase, cleaves the lipid from the protein; the lipid is then picked up by another protein called a lipid binding protein and is carried into the interior of the cell for storage. The β-globulin protein carrier, once free of its lipid, returns to the liver or intestinal mucosa and is recycled.

The plasma lipids, phospholipids, acylglycerides, cholesterol, cholesterol esters, and "free" fatty acids are usually transported as loosely associated lipid-protein complexes (see Unit 6). At least three different proteins have been identified. Albumin usually transports the free fatty acids, whereas the α- and β-globulins transport the phospholipids, acylglycerols, and cholesterols. The different lipoprotein complexes can be separated and identified on the basis of their antigenicity, their electrophoretic mobility, and their density. The low density or β-lipoproteins contain the β-peptide, cholesterol, and some phospholipids. The majority of the phospholipids are carried as α-lipoproteins. With age, the lipid content of the plasma tends to rise and the rise is reflected almost entirely as an increase in β-lipoproteins. As the density of the lipoproteins decreases, the molecular weight and complexity of the lipid it carries decreases. The β-lipoproteins carry mainly (up to 60%) acylglycerides. These glycerides are usually those synthesized in the body rather than coming from the diet. The dietary acylglycerols are usually carried as chylomicrons. These particles are the largest and least dense of the lipid-protein complexes.

In addition to serving as carriers of lipids, some of the globulins in the plasma can combine stoichiometrically with iron and copper as well as with other divalent cations. These combinations are called metalloproteins. The globulins serve to transport these cations from the gut to the tissues where they are used. The monovalent cations, sodium and potassium, do not need carriers but most other minerals do.

Many hormones and vitamins require transport or carrier proteins to take them from their point of origin to their active site. In addition, there are intracellular transport proteins such as the lipid binding protein mentioned above that are responsible for the transport of materials between the various cellular compartments. Lastly, there are transport proteins which carry single molecules. The classic example, of course, is hemoglobin, the red cell protein responsible for the transport of oxygen from the lungs to every oxygen-using cell in the body.

C. PROTEINS AS REGULATORS OF WATER BALANCE

As substrates and solutes are transferred or exchanged across membranes, water has a tendency to follow to maintain equal osmotic pressure on each side of the membrane. If osmotic pressure is not maintained, the individual cells either shrink from lack of internal water or burst from too much. The balance of water between the intracellular and extracellular compartments is closely regulated (see Unit 2).

One of the most carefully controlled points of water balance is across the capillary membrane where a close balance is maintained between the osmotic pressure of the blood plasma, the interstitial fluids, and the cells and the hydrostatic pressure exerted by the pumping action of the heart. The total osmotic pressure of the plasma and of the intra- and extracellular fluids is the result of its content of inorganic electrolytes, its organic solutes, and its proteins. The concentrations of the electrolytes and organic solutes in plasma, interstitial fluid, and cells are substantially the same so that the contribution to the osmotic pressure by these substances is practically equal. However, since there are more proteins in plasma than in the cells, plasma exerts an osmotic pressure on the tissue fluids. The result of this inequity of solutes is the drawing of fluids from the tissue spaces and from the cells into the blood. Opposing this force is the hydrostatic pressure, exerted by the pumping action of the heart, which moves fluids from the blood into the tissue spaces and into the cells. The hydrostatic pressure is greater on the arterial side of the capillary loop than on the venous side. There is an interplay between these four kinds of pressure — blood osmotic pressure, tissue osmotic pressure, blood hydrostatic pressure, and tissue hydrostatic pressure. This interplay results in a filtration of solutes and metabolites and the transfer of oxygen from the arterial blood into the tissues and cells it supplies, and on the venous side, a resorption from the tissue space of CO_2, metabolites, and solutes back into the blood supply.

Albumin plays a more significant role in maintaining the osmotic pressure than the other blood proteins because of its size and abundance. It is a small molecule and will have a greater number of particles per unit volume than the other larger serum proteins. With fewer proteins in the serum, water leaks out into the interstitial space and accumulates. The condition known as edema results. The edema of protein deficiency may also be the result of the body's inability to regulate the protein hormone, particularly ADH (see Unit 2). This hormone plays a role in controlling water balance. Edema not involving protein deficiency can also result from other factors such as increased blood pressure or renal disease, but the edema which results in these situations is a result of increased body water. The effect of protein is on the distribution of water amongst the various body compartments rather than on the total body water.

D. PROTEINS AS BIOLOGICAL BUFFERS

Proteins have the ability to accept or donate hydrogen ions, and by so doing they serve as biological buffers. In blood, there are three important buffering systems: plasma proteins, hemoglobin, and carbonic acid-bicarbonate. The equilibrium reactions for each of these buffering systems follows:

$$HProtein \rightleftarrows H^+ + Protein^-$$

$$H_2CO_3 \rightleftarrows H^+ + HCO_3^-$$

$$HHb \rightleftarrows H^+ + Hb^-$$

The first of these buffering systems, the plasma proteins, can function as a weak acid/salt buffer when the free carboxyl groups on the protein dissociate, or as a weak base/salt buffer when the free amino groups dissociate. Although the buffering ability of the plasma protein is extremely important in maintaining blood pH, it is not as important as the other two systems.

The second buffering system, carbonic acid-bicarbonate, is extremely effective because there are reactions which follow this equilibrium which will regulate either acids or bases. The H_2CO_3 level in plasma never goes too high because it is in equilibrium with CO_2 ($H_2CO_3 \rightleftarrows CO_2 + H_2O$), which is expired by the lungs. In blood, this equilibrium proceeds very quickly because of the presence of carbonic anhydrase, an enzyme found in red blood cells which catalyze it. If the carbonic acid-bicarbonate reaction goes in the opposite direction, the concentration of the HCO_3^- so formed will be regulated by the kidneys.

The third important buffering system in blood results from hemoglobin. Hemoglobin has six times the buffering power of the plasma proteins. It functions well as a buffer for three reasons. First, it is present in large amounts. Second, it contains 38 histidine residues. Histidine residues are good buffers because they can dissociate to H^+ and the imidazole group. Third, hemoglobin exists in blood in two forms, reduced hemoglobin and oxyhemoglobin. The imidazole groups of reduced hemoglobin dissociate less than those of oxyhemoglobin; it is, thus, a weaker acid and a better buffer.

Hemoglobin's role in maintaining blood pH is extremely important and is best appreciated by understanding the transport of oxygen and carbon dioxide during respiration through the blood. Oxyhemoglobin is formed when each of the four ferrous ions in hemoglobin reversibly combines with one O_2 molecule. The reaction between oxygen and hemoglobin is written as $Hb + O_2 \rightarrow HbO_2$. The combination is not an oxygenation reaction because iron stays in the positive two-oxidation state. Instead, there is a loose association that exists between the oxygen and hemoglobin molecules.

At an oxygen tension of at least 100 mmHg hemoglobin is almost completely saturated with oxygen. This curve has a sigmoid shape rather than being linear because after the first oxygen molecule is added to the hemoglobin the affinity for the second is increased, the second increases the affinity for the third, etc. This increase in affinity results because as the O_2 is taken up the two β chains move closer together. As O_2 is given up they move further apart. When fully saturated, as it is at normal physiologic conditions, each gram of hemoglobin contains 1.34 mL of oxygen. In a normal 100 mL of blood there are about 15 g of hemoglobin and, hence, 20 mL of oxygen.

In addition to the oxygen carried in the blood in association with hemoglobin, there is additional oxygen present that is dissolved in the blood. Henry's law states that this concentration is a linear function of the pressure of the oxygen. Only 0.4 mL of oxygen is in blood by being dissolved there, thus, the major source of oxygen in the blood is hemoglobin.

As the cells consume the oxygen carried to them by hemoglobin the oxygen tension falls, the oxyhemoglobin more readily dissociates, and the saturation of the hemoglobin falls. At about 50 mmHg, hemoglobin rapidly "unloads" its oxygen. In the tissues, oxygen tension is about 40 mmHg. This tension is below that necessary for unloading to occur and a gradient of high to low oxygen tension exists which facilitates the passage of oxygen to the tissues. This gradual change in oxygen in the blood can be followed visually. Leaving the lungs, the blood is bright red. As it moves through the vascular system towards the periphery, the blood gradually darkens, and by the time it returns to the lungs it has a bluish hue. This bluish hue is a characteristic of deoxygenated hemoglobin and the reason why persons lacking good respiratory exchange have a bluish tinge to their skin.

The CO_2 that is expired by the cells is transported in three forms. That which diffuses into the red blood cells is rapidly hydrated to H_2CO_3 by the presence of the carbonic anhydrase. The H_2CO_3 then dissociates into H^+ and HCO_3^-. The H^+ is neutralized primarily by hemoglobin, and the bicarbonate diffuses into the plasma; this is the form in which most expired CO_2 is carried. Some CO_2 that diffuses into red blood cells is not converted into bicarbonate ion but instead reacts with the amino groups of proteins, principally hemoglobin, to form carbamino compounds:

$$CO_2 + R-N\begin{matrix} H \\ \\ H \end{matrix} \rightleftharpoons R-N\begin{matrix} H \\ \\ COOH \end{matrix}$$

Reduced hemoglobin forms the carbamino compounds more readily than does oxyhemoglobin. The third form of CO_2 is that which is dissolved; it will exist as carbonic acid. It makes up only a small fraction of the total amount of CO_2 present. CO_2 present as carbonic acid will lower the blood pH.

That CO_2 which diffuses into the plasma also exists in these three forms. The carbamino compounds will react with the plasma proteins. Much less CO_2 is hydrated to form carbonic acid in plasma than in red blood cells because the carbonic anhydrase enzyme is located only in red blood cells. And, finally, a small amount of dissolved CO_2 is present.

There is a much greater rise in the HCO_3^- concentration in red blood cells than in plasma. As a result, HCO_3^- will diffuse into the plasma. This represents a problem of maintaining electrochemical neutrality. It is accompanied by a diffusion of chloride ions from the plasma to the red blood cells. This phenomenon is known as the chloride shift. Since CO_2 transport will occur primarily in venous blood, the chloride content of venous blood is higher than that of arterial blood. At the lungs, when venous blood becomes arterial, all these reactions are reversed. Occasionally, these reactions are perturbed and the acid-base balance is not maintained. Under normal conditions, the carbonic acid:bicarbonate ratio is maintained at 1:20. When the CO_2 levels rise, carbonic acid levels rise and respiratory acidosis occurs. Conversely, when CO_2 levels fall, respiratory alkalosis occurs. By adjusting inspiration and expiration, respectively, small rises and falls in CO_2 levels can be adjusted, and the ratio of carbonic acid to bicarbonate remains constant. The kidney, through increasing its resorption of bicarbonate, can also assist in the regulation of this buffer system.

Large shifts in the acid-base balance which originate not in the respiratory system but rather as a result of metabolic alterations also occur. The prime example is the metabolic acidosis which occurs in the severe, uncontrolled diabetic. As a result of the lack of insulin the metabolic fuel, glucose, cannot be used. The body then uses the alternate fuel, fatty acids. The initial steps of fatty acid oxidation do not require insulin. However, the final steps do. Since there is an insulin deficiency, the body begins to accumulate the ketone bodies — acetone, acetoacetate, and β-hydroxybutyrate. Normally, these substances are further oxidized to produce CO_2 and water. However, in this instance, further oxidation is not possible. Acetoacetate and β-hydroxybutyrate are acidic and they must be neutralized. All of the buffering systems are mobilized but eventually they will not be able to compensate for this gradual increase in ketone bodies. The pH will fall, the enzymes which work at pH 7.4 will be appreciably less active, and hemoglobin will become less able to carry oxygen. Unless treated with insulin, the patient will become comatose (lack of oxygen to the brain) and die.

Metabolic alkalosis is not nearly as common as metabolic acidosis. However, it can occur in persons having prolonged bouts of both diarrhea and vomiting. This is a result of the loss of the stomach acid, hydrochloric acid (the chloride ion), and the loss of potassium ions. Alkalosis can also occur in individuals who consume large quantities of alkali, as might occur in persons with peptic ulcers who self medicate with antacids. In any event, the elevated blood pH may result in slow and shallow breathing, lowered serum calcium and potassium levels, and muscle tetany (prolonged contractions). Buffering activity is not limited to the blood. The carbonic acid/bicarbonate buffering system is active in interstitial fluids. Intracellular buffers include the proteins and organic phosphates.

While the blood pH is maintained within a fairly narrow range through the systems just described, the urine pH can vary considerably depending on the metabolic state of the individual. The kidney and the urinary tract can tolerate a greater fluctuation in pH than can other tissues. Nonetheless, a number of buffer systems are also active in this tissue. In the kidney, although little buffering is done by the proteins, the bicarbonate buffer system is particularly active in the extracellular fluid. Once urine is produced, little effort is made to buffer its pH; it can vary from 4.7 to 8.0. The bladder and urinary tract are constructed so that this broad pH range is tolerated with little effect on the metabolism that occurs in these tissues.

E. PROTEINS AS STRUCTURAL ELEMENTS AND STRUCTURAL UNITS

In Unit 6, the lipid component of the membrane is discussed. Analysis of the liver cell membrane has shown that this membrane contains 50 to 60% protein, 35% lipid, and 5% carbohydrate. The carbohydrate present is joined primarily to the protein forming glycoproteins, compounds which constitute the receptor sites of several hormones. The protein portion of the membrane is so oriented that its hydrophilic aspects are also in close proximity to the intracellular and extracellular fluids. The protein molecules are interspersed within the lipids and lend both structural stability and fluidity to the membrane.

Membrane function depends on how the proteins are placed in the membrane and on the fluidity which results from the combination of proteins in a lipid mixture. As indicated earlier, the lipid portion of the membrane needs to be fairly unsaturated. If saturated, a more rigid crystalline structure will form. By being fluid and less rigid, these lipids can allow the proteins to change their shape in response to ionic changes and thus these proteins can function as enzymes, carriers, binding or receptor sites, or entry ports for the large variety of materials binding, entering, or leaving the cell. How can these proteins serve in this fashion? Recall the protein conformation. The R groups of the amino acids project both in and out from the conformation and interact to form hydrogen bonds and disulfide bridges, however briefly, with compounds in close proximity to them. Proteins which react with materials external to the cell may change their conformation and, in so doing, change their position within the membrane structure so that the reactive site changes from facing outward to the extracellular environment to facing inward, toward the intracellular environment. Once facing inward, the material temporarily attracted to the membrane protein might be more attracted to another protein within the cell and "let go" of the membrane protein. Of course, this explanation is very simplistic. Transport into and out of cells probably involves many other reactions, a source of energy, and cations and/or anions for exchange. Yet, this simplified explanation may be sufficient to explain the passage of a number of materials through the cell membrane. The reactive groups of the amino acid side chains, the R groups, of the "structural" membrane proteins may also serve as identifiers or facilitators of reactive sites and comprise the receptor site for materials, such as insulin, which do not usually enter the cell. Insulin, also a protein, has reactive side chains protruding from it just as reactive side chains protrude from the proteins in the membrane. These two reactive groups interact and the binding of the insulin to the receptor site occurs. Again, this is a very simplistic explanation of receptor site action. In the instance of insulin, the receptor site is probably a glycoprotein.

Some receptor sites are specific for one compound while other receptor sites react to classes of similar compounds. It is thought that glucagon and insulin may have overlapping receptor sites since the effect of one of these hormones can be blunted if cells are exposed to the other hormone first. If this blunting occurs because the receptor sites overlap and one hormone already occupies the site, then the second hormone cannot adequately bind. Once binding occurs, the hormone's effects on the cell can be observed.

In addition to the function of proteins in the cell membrane as a structural element and as functional units, proteins are important intracellular structural units. Muscle is 20% protein, 75% water, and 5% inorganic material, glycogen, and other organic compounds. The major proteins in muscle are myosin, a large globular protein, and actin, a smaller globular protein. These two proteins, plus the filamentous tropomyosin and troponin, are the molecular components of the muscles. The muscle proteins are characterized by their elasticity, which in turn contributes to the contractile power of this tissue.

Perhaps one of the most important structural functions of protein is that related to skin and connective tissue. The skin is composed of epithelial tissue which covers not only the exterior of the body but lines the gastrointestinal tract, the respiratory tract, and the urinary tract. One of the major proteins found in the skin is melanin. It gives the skin its characteristic color. Keratin is the protein which forms hair, nails, hooves, feathers, or horns. Each of these structures is slightly different but all contain keratin. This protein is insoluble in water and is resistant to most digestive enzymes. It has a high percentage of cystine. Melanin is a tyrosine derivative and provides the pigmentation or color to the skin. Persons unable to form this pigment are albinos and their disease is called albinism. Three separate genetic errors have been identified as causes for albinism.

Connective tissue is that tissue which holds all of the various cells and tissues together. In the broadest definition, connective tissue includes the bones and teeth as well. Bones and teeth start out with a matrix protein ("ground substance") into which various amounts of minerals are deposited. Connective tissue contains two distinct types of proteins: collagen and elastin. Collagen is the principal solid substance in white connective tissue. It contains a high percentage of proline, hydroxyproline, and glycine. It is difficult to degrade this protein and, like hair, it is relatively inert metabolically. Even in protein deficient states, the body will synthesize collagen and elastin and these proteins will not be catabolized for needed amino acids. Incidentally, although the body does not readily catabolize collagen, this protein can be degraded to a limited degree by boiling in acid. It is then converted to gelatin. The collagen of bone, skin, cartilage, and ligaments differ in chemical composition from that of the white fibrous tissue which holds individual cells together within muscle, liver, and other organs. Elastin and chondroalbumoid are two other proteins in the connective tissue. They are present in small amounts and serve as part of the structural protein.

F. PROTEINS AS LUBRICANTS

The mucus of the respiratory tract, the oral cavity, the vaginal tract, and the rectal cavity reduces the irritation which might be caused by materials moving through these passages. This mucus is a mucoprotein, a conjugated protein which contains hexosamine. Proteins, as lubricants, also surround the joints and facilitate their movement. Should these lubricants not be present, or present but with substantial decreases in their fluidity through the deposition of minerals, skeletal movement may be difficult and painful.

G. PROTEINS IN THE IMMUNE SYSTEM

Proteins such as γ-globulin serve to protect the body against foreign cells. The immunoglobins produced by lymphocytes are large polypeptides having more than one basic monomeric unit. These proteins differ in their amino acid structure which, in turn, affects their secondary, tertiary, and quaternary structures. Just as the amino acid sequence of an enzyme determines substrate specificity, the amino acid sequence of the immunoprotein assures antigen-antibody specificity. The synthesis of particular immunoglobulins has been much studied. It is now well accepted that initiation of synthesis by the lymphocyte requires the binding of an antigen (a foreign protein) to the cell surface at particular locations called antigen receptors. As with other receptor sites on other cells, there must be a good conformational "fit" between the site and the antigen. Once the immunoglobulin is synthesized, it will bind with the foreign protein, immobilizing it, and the complex antigen-antibody will be formed.

VIII. PROTEIN REQUIREMENTS

Human protein and amino acid requirements have been studied for well over 100 years using a variety of techniques. Nutrition scientists have collected data on the quantity of protein foods consumed vs. health, growth, and weight gain of various populations. The assumption was made that whatever "healthy" people ate was probably what kept them "healthy" and should, therefore, be used as a standard of comparison for other diets. These standards, with respect to protein, were invariably high for populations having an abundance of meat, milk, poultry, and fish in their diets. Voit and Atwater, around the turn of the century, found intakes of 118 and 125 g protein/day, respectively, for an adult man.

As nutrition developed as a science, more accurate methods for assessing nutrient needs were developed. Among these methods were those for assessing the intake and excretion of nitrogen compounds. The Kjeldahl method, described in an earlier section, as well as methods for determining the nitrogenous end products of metabolism were devised. These methods made possible the development of the concepts which today's scientists use to determine the nutrient requirements of humans as well as other species. In protein nutrition, it was realized that the body consists of two pools of protein: one which has a short half-life and which must be constantly renewed and one which is slowly broken down and rebuilt. If one assumes that over a short period of time the pool having the long half-life contributes almost nothing to the nitrogenous metabolic end products, then a measure of the amount of nitrogen excreted will reflect only the turnover of the short-lived proteins. These proteins have to be replaced by proteins newly synthesized from the amino acids provided by the diet. Hence, the term protein requirement (or the requirement for any nutrient) means that amount of protein which must be consumed to provide the amino acids for the synthesis of those body proteins irreversibly catabolized in the course of the body's metabolism. The intake of nitrogen from protein must be sufficient to balance that excreted; this basic concept is called nitrogen balance and has been discussed in Section V.C.2. While this concept is useful in understanding why we have a minimal need for protein in the diet, its application is fraught with difficulty. In Section V.C.2 the possible sources of error in the nitrogen balance technique were discussed in terms of their contribution to the accuracy and precision of the methods available for comparing various food proteins. These same sources of errors also apply when using the nitrogen balance technique for assessing protein and amino acid requirements. Lastly, the need for dietary protein is influenced by age, environmental temperature, energy intake, gender, micronutrient intake, infection, activity, previous diet, trauma, pregnancy, and lactation.

A. AGE

Protein in excess of maintenance needs is required when new tissue is being formed. Certain age periods, when growth is rapid, require more dietary protein than other periods. Age differences in protein turnover (protein flux) as well as protein synthesis explain some of the effects of age on protein need. Table 17 gives figures for humans at different ages. Premature infants (those infants born before their 10 lunar month gestation time) grow at a very rapid rate and require between 2.5 to 5 g/protein/kg/day if they are to survive.

Studies of full-term infants have indicated that a protein intake of 2 to 2.5 g/kg/day resulted in a satisfactory weight gain and that further increases in protein intake did not measurably improve growth. Older infants and children, whose growth rate is not as rapid as the premature

TABLE 17
Age Effects on Nitrogen Flux Which Reflects Protein Flux and Protein Synthesis Rate Per Day

Age	Protein (N) flux (mg N/kg/hr)	Total body protein synthesis, (g/kg/day)
Newborn	124 ± 46	17.4 ± 9.9
Infant	65 ± 7	6.9 ± 1.1
Young adult	26 ± 2	3.0 ± 0.2
Elderly	19 ± 2	1.9 ± 0.15

or newborn infant, require considerably less protein (~1.25 g/kg/day). As growth rate increases during adolescence, the protein need increases. Again, this can be related to the demands for dietary amino acids to support the growth process. As the human completes his/her growth, the need for protein decreases until it arrives at a level which is called the maintenance level. It is at this level that the concept of body protein replacement by dietary protein applies. During the growth period, it is very difficult to separate the requirements for maintenance from those of growth. The impulse for growth is so strong that it will occur in many instances at the *expense* of the maintenance of body tissues. For example, protein-malnourished children will continue to grow taller *even though* their muscles as well as other tissues show evidence of wastage due to dietary protein deficiency.

Growth carries with it not only a total nitrogen requirement but also a particular amino acid requirement. Maintenance, on the other hand, appears to have only a total protein requirement. The adult can make a number of short-term adjustments in his/her protein metabolism that can compensate for possible inequities or imbalances in amino acid intake as long as the total protein requirement is met. The young growing animal is not that flexible. The essential amino acid requirements are age dependent. Histidine, although it can be synthesized in sufficient quantities by the adult to meet maintenance needs, is not synthesized in great enough amounts to support growth or tissue repair. Thus, histidine is an essential amino acid for the infant, growing child, and injured adult. This is due to the nature of the growth and repair processes.

B. ENVIRONMENTAL TEMPERATURE

As environmental temperatures rise or fall above or below the range of thermic neutrality, animals begin to increase their caloric expenditure to maintain their body temperature. In environments that are too warm, vasodilation occurs along with sweating and increased respiration. All of these mechanisms are designed to cool the body and all require an increase in the basal energy requirement as expressed per unit of body surface area. In cool environments, vasoconstriction and shivering occur in an effort to warm the body and prevent undue heat loss. Again, an increase in basal energy requirement is observed. Smuts, in 1934, found that nitrogen requirements were related to basal energy requirements. Through the study of a large number of species, he concluded that 2 mg nitrogen were required for every basal kilocalorie required when the energy requirement was expressed on a surface area basis. Thus, any increase in basal energy needs due to a change in environmental temperature will, because of the relationship between protein and energy, be accompanied by an increase in the protein requirement for maintenance. In addition, profuse sweating as occurs in very warm environments carries with it a nitrogen loss which must be accounted for in the determination of minimal protein needs.

C. PREVIOUS DIET

The effects of previous diet on the determination of protein requirements may be rather profound. If, for example, the subjects selected for studies on protein needs have been poorly nourished prior to the initiation of the study, their retention of the protein during the study will be greater than would be observed in subjects who have been well nourished prior to the initiation of the study. In other words, malnourished subjects have a higher protein requirement than well-nourished subjects. This, of course, raises the issue of whether there are body protein reserves. Voit, Wilson, Cuthbertson, Fisher, and others observed that animals fed a protein-free diet exhibit a "lag" before their nitrogen excretion level is minimized; during this phase the animal is metabolizing his protein reserve. Other investigators maintain that there is no such thing as a protein reserve or store. These investigators maintain that every protein in the body has a function, and if some of these proteins are lost there is a loss in body function. Support for this concept is seen in the reduced ability of protein-depleted animals to fight infection or respond to the metabolic effects of trauma. Whether one believes that there is such an entity as a protein reserve may depend upon whether one perceives a difference between an optimal protein intake and a minimum protein intake. This difference may relate more to a personal opinion on how nutrient requirements should be defined. Some nutritionists believe in stating the absolute minimum requirement to sustain life and then adding on increments for each body function above mere survival; this is known as the particulate approach. Other nutritionists believe that one cannot separate and quantitate the individual requirements of each function beyond survival. They advocate a protein intake sufficient for optimal function of the animal; this is known as the integrative approach. The particulate and integrative approaches each have their merits when argued intellectually. However, since humans do not merely exist, many human nutritionists tend to take the integrative approach to human nutrition requirements in their determination of protein needs.

D. PHYSICAL ACTIVITY

Research on protein needs for muscular work had its beginning in 1863 when Von Leiberg postulated that muscle protein was destroyed with each contraction of the muscle. On this basis, he recommended that heavy muscular work required a heavy protein diet. This theory has been amply disproved, yet even today many believe that a protein-rich diet will contribute to athletic prowess. Today, we know that muscle contraction does not result in destruction of the muscle. It does, however, require energy in the form of ATP, glucose, and fatty acids, and does result in the breakdown of creatine-phosphate to creatine which is then converted to creatinine, a nitrogenous waste product excreted in the urine.

As the energy requirement is increased to support the increase in muscular activity, so too is the protein requirement in much the same manner as described above for the effects of temperature. In a number of studies, the athletic performance of subjects could not be directly related to the quantity of protein consumed above that determined to be the requirement for those subjects. When subjects were fed less than their respective protein requirements, their muscular efficiencies were reduced unless a vigorous training program was included as part of the experiment's protocol. Since most of the studies were of short duration and since muscle protein has a relatively long half-life, the lack of any demonstrable effect of protein intake on muscle performance (aside from the energy/protein relationship) is not surprising.

Other factors such as *sex*, *pregnancy*, *lactation*, and *trauma* affecting the protein requirement have been studied. As can be anticipated, males, due to their greater physical activity and larger body size have a larger protein requirement than females; pregnancy, lactation, and trauma all increase the protein requirement.

E. RECOMMENDED DAILY INTAKES (RDA)

The minimum daily requirement, that is the minimum amount of dietary protein which will provide the needed amounts of amino acids to optimally maintain the body, is impossible to determine for each individual without expending a good deal of time and effort for each person. With a U.S. population of over 230 million, the task would be monumental. To eliminate the necessity of determining individual nutrient requirements, a system called the recommended daily allowance (RDA) has been devised. As research accumulates for each of the many essential nutrients, its associated RDA is revised. How is the RDA established? Ideally, sufficient research is conducted to show (1) that a given nutrient is needed by the human, (2) that certain deficiency signs can be produced, (3) that these signs can be avoided or reversed if the missing nutrient is administered, and (4) that no further improvement is observed if the nutrient is administered at levels above that which reversed the deficiency symptoms. Next, studies are conducted on a variety of subjects to determine their minimal need. Since humans vary so much, it is not possible to measure the requirements over a broad range of human variability. To allow for this variability, a safety factor is added on to the determined minimum needs of the group of subjects studied. As more subjects are studied and more data accumulated, the added safety factor becomes smaller.

In the case of protein and amino acid requirements, the RDA was set at twice the minimum value of the subject who required the most protein and/or amino acid in all the studies conducted. By greatly increasing the recommended intake figure over that experimentally determined, it was hoped that the protein and amino acid needs of the majority or 95% of the U.S. population would be met. The RDA for protein was originally quite high. For many years, it was set at 1 g/kg body weight for the average adult male. The average adult male was assumed to weigh 70 kg (about 155 pounds) so the RDA was 70 g/day. With an ever-increasing data base which the Nutrition Board of the National Research Council can use for its recommendations, the RDA for protein has been adjusted downward every 5 years. At present, 1993, the protein RDA for an adult male has been set at 56 g/day. This presumes that the dietary protein is coming from a mixed diet containing a reasonable amount of good-quality proteins. For persons subsisting on mixtures of poor-quality proteins, this RDA may not be adequate.

RDAs are set for all of the nutrients in the human diet for which there are adequate data on which to base a recommendation. Some of the newer micronutrients, while shown to be needed in test animals, have not yet been established as needed nutrients for humans. As the data base for these nutrients expands, RDAs will be forthcoming. RDAs are set not only for the individual nutrients but also for age groups within each nutrient. For some age groups the data base is very poor, e.g., preadolescents, toddlers, young children, and pregnant females; there is continual revision as data become available. Table 18 gives the current RDA for protein for different age groups.

IX.   PROTEIN DEFICIENCY

One of the most common nutritional disorders in the world today is the deficiency of protein. Both adults and children are affected as the populations in the less developed nations of the world exceed their food supply. Instances of deficiency in the U.S. have also been observed. Due to the ubiquitous nature of protein and its role in bodily function, protein deficiency is characterized by a number of symptoms. In many situations, not only is protein lacking in the diet but calories are also insufficient. For this reason, it is difficult to segregate symptoms due solely to protein deficiency from those due solely to energy deficit. In children, one may observe the different symptoms and visualize them all as parts of a continuum called protein-energy or protein-calorie malnutrition (PEM or PCM) rather than distinctly different nutritional disorders. Kwashiorkor, a disease first observed in Africa, at first was regarded as a dietary state where only protein was deficient, not energy. Marasmus, on the other hand, was regarded as a dietary state where both protein and energy are deficient. Today, as mild and moderate cases of these two diseases are treated, it has become apparent that the symptoms of one of them may intermingle with the other so that a clear-cut diagnosis is impossible. For every person with a severe case of either kwashiorkor or marasmus that is identified, treated, and cured, there are probably another 99 who are not diagnosed and treated and who will, if they survive, experience life-long effects of their early nutritional deprivation.

TABLE 18
Recommended Daily Allowances for Protein
(1993)

Age group		Recommended protein intake g/day
Infants to 6 months		kg × 2.2
Infants, 6 months to 1 year		kg × 2.0
Children	1 to 3	23
	4 to 6	30
	7 to 10	34
Males	11 to 14	45
	15 to 18	56
	19 to 22	56
	23 to 50	56
	51+	56
Females	11 to 14	46
	15 to 18	46
	19 to 22	44
	23 to 50	44
	51+	44
Pregnant		add 30
Lactating		add 20

A. KWASHIORKOR

Kwashiorkor usually affects the young child after he/she is weaned. The child is usually between 1 and 3 years old and is weaned because the mother has given birth to another child or is pregnant and cannot support both children. If the child has no teeth, he/she is given a thin gruel. This may be a fruit, vegetable, or cereal product mixed with water; it is not usually a good protein source. Cultural food practices or taboos may further limit the kinds and amounts of protein given to the child. Concurrent infections, parasites, seasonal food shortages, and poor distribution of food amongst the family members may also contribute to the development of kwashiorkor. The deficiency develops not only because of inadequate intake but also because at this age the growth demands for protein and energy are high.

Growth failure is the single most outstanding feature of protein malnutrition. The child's height and weight for his age will be less than that of his well-nourished peer. *Tissue wastage* is present but may not be apparent if edema is present. The *edema* begins with the feet and legs and gradually presents itself in the hands, face, and body. If edema is advanced, the child may not appear underweight but many appear "plump". This plumpness can be ascertained as edema by feel. If one were to press a thumb on the surface of the foot or ankle and then remove the thumb, the depression would remain for a short time. This is edema. The edema is thought to result from insufficient ADH production and insufficient serum and tissue proteins needed to maintain water balance. The protein deficient child is usually *apathetic*, has little interest in his/her surroundings, and is listless and dull. This child is usually "fussy" and irritable when moved. Mental retardation may or may not result. *Hair changes* are frequently observed. Texture, color, and strength are affected. Black, curly hair may become silkier, lusterless, and brown or reddish-brown in color. *Lesions of the skin* are not always present, but if present they give the appearance of old flaky paint. Depigmentation or darkly pigmented areas may develop with a tendency for these areas to appear in places of body friction such as the backs of legs, groins, and elbows. *Diarrhea* is almost always present. The diarrhea may be a result of the inability of the body to synthesize the needed digestive enzymes so that the food that is consumed can be utilized, and/or it may be the result of concurrent infections and parasites. In rats fed protein-free diets, significantly less intestinal enzyme activity has been measured. *Anemia* due to an inability to synthesize hemoglobin as well as red blood cells is invariably present. *Hepatomegaly* (enlarged liver) is usually observed.

In children consuming energy sufficient-protein insufficient diets, the enlarged liver is usually fatty because the child is unable to synthesize the proteins needed to make the transport proteins which, in turn, are needed to transport the lipids out of the liver. Studies with rats and chickens have shown that protein deficiency also results in decreases in a variety of hepatic enzymes, a decrease in hepatic RNA and DNA content, a reduction in spleen size, a decrease in antibody formation, a decrease in urea enzyme activity and urea production, and a decrease in the levels of plasma amino acids. All of the above symptoms can be related to the various functions of proteins as discussed in the earlier section.

B. MARASMUS

Although children of all ages and adults can suffer from a deficiency of both energy and protein, the marasmic child is usually less than one year old. In developing countries, a common cause for marasmus is a cessation of breast feeding. Milk production by the mother may have stopped because of the mother's poor health, or the mother may have died, or there may be a desire on the part of the mother to bottle feed her infant rather than breast feed. This decision to bottle feed may be made for a variety of reasons. The mother may view bottle feeding as a status symbol, or she may be forced to work to earn a living and may be unable to have her baby with her, or she may not be able to lactate. While under optimal conditions of economics and sanitation the bottle-fed child may be well fed, in emerging nations this is not always true. The mother may not be able to buy the milk formula in sufficient quantities to adequately nourish the child, she may overdilute the milk, or she may use unsafe water and unsanitary conditions to prepare the formula for the child. This, plus the insufficient nutrient content, often precipitously leads to the development of marasmus, a form of starvation characterized by *growth failure* with prominent ribs, a characteristic monkey-like face, and matchstick limbs with little muscle or adipose tissue development; *tissue wastage* but not edema is present. Whereas the kwashiorkor child has a poor appetite, the marasmus child is *eager to eat*. The child is *mentally alert* but not irritable. *Anemia* and *diarrhea* are present for the same reasons as in kwashiorkor. The skin and hair appear to be of normal color.

The treatment of both kwashiorkor and marasmic children must be approached with due care and caution. Because their enzymes for digestion and their protein absorption and transport systems are less active; feeding these children with large quantities of good-quality protein would be harmful. Their diets must be gradually enriched with these proteins to allow their bodies sufficient time to develop the appropriate metabolic pathways to handle a better diet. Giving these children solutions of either predigested proteins or solutions of amino acids may be of benefit initially, but these solutions, too, must be used with care. If the amino acids in excess of immediate use are deaminated and if the pathway for synthesizing urea is not fully functional, ammonia can accumulate in the child and become lethal. Schimke has shown that in the rat up to 3 days are needed to increase the activities of the urea cycle enzymes. The rat has a much faster metabolic rate than the human so one would anticipate that a much longer period of time would be necessary for a similar induction in humans.

Not only must one be concerned about the enzymes of the malnourished child, the protein-depleted child is also unable to synthesize adequate amounts of the protein hormones which regulate and coordinate his/her use of dietary nutrients. In addition, protein deprivation affects the structures of the cell hormone receptor sites thus further dampening the effectiveness of those hormones produced. Children with marasmus or kwashiorkor have been shown to have decreased blood sugar levels, decreased serum insulin and growth hormone levels and, in marasmus, decreased thyroid hormone levels. Additional hormonal changes have been observed, but their relevance to treatment has not been ascertained. Most probably, these changes in the levels of the protein, peptide, or amino acid derived hormones are reflective of reduced synthesis of them as a result of a shortage of incoming amino acids. Changes in the steroid hormones probably reflect the response of the child to the stress of deprivation.

X. INTEGRATION OF THE METABOLIC FEATURES OF PROTEIN NUTRITION

In the preceding section, protein malnutrition and protein-energy malnutrition or starvation has been characterized. Throughout this unit the chemical and biochemical nature of the proteins has been discussed in detail. The individual catabolic pathways for the amino acids have been given as well as the process by which new body proteins are synthesized. But how does the body "know" when to synthesize a new protein or degrade a resident one? What messages are sent and received that integrate these anabolic and catabolic processes? How does the body cope with its everchanging environment of which nutrition is but a part?

Recall that some of the amino acids that are contained by the dietary protein can be decarboxylated and converted to amines. These amines are potent neurotransmitters. That is, they are capable of eliciting system responses via activation of certain neurons or neuronal pathways. Some of these systemic responses include the release of hormones which have positive effects on protein synthesis. An example might be the signals to the pituitary to release growth hormone which, when bound to its cognate membrane receptor, elicits a cascade of intracellular signals which, in turn, migrate to the nucleus and serve as instigators of protein synthesis. Providing that sufficient ATP and amino acids are available, protein synthesis will be stimulated. Another example might be the chronic ingestion of a high-sugar diet that stimulates insulin release. The insulin plus the glucose plus several other factors instigate the synthesis of enzyme proteins needed to metabolize this sugar load. Initiation and cessation of feeding is an example of a system response to changing levels of the neurotransmitter, serotonin. Likely, other neurotransmitters are involved as well (see Unit 3 Section IV). Through the action of neurotransmitters, other systems can be activated or suppressed and these systems might include sleep or voluntary activity or other such whole-body actions. These responses will have effects on the need for energy, and because the energy need is tightly linked to the protein need, effects on the latter should be expected.

The dietary protein, once consumed, stimulates the release of a variety of gut hormones and these hormones likewise elicit systemic responses as outlined in Sections VI.A and VI.B of this unit. Further, once amino acids are liberated through the action of the digestive enzymes, these amino acids, as substrates for enterocyte carriers (see Section VI.B), stimulate not only the carrier activity (substrate activation) but also are involved in the synthesis of the carrier itself by the enterocyte. This is not an uncommon phenomenon. A number of high-turnover proteins, i.e., enzymes, carriers, and hormones, have their synthesis dictated by rising levels of the substrates upon which they act. Hence, rising levels of cytosolic citrate in the cell might be expected to instigate the transcription of the messenger RNA for ATP citrate lyase, the enzyme which catalyzes the formation of acetyl CoA and oxalacetate from citrate and CoA, with a concomitant hydrolysis of ATP to ADP and phosphate. So, too, might one expect to find in the enterocyte an increase in the mRNAs for those proteins which are responsible for the transport of the amino acids into the enterocyte via carrier-mediated mechanisms.

Thus, we see multiple roles for the amino acids found in the dietary proteins and these roles are not restricted to just the enterocyte. Other cells, tissues, and organs also are affected. The enzymes which are responsible for amino acid metabolism are likewise synthesized or degraded in response to the levels of those amino acids on which they work. The expression of the genes which encode these enzymes may be unique to a given cell type, tissue, or organ, or may be universal. Uniqueness of gene expression means that factors other than the substrate are operative in the regulation of that expression. For example, muscle cells cannot complete the oxidation of histidine. Histidine is liberated as muscle protein is degraded during muscle contraction and relaxation. Even though the muscle cell contains the same DNA as every other cell type, the expression of those genes responsible for the complete deamination and oxidation of histidine (see Figure 21) does not occur despite the rising levels of histidine. Instead, this histidine is methylated and excreted in the urine. In few other cell types does this methylation occur; histidine is usually metabolized as shown in Figure 21. However, expression of the gene for the enzyme responsible for histidine methylation is "turned on" by its substrate, histidine, and its affinity for this substrate as well as its activity as a catalyst exceeds that of any other enzyme in the muscle cell which might use histidine.

As the muscles are increased in activity and size, the amount of methylated histidine found in the urine also increases. Here, then, is a complete loop. The histidine in the food is transported to the muscle which uses it to synthesize myosin and actin, and when that muscle is actively working, myosin and actin are degraded with 3-methyl-histidine appearing in the urine. Histidine has acted as both a signal for the expression of genes coded for its transport, for its incorporation into muscle protein, and for its methylation and excretion. It has also served as a substrate for all of these processes plus those outlined in Figure 21.

Each of the amino acids as well as every other nutrient consumed as part of the diet likewise have multiple roles. Amino acids serve as signals in and of themselves of metabolic processes, or they can serve as substrates for the synthesis of proteins that act as carriers or receptors, enzymes, hormones, or structural materials.

The complexity of these interacting roles of amino acids as neurotransmitters, as enzyme activators, as inducers of gene expression, and as substrates for a multitude of synthetic and degradative reactions is enormous. Yet the brain and other vital organs signal each other such that integration of function occurs and a comprehensive metabolic pattern emerges. When without sufficient nutrient intake to sustain normal body function, the body has a hierarchy in place which controls amino acid use such that more important functions are maintained at the expense of less important ones. Hence, in the protein malnourished child, the symptoms of weight loss, skin lesions, and hair changes are observed while the activity of energy-producing processes are conserved. Protein synthesis is energetically very expensive as well as being dependent on amino acid availability. Thus, protein synthesis is also suppressed in a hierarchical manner. Skin cells and hair cells are not replaced, due to this decreased protein synthesis, as rapidly as in the well-nourished individual. Hence, the skin lesions and hair changes that typify protein malnutrition.

Energy conservation and protein conservation similarly are preserved. The synthesis and release of hormones which accelerate protein breakdown and use are suppressed via effects of diet deprivation on the brain; peptides which signal food-seeking behavior are maintained; gut motility is suppressed so as to retard the passage of food from mouth to anus and extract as much nourishment as possible from that food; body activity is reduced to reduce energy expenditure (the symptom of lethargy); sleep time is increased for the same reason. All of these defenses against death due to starvation are directed by the central nervous system and executed by the secretions of the endocrine organs. In turn, these defenses are activated when the body senses, via the gut cells, that insufficient food has been consumed.

Some of these defenses can be compromised by additional problems in the environment. If the drinking water is contaminated, the reduction in gut passage time as a defense is negated by pathogen-induced diarrhea. This results in a loss of gut contents and abrasion of the cells lining of the intestinal tract. In this instance, the person is less able to cope with an inadequate food supply. The coordination of the defense against death due to starvation is disrupted by the stress response (also coordinated by hormones) to the invading pathogens. Such stress elicits a signal from the pituitary which stimulates an outpouring of the catecholamines and steroidal hormones by the adrenals. These hormones mobilize muscle protein, body fat stores, and glycogen stores needed for the synthesis of antibodies to the pathogens as well as for the synthesis of replacement enterocytes and the conservation of electrolytes and water. Because such syntheses require energy, amino acids, and a number of micronutrients, all of which may be in short supply, one can now understand why malnourished individuals are more vulnerable to environmental contaminants and why the resultant disease is far more severe.

The interaction of disease and nutritional state can have lasting effects on body function. Hence, it is not uncommon to observe short stature in populations whose food supply is inadequate. Growth, a reflection of protein synthesis, which in turn is dependent on nutrient intake, is suppressed because growth is lower on the hierarchical scale of body functions that are preserved in times of need. When the food supply changes and becomes reliably abundant with a variety of foods, including sources of good-quality protein, then the genetic potential for body size is fully realized. The average height of the population increases from one generation to the next and the body fat stores are maintained at capacity. The latter feature may not be deemed to be desirable (see Unit 3, Section III).

SUPPLEMENTAL READINGS

ARTICLES

Aragon, J. and Sols, A. 1991. Regulation of enzyme activity in the cell: effect of enzyme concentration, *FASEB J.,* 5:2945–2950.

Bach, L. A. and Rechler, M. M. 1992. Insulin like growth factors and diabetes, *Diabetes Metab. Rev.,* 8:229–257.

Benevenga, N. J., Gahl, M. J., and Blemings, K. P. 1993. Role of protein synthesis in amino acid catabolism, *J. Nutr.,* 123:332–336.

Baumann, G. 1993. Growth hormone binding proteins, *Proc. Soc. Exp. Biol. Med.,* 202:392–400.

Clarke, S. D. and Abraham, S. 1992. Gene expression: nutrient control of pre and posttranscriptional events, *FASEB J.,* 6:3146–3152.

Freedman, L. P. and Luisi, B. F. 1993. One of the mechanisms of DNA binding by nuclear hormone receptors: a structural and functional perspective, *J. Cell. Biochem.,* 51:140–150.

Gietzen, D. W. 1993. Neural mechanisms in the responses to amino acid deficiency, *J. Nutr.,* 123:610–625.

Glenney, J. R. 1992. Tyrosine-phosphorylated proteins: mediators of signal transduction from tyrosine kinases, *Biochem. Biophys. Acta,* 1134:113–127.

Greenberg, C. S., Birckbichler, P. J., and Rice, R. H. 1991. Transglutaminases: multifunctional cross-linking enzymes that stabilize tissues, *FASEB J.,* 5:3071–3077.

Harper, A. E. and Yoshimura, N. N. 1993. Protein quality, amino acid balance, utilization and evaluation of diets containing amino acids as therapeutic agents, *Nutrition,* 9:460–469.

Hartree, A. S. and Renwick, A. G. 1992. Molecular structures of glycoprotein hormones and functions of their carbohydrate components, *Biochem. J.,* 287:665–679.

Kilberg, M. S., Stevens, B. R., and Novak, D. A. 1993. Recent advances in mammalian amino acid transport, *Ann. Rev. Nutr.,* 13:137–166.

Kollmar, R. and Farnham, P. J. 1993. Site specific utilization of transcription by RNA poymerase II, *P.S.E.B.M.,* 203:127–139.

Lea, M. A. 1993. Regulation of gene expression in hepatomas, *Int. J. Biochem.,* 25:457–469.

Lobley, G. E. 1993. Species comparisons of tissue protein metabolism: effects of age and hormonal action, *J. Nutr.,* 123:337–343.

Maltese, W. A. 1990. Post translational modifications of proteins by isoprenoids in mammalian cells, *FASEB J.,* 4:3319–3328.

Muller, H. and Scott, R. 1992. Hereditary conditions in which the loss of heterozygosity may be important, *Mutation Res.,* 284:15–24.

Olson, E. N. 1988. Modification of proteins with covalent lipids, *Prog. Lipid Res.,* 27:177–197.

Putney, J. W. and Bird, G. 1993. The inositol phosphate-calcium signaling system in non excitable cells, *Endocrine Rev.,* 14:610–631.

Rapoport, T. A. 1991. Protein transport across the endoplasmsic reticulum membrane: facts, models, mysteries, *FASEB J.,* 5:2792–2798.

Reichel, R. R. and Jacob, S. T. 1993. Control of gene expression by lipophilic hormones, *FASEB J.,* 7:427–436.

Van der Rest, M., and Garrone, R. 1991. Collagen family of proteins, *FASEB J.,* 5:2814–2823.

Vedeckis, W. Y. 1992. Nuclear receptors, transcriptional regulation and oncogenesis, *Proc. Soc. Exp. Biol. Med.,* 199:1–12.

Wolfe, R. R., Jahoor, F., and Hartl, W. H. 1989. Protein and amino acid metabolism after injury, *Diabetes Metab. Rev.,* 5:149–164.

Young, V. R. and Marchini, J. S. 1990. Mechanisms and nutritional significance of metabolic responses to altered intakes of protein and amino acids with reference to nutritional adaptation in humans, *Am. J. Clin. Nutr.,* 51:270–289.

BOOKS

Berdanier, C. D. and Hargrove, J. L., Eds. 1993. *Nutrition and Gene Expression*, CRC Press, Boca Raton, FL, 579 pages.

CARBOHYDRATES

TABLE OF CONTENTS

I. INTRODUCTION

The carbohydrates provide as much as 60% of the daily energy intake. The percentage of the diet that is carbohydrate varies inversely with economic conditions and with the percentage of the diet that is fat and protein. As a general rule, the carbohydrate-rich foods are less expensive than the fat- and protein-rich foods. Hence, as people have more disposable income they tend to buy and consume fewer cereals, breads, fruits, and vegetables and buy more meat, butter (or margarine), milk, and eggs. This is not always true, however. Over the last decade, education about the possible health risks of high intakes of fatty foods and the health benefits of high-fiber intakes, as well as the benefits of consuming fruits and vegetables, has altered the eating habits of many consumers. This, in turn, has had an impact on the percent of the energy intake provided by the carbohydrates.

The term carbohydrate originated in the late 1800s from the idea that there existed naturally occurring compounds composed of carbon, hydrogen, and oxygen which could be represented as hydrates of carbon. For instance, glucose ($C_6H_{12}O_6$), sucrose ($C_{12}H_{22}O_{11}$), and starch ($C_6H_{10}O_5$)$_n$ could all be represented by the general formula $C_x(H_2O)_y$. This definition proved to be too rigid because it excluded such common carbohydrate compounds as deoxyribose ($C_5H_{10}O_4$) and ascorbic acid ($C_6H_8O_6$) but included the compound acetic acid ($C_2H_4O_2$), which is not a carbohydrate. A more comprehensive definition evolved: carbohydrates are polyhydroxy aldehydes or ketones and their derivatives.

II. CLASSIFICATION

The carbohydrates are divided into three major classes: monosaccharides, oligosaccharides, and polysaccharides. A monosaccharide consists of a single polyhydroxy aldehyde or ketone unit. An oligosaccharide contains two to ten monosaccharide units. Disaccharides, composed of two monosaccharides, are the most prevalent oligosaccharides. A polysaccharide is composed of very long chains of monosaccharides.

III. STRUCTURE AND NOMENCLATURE

A. MONOSACCHARIDES

Monosaccharides, called simple sugars, have the empirical formula (CH_2O)$_n$, where n is 3 or more. Although monosaccharides may have as few as three or as many as nine carbon atoms, the ones of interest to the nutritionist have five or six. The carbon skeleton is unbranched and each carbon atom, except one, has a hydroxyl group and a hydrogen atom. At the remaining carbon atom there is a carbonyl group. If the carbonyl function is on the last carbon atom, the compound is an aldehyde and is called an *aldose*; if it occurs at any other carbon, the compound is a ketone and is called a *ketose*. These structures are illustrated in Figure 1.

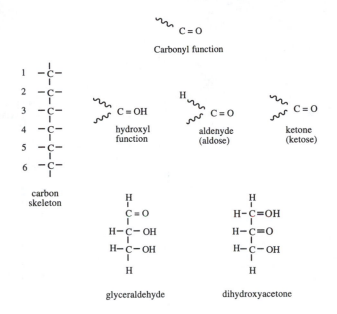

FIGURE 1.   Structures of monosaccharides.

The simplest monosaccharide is the three-carbon aldehyde or ketone, *triose*. Glyceraldehyde is an aldotriose; dihydroxyacetone is a ketotriose. Successive chain elongation of trioses yields *tetroses*, *pentoses*, *hexoses*, *heptoses*, and *octoses*. In the aldo-series these are called: aldotriose, aldotetrose, aldopentose, aldohexose, etc.; in the keto-series, ketotriose, ketotetrose, ketopentose, ketohexose, etc. Figure 2 shows the D-aldose monosaccharides which have three to six carbons.

Figure 3 illustrates the corresponding D-ketoses. Within a given series of the same number of carbon atoms, these molecules differ only in the arrangement of the hydrogen atom and the hydroxyl group about the carbon atoms. Compare, for example, glucose and mannose: the configuration of the hydrogen and hydroxyl group about each of the carbons is the same except for the second carbon down from the top. In glucose, the hydroxyl function is to the right; in mannose it is to the left. Two sugars which differ only in the configuration about one carbon atom are referred to as epimers. D-glucose and D-mannose are epimers with respect to the number two carbon atom; D-mannose and D-tallose are epimers with respect to the number four carbon atoms.

Configuration and conformation are two terms that are used frequently and are easily confused. Configuration is the arrangement in space of atoms or groups of atoms of a molecule that can be changed only by breaking and making bonds. Conformation is the arrangement in space of atoms or groups of atoms of a molecule that can arise by rotation about a single bond and that is capable of a finite existence. Picture a one-legged pirate; his configuration is fixed:

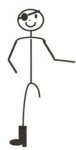

configuration of a one-legged pirate

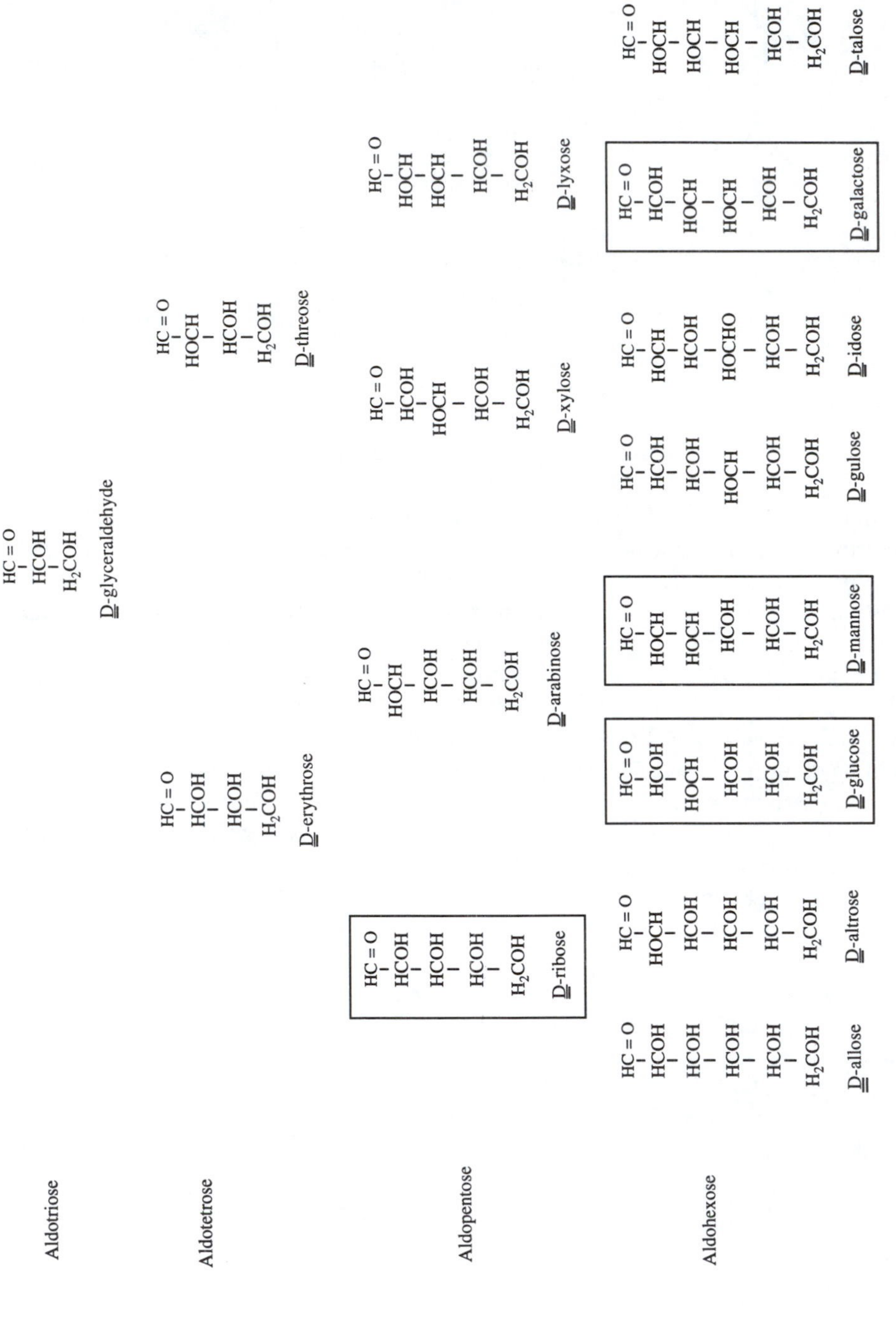

Aldotriose

Aldotetrose

Aldopentose

Aldohexose

HC=O
HCOH
H₂COH
D-glyceraldehyde

HC=O
HCOH
HCOH
H₂COH
D-erythrose

HC=O
HOCH
HCOH
H₂COH
D-threose

HC=O
HCOH
HCOH
HCOH
H₂COH
D-ribose

HC=O
HOCH
HCOH
HCOH
H₂COH
D-arabinose

HC=O
HCOH
HOCH
HCOH
H₂COH
D-xylose

HC=O
HOCH
HOCH
HCOH
H₂COH
D-lyxose

HC=O
HCOH
HCOH
HCOH
HCOH
H₂COH
D-allose

HC=O
HOCH
HCOH
HCOH
HCOH
H₂COH
D-altrose

HC=O
HCOH
HOCH
HCOH
HCOH
H₂COH
D-glucose

HC=O
HOCH
HOCH
HCOH
HCOH
H₂COH
D-mannose

HC=O
HCOH
HCOH
HOCH
HCOH
H₂COH
D-gulose

HC=O
HOCH
HCOH
HOCHO
HCOH
H₂COH
D-idose

HC=O
HCOH
HOCH
HOCH
HCOH
H₂COH
D-galactose

HC=O
HOCH
HOCH
HOCH
HCOH
H₂COH
D-talose

FIGURE 2. D-Aldoses having from three to six carbon atoms. Those of the greatest biological significance are enclosed in boxes.

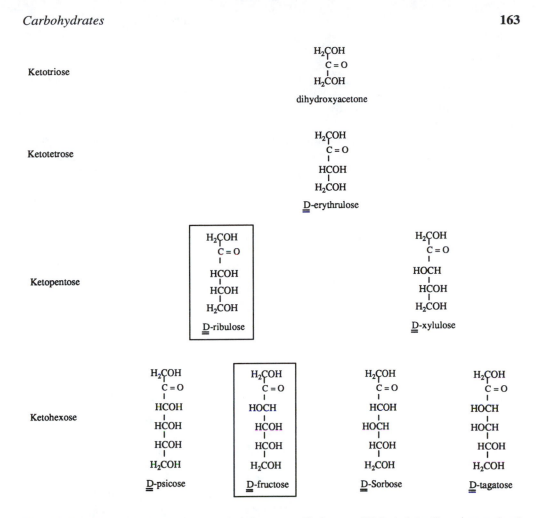

FIGURE 3. D-Ketoses having from three to six carbon atoms. The ketoses of biological significance are enclosed in boxes. Ketoses are sometimes named by inserting a "-ul" into the name of the corresponding aldose. D-Ribulose is the ketopentose corresponding to aldopentose D-ribose.

However, his conformation can change—he can stand, sit or lie:

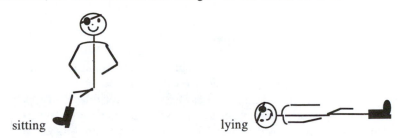

sitting   lying

Hexoses are white crystalline compounds, freely soluble in water but insoluble in such nonpolar solvents as benzene and hexane. Most of them have a sweet taste and are by far the most abundant of the monosaccharides. Of these, glucose, fructose, and galactose are most often found in foods, frequently as compounds of disaccharides or polysaccharides. Mannose is occasionally found, but only in complexes that are poorly digested. Aldopentoses are important components of nucleic acid (see Section VI); derivatives of triose and heptose are intermediates in carbohydrate metabolism.

1. Stereoisomeric Forms

All of the monosaccharides (except for dihydroxyacetone) contain at least one asymmetric carbon atom. An asymmetric carbon atom, in the simplest sense, is one to which four different constituents are attached. Molecules which possess an asymmetric center can exist in *stereoisomeric* forms.

Stereoisomers have the same structural framework but differ in the spatial arrangement of the various substituent groups. Stereoisomers include *cis* and *trans* forms, chair and boat forms, and epimers. They are to be distinguished from *structural isomers*. Structural isomers have different structural frameworks; the bonding arrangements for the component atoms are different. C_4H_8 is the molecular formula for the four structural isomers which follow:

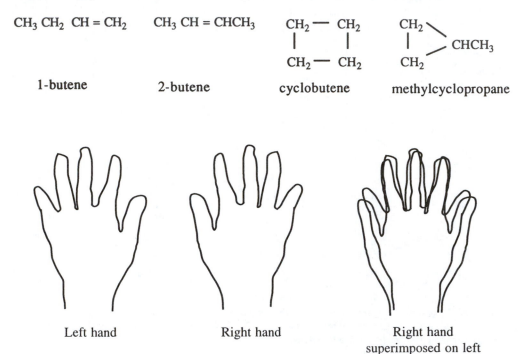

$CH_3\ CH_2\ CH = CH_2$ $CH_3\ CH = CHCH_3$

1-butene   2-butene   cyclobutene   methylcyclopropane

Left hand   Right hand   Right hand
                                                                                        superimposed on left

For example, glyceraldehyde may occur in either the D or the L stereoisomer. D and L stereoisomers bear the same relationship to each other as one's right and left hands: if both hands are laid flat on a table and the right hand slid onto the top of the left hand, the right hand does not cover the left (note that thumbs stick out in opposite directions). When the chemical structure for each of these molecules is written as projection formulas, their differences are obvious: the hydroxyl group and the hydrogen atom on the asymmetric carbon reverse positions; these two compounds are mirror images of each other. Mirror image forms of the same compound are called enantiomers. Pairs of enantiomers (the D and L stereoisomers of a molecule) possess the same chemical and physical properties except for rotating plane-polarized light in opposite but equal directions; i.e., the values of their specific rotations have opposite signs. A note of caution, however, a D or an L used in the name of a sugar molecule does not refer to the sign of its optical rotation; these letters specify the absolute configuration of the molecule. If one desires to include the sign of optical rotation in the molecular name, a (+) for dextrorotary, rotation to the right, or (–) for levorotary, rotation to the left, is used. For example, the specific rotation of the D-glyceraldehyde is 14°; hence, its name is D-(+)-glyceraldehyde; D-lactic acid has a specific rotation of –3.8°, and is called D-(–)-lactic acid.

By convention, a carbohydrate belongs to the D series if, when it is written in the projection formula with the aldehyde or hydroxyketone group at the top, the hydroxyl group on the next to the last carbon is to the right; conversely, if the molecule is written exactly as just described except for the fact that the hydroxyl group on the next to the last carbon is written to the left, it belongs to the L series. A molecule which possesses n asymmetric carbons has 2^n as the upper limit of the number of stereoisomers. The aldohexose series has 4 asymmetric carbon atoms; thus, it has 16 stereoisomers or 8 pairs of enantiomers. One of these pairs is α-D-glucose, and α-L-glucose.

In nature, D monosaccharides are much more abundant than L. Most mammalian cells require D sugar because they are unable to metabolize the L form. However, a few L monosaccharides can be found; among the most important are L-rhamnose and L-sorbose. Glucose is often called dextrose because the stereoisomer almost always found in nature rotates plane-polarized light to the right; it is dextrorotary. Similarly, fructose is often called levulose because its most common natural form is levorotary.

2. Anomeric Forms

In the section above on stereoisomeric forms, glucose was referred to as α-D-glucose instead of D-glucose as was done in Figure 2. The presence of the Greek letter alpha (α) adds another dimension to the structure of carbohydrates. This feature can be more readily understood if first there is a review of specific reactions that aldehydes and ketones undergo.

Aldehydes and ketones can add hydroxyl groups at the carbonyl function. If water is added, the unstable hydrate of the aldehyde is formed. If alcohol is added to the hydrate a *hemiacetal* is formed. If alcohol is added to the hemiacetal, a full *acetal* (or simple acetal) is formed by the elimination of water.

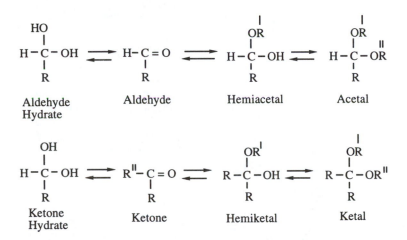

Ketones undergo similar reactions but form hemiketals or ketals; however, the hemiketal or ketal is frequently referred to as the hemiacetal or acetal. The hemiacetal, having four different constituents, is an asymmetric carbon atom; it exists in one of two stereoisomeric forms.

In the case of carbohydrates, the same hemiacetal formation can occur, but it will be an intramolecular reaction and a ring is produced. A six-membered ring, containing five carbon atoms and one oxygen atom is called a pyranose (after pyran). A five-membered ring, containing four carbons and one oxygen, is called a furanose (after furan). Figure 4 illustrates these two structures. As with aldehydes, this additional reaction in a carbohydrate produces an asymmetric carbon atom; it is referred to as the anomeric carbon. One now has two monosaccharides that differ only in their configuration about the anomeric carbon; they are called anomers and are referred to as α and β forms. In the α form the hydroxyl group is below the plane of the ring to which it is attached. In the β form it is above. This ring closure is illustrated for D-glucose and D-fructose in Figure 5.

The monosaccharides in the body undergo a number of reactions which will be detailed in Section VI. These reactions produce five general groups of products as shown in Table 1.

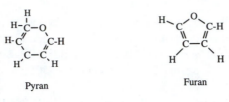

FIGURE 4. Structural representations of a pyran and furan ring.

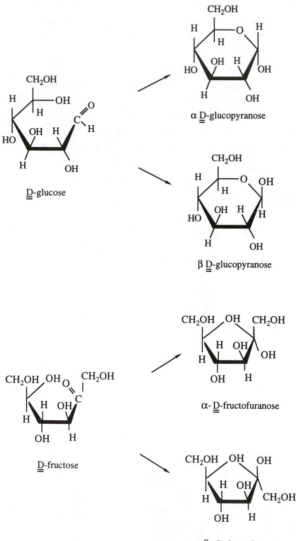

FIGURE 5. Ring closure of D-glucose and D-fructose to make the pyranose and furanose forms.

B. OLIGOSACCHARIDES

Oligosaccharides consist of two to ten monosaccharides joined with a glycosidic bond. The bond is formed between the anomeric carbon of one sugar and any hydroxyl function of another sugar. If two monosaccharides are bonded in this manner, the resulting molecule is a disaccharide; if three, a trisaccharide; if four, a tetrasaccharide, etc.

TABLE 1

Product	Example
Phosphoric acid esters	Glucose-6-phosphate
Polyhydroxy alcohols	Sorbitol
Deoxy sugars	Deoxyribose
Sugar acids	Gluconic acid
Amino sugars	Glucosamine

1. Disaccharides

Of the oligosaccharides, by far the most prevalent in nature are the disaccharides. Of dietary significance are the disaccharides lactose, maltose, and sucrose.

Lactose, the sugar found in the milk of most mammals (it is lacking in the milk of the whale and the hippopotamus), consists of a D-galactose and D-glucose joined with a glycosidic linkage at carbon one of galactose and carbon four of glucose. The glucose residue of lactose possesses a free anomeric carbon; the α form is the most predominant. Lactose is a reducing sugar. The glycosidic linkage between galactose and glucose is symbolized by α (1→4).

An important characteristic of lactose is its ability to promote in the intestinal tract the growth of certain beneficial lactic acid-producing bacteria. These bacteria have a possible role in the displacement of undesirable putrefactive forms of bacteria. Lactose also appears to enhance the absorption of calcium.

Maltose, also known as malt sugar, contains two glucose residues. The glycosidic linkage is α (1→4).

Celiobiose, the repeating disaccharide unit of cellulose, and gentiobiose are two other disaccharides that have as their repeating units D-glucose. In celiobiose the glycosidic linkage is β (1→4); in gentiobiose it is β (1→6). Since all have free anomeric carbons, they are reducing sugars.

Sucrose, also known as table sugar, cane sugar, beet sugar, and grape sugar, is a disaccharide of glucose and fructose linked through the anomeric carbon of each monosaccharide. Because neither anomeric carbon is free, sucrose is a nonreducing sugar. It is not a hemiacetal and does not undergo mutarotation. In dilute acid or in the presence of the enzyme invertase, sucrose hydrolyzes into its constituent monosaccharides. The hydrolysis of sucrose ($[a]_D^{20} = -65.5°$) to D-glucose ($[a]_D^{20} = +52.5°$) and D-fructose ($[a]_D^{20} = -92°$) is called inversion because it is accomplished by a change in the sign of specific rotation from dextro (+) to levo (−) as the equimolar mixture of glucose and fructose is formed; this mixture is called *invert sugar*. Invert syrups, which are available commercially at varied levels of inversion, are sweeter than sucrose at comparable concentrations. This greater sweetness reflects the D-fructose component which is sweeter than either sucrose or glucose.

When sucrose is used in the preparation of acidic foods, some inversion invariably takes place. For instance, if it is used to sweeten fruit drinks, it is completely inverted within a few hours. In soft drinks there is also a considerable amount of inversion. Honey, in large part, is invert sugar. The bees primarily collect sucrose from flowers. Enzymes invert sucrose in their bodies. Honey, however, is not pure glucose and fructose; its other major constituents are sucrose, water, and small quantities of flavor extract peculiar to the flower from which it is obtained. The development of an enzyme which will isomerize D-glucose to D-fructose has proved to be commercially valuable. It provides a method of obtaining a product known as high-fructose corn syrup.

In general, the disaccharides, while of importance as dietary sources of carbohydrates, have few metabolic functions. They are hydrolyzed into their component monosaccharides in the enterocyte and converted to glucose, which is the body's primary metabolic fuel.

A few oligosaccharides with more than two monosaccharide moieties are of nutritional significance. Stachyose, a tetrasaccharide composed of two molecules of D-galactose, one of D-glucose, and one of D-fructose is found in certain foods, particularly those of legume origin. It is usually found with raffinose (fructose, glucose, and galactose) and sucrose. The human digestive tract does not possess an enzyme which can hydrolyze stachyose or raffinose. Evidently, however, these sugars are fermented in the lower intestinal tract by the intestinal flora. This further metabolism is thought to be responsible for the unwanted flatus (gas produced and released by the intestinal tract) that frequently follows the ingestion of legumes.

2. Polysaccharides

Polysaccharides (also known as glycans) are compounds consisting of large numbers of monosaccharides linked by glycosidic bonds; they are analogous in structure to oligosaccharides. Some possess low molecular weights, corresponding to 30 to 90 monosaccharides. However, most of the carbohydrates found in nature which exist as polysaccharides have a high molecular weight; they may contain several hundred or even thousands of monosaccharide units. Polysaccharides differ from one another in the nature of their repeating monosaccharide units, in the number of such units in their chain, and in the degree of branching.

The polysaccharides which contain only a single kind of monosaccharide or monosaccharide derivative are called *homopolysaccharides*; those which have two or more different monomeric units are called *heteropolysaccharides*. Often homopolysaccharides are given names which indicate the nature of the building blocks: for example, those which contain mannose units are mannans; those which contain fructose units are called fructans. The important biological polysaccharides are the *storage polysaccharides*, the *structural polysaccharides*, and the *mucopolysaccharides*.

a. Storage Polysaccharides

Among plants the most abundant storage polysaccharide is starch. It is deposited abundantly in grains, fruits, and tubers in the form of large granules in the cytoplasm of cells; each plant deposits a starch characteristic of its species. Starch exists in two forms: α-amylose and amylopectin. α-Amylose makes up 20 to 30% of most starches and consists of 250 to 300 unbranched glucose residues bonded in α (1→4) linkages. The chains vary in molecular weight from a few thousand to 500,000. The molecule is twisted into a helical coil. Amylopectin, which comprises the remainder of the starch in a plant, is highly branched. Its backbone consists of glucose residues with α (1→4) glycosidic linkages; its branch points are α (1→6) glycosidic bonds. Although the structure of amylopectin is shown in Figure 6 as being linear it, too, exists as a helical coil.

When amylose is broken down in successive stages by either the enzyme amylase or by the action of dry heat, as in toasting, the resulting polysaccharides of intermediate chain length are called *dextrin*. Amylopectin, when broken down by the same methods, does not cleave at its branch points. This end product is a highly branched product called *limit dextrin*.

Other homopolysaccharides are found in plants, bacteria, yeast and mold as storage polysaccharides. Dextrans, found in yeast and bacteria, are branched polysaccharides of D-glucose with their major backbone linkage α (1→6). Inulin, found in artichokes, consists of D-fructose monomers with β (2→1) glycosidic linkages. Mannans are composed of mannose residues and are found in bacteria, yeasts, mold, and higher plants.

Among animals, the storage polysaccharide is glycogen. Glycogen is stored primarily in the liver and muscles. Like amylopectin, glycogen is a branched polysaccharide of D-glucose with a backbone glycosidic linkage of α (1→4) and branch points of α (1→6). However, its branches occur every 8 to 10 residues, as compared to every 12 for amylopectin. For muscle glycogen, the molecular weight has been estimated to be about 10^6; for liver, 5×10^6 (corresponding to about 30,000 glucose residues). Glycogen is of no importance as a dietary

The helical coil of amylose.

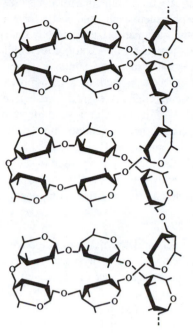

An α (1→6) branch point in amylopectin

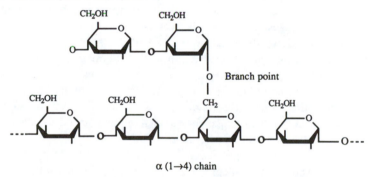

α (1→4) chain

FIGURE 6.   Structures of storage polysaccharides.

source of carbohydrate. The small amount of glycogen in an animal's body when it is slaughtered is quickly degraded during the post-mortem period.

b.   *Structural Polysaccharides*

Cellulose is the most abundant structural polysaccharide in the plant world; 50% of the carbon in vegetables is cellulose; wood is about one half cellulose and cotton is nearly pure cellulose. It is a straight chain polymer of D-glucose with β (1→4) glycosidic linkages between the monosaccharides. Cellobiose, a disaccharide, is obtained on partial hydrolysis of cellulose. The molecular weight of cellulose has been estimated to range from 50,000 to 500,000 (equivalent to 300 to 3000 glucose residues). Cellulose molecules are organized in bundles of parallel chains, called fibrils, which are cross linked by hydrogen bonding; these chains of glucose units are relatively rigid and are cemented together with hemicelluloses, pectin, and lignin.

Hemicellulose bears no structural relation to cellulose. It is composed of polymers of D-xylose with β (1→4) glycosidic linkages and side chains of arabinose and other sugars.

Pectin is a polymer of methyl D-galacturonate. Pectin is found in fruit and is the substance needed to make jelly out of cooked fruit. The juice plus sucrose plus the pectin form a gel that is stable for many months at room temperature. Pectin is a nonabsorbable carbohydrate that has pharmacological use as well. It is a key component together with kaolin of an antidiarrheal remedy.

There are other structural polysaccharides found in nature. Chitin is a polysaccharide which forms the hard skeleton of insects and crustaceans and is a homopolymer of *N*-acetyl-D-glucosamine. Agar, derived from sea algae, contains D- and L-galactose residues, some esterified with sulfuric acid, primarily with 1→3 bonds; alginic acid, derived from algae and kelp, contains monomers of D-mannuronic acid; and vegetable gum (gum arabic) contains D-galactose, D-glucuronic acid, rhamnose, and arabinose. These are used as food stabilizers by the food processing industry. Algin derivatives, for example, are used to stabilize the emulsions made in salad dressings; gum arabic is frequently used to stabilize processed cheese products, where it acts to retard the separation of the solids from the fluid component in such products.

3. Mucopolysaccharides

The mucopolysaccharides are heteropolysaccharides which are components of the structural polysaccharides found at various places in the body. Mucopolysaccharides consist of disaccharide units in which glucuronic acid is bound to acetylated or sulfurated amino sugars with glycosidic β (1→3) linkages. Each disaccharide unit is bound to the next by a β (1→4) glycosidic linkage. Thus, they are linear polymers with alternating β (1→3) and β (1→4) linkages.

Hyaluronic acid is the most abundant mucopolysaccharide. It is the principal component of the ground substance of connective tissue and is also abundant in the synovial fluid in joints and the vitreous humor of the eye. The repeating unit of hyaluronic acid is a disaccharide composed of D-glucuronic acid and *N*-acetyl-D-glucosamine; it has alternating β (1→3) and β (1→4) glycosidic linkages. The molecular weight is several million.

Another mucopolysaccharide which forms part of the structure of connective tissue is chondroitin. It differs from hyaluronic acid only in that it contains *N*-acetyl-D-galactosamine residues rather than *N*-acetyl-D-glucosamine ones. The sulfate ester derivatives of chondroitin, chondroitin sulfate A and chondroitin sulfate C, are major structural components of cartilage, bone, cornea, and other connective tissue. Types A and C have the same structure as chondroitin except for a sulfate ester at carbon atom 4 of the *N*-acetyl-D-galactosamine residue on type A and one at carbon atom 6 of type C.

Heparin (β-heparin) is a mucopolysaccharide which is similar in structure to hyaluronic acid for it contains residues of D-glucuronic acid. However, in heparin these residues contain varying portions of both sulfate and acetyl groups. Its structure is not entirely known. It is a blood anticoagulant.

IV.   SOURCES OF CARBOHYDRATE

Carbohydrates are constituents of all living cells. As such, one could anticipate finding one or more carbohydrates in almost all foods of importance to humans. Practically speaking, however, foods from animal sources contain few carbohydrates. Milk, with its high lactose content, is the only animal source of any significance. Cow's milk contains 4.8% lactose; human milk, 7%. Eggs, scallops, and oysters contain small amounts of carbohydrate. The percentage of carbohydrate in several common foods can be seen in Table 2.

Foods from plant sources, on the other hand, contain large amounts of carbohydrates. Oranges, bananas, and apples are good sources of fructose. Potatoes and cereal grains are good sources of starch.

The sugar content of several fresh fruits and vegetables is given in Table 3. The starch content is not shown. Canned and frozen fruits contain additional sugar which is added as part of the syrup needed to preserve the structure of the fruit. This syrup may be either a sucrose syrup or a high-fructose syrup made using an enzymatic process that starts with cornstarch.

TABLE 2
Percent Carbohydrates in Common Foods

Food	% CHO
Fruits and vegetables	5 to 20%
Milk	5%
Shellfish	<1%
Fish	<1%
Lean pork	<1%
Ice cream, cake, pie	40 to 50%
Lunch meat	<5%
Cheese, roast beef	<1%
Peanut butter, bacon	<10%
Nuts	<10%
Butter, margarine	0%
Salad oil	0%
Sugar	100%

TABLE 3
Free Sugar Content (g/100 g Fresh Weight) in Fruits and Vegetables

Item	Glucose	Fructose	Sucrose	Maltose	Raffinose	Stachyose
Apple	1.17	6.04	3.78	Trace		
Beans, lima	0.04	0.08	2.59		0.20	0.59
Beans, pole snap	0.48	1.30	0.28		0.26	
Broccoli	0.73	0.67	4.24			
Peach	0.91	1.18	6.92	0.12		
Strawberry	2.09	2.40	1.03	0.07		

Adapted from R.S. Shallenberger, in *Sugars in Nutrition,* H. L. Stipple and K. W. McNutt, Eds., Academic Press, New York, 1974, 112–126.

This syrup varies in its fructose and glucose content and is used because of its intense sweetness and low cost. Thus, canned and frozen fruits may have more sugar in them than when eaten fresh and unprocessed. These high-fructose corn syrup solutions of glucose or glucose and fruit are also used in soft drinks to add body without affecting or masking flavors. Canners and preservers like to use these syrups because they penetrate the fruit easily and preserve its natural form, flavor, and color.

In addition to the sugars and starches, plants contain cellulose, hemicellulose, pectin, and lignin. These carbohydrates provide the fiber or indigestible residue. The exact amount of fiber which a food can provide is the subject of some dispute. In the past, chemical analyses of foods have given their crude fiber content. Crude fiber is the residue of plant food left after extraction by dilute acid and alkali. The data in Table 4 are the amounts of crude fiber in many common foods. However, the term crude fiber does not include all the undigested material which may prove to have nutritional value to man. While cellulose, plant fibers, and other so-called nondigestible carbohydrates are not digestible by the enzymes located in the upper portion of the intestine, the intestine contains flora which can partially degrade some of these food components. This degradation provides fatty acids and other useful compounds which are then absorbed by the lower small intestine and colon. Dietary fiber is thus the residue of foods from plants that is resistant to hydrolysis and human bacterial digestive enzymes.

Data on the dietary fiber content of foods are needed; the values for dietary fiber are not identical to those for crude fiber. Several methods of analysis for dietary fiber are being

TABLE 4
Fiber Content in Common
Foods

Item	Fiber (g/100 g)
Almonds	2.6
Apples	0.9
Beans, lima	1.8
Beans, string	1.0
Broccoli	1.5
Carrots	1.0
Flour, whole wheat	2.3
Flour, white wheat	0.3
Noodles, dry	0.4
Oat flakes	1.4
Pears	1.5
Pecans	2.3
Popcorn	2.2
Strawberries	1.3
Walnuts	2.1
Wheat germ	2.5

Adapted from Tables of Food Composition, *Scientific Tables,* K. Diem and C. Letner, Eds., 7th ed., CIBA-Geigy, Ardsley, New York, 1974.

investigated. One method obtains a value of the fiber content of food by difference. The amount of fiber is estimated to be that part of the food left in the fat-free, alcohol-insoluble residue after subtraction of available carbohydrate and protein. Southgate has developed a detailed and time-consuming method for the determination of cellulose, hemicellulose, and lignin in foods consumed by humans. Van Soest and Goering have developed a simpler method, but their method was originally designed for animal feeds. Table 5 lists values of fiber in foods obtained by these different methods. They indicate that only one fifth to one half of the total dietary fiber is crude fiber.

Fruits and vegetables have higher values of the total dietary fiber determined as crude fiber than do cereals and legumes.

V. DIGESTION AND ABSORPTION

Once a carbohydrate-rich food is consumed, digestion begins. As the food is chewed it is mixed with saliva which contains α-amylase. This amylase begins the digestion of starch by attacking the internal α-1,4-glucosidic bonds. It will not attack the branch points having α-1,4- or α-1,6-glucosidic bonds, hence the salivary α-amylase will produce molecules of glucose, maltose, α-limit dextrin, and maltotriose. The α-amylase in saliva has an isozyme with the same function in the pancreatic juice. The salivary α-amylase is denatured in the stomach as the food is mixed and acidified with the gastric hydrochloric acid.

As the stomach content moves into the duodenum, it is called chyle. The movement of chyle into the duodenum stimulates pancreazymin release. This gut hormone acts on the exocrine pancreas stimulating it to release pancreatic juice into the duodenum. Pancreazymin has another name, cholecystokinin. The two names were given before it was realized that the two different functions, the stimulation of the release of pancreatic juice from the exocrine pancreas and bile from the gall bladder, were performed by the same hormone. This hormone is secreted by the epithelial endocrine cells of the small intestine, particularly the duodenum.

TABLE 5

Extraction Method Effects on the Fiber Content of Food (g/100 gm)

| Food | Crude fiber | Southgate method | | | Van Soest method | | Indigestible residue | |
		Cellulose	Hemicellulose	Lignin	Acid-detergent fiber	Lignin	Enzymatic	By difference
Apple	0.66–1.0	0.47	0.66	0.18	0.18	0.18	1.15	1.7–2.4
Carrots	1.0	0.81	0.29	0.08	—	—	1.64	2.9–3.1
Peas	0.57–2.0	3.06	1.42	0.33	—	—	3.29	5.2
Wheat bran	9.1	9.3	21.7	4.3	12.2	2.8	48.8	—

Adapted from J. L. Kelsay, *Am. J. Clin. Nutr.*, 31(1978):142.

Its release is stimulated by amino acids in the lumen and by the acid pH of the stomach content as it passes into the duodenum. The low pH of the chyle also stimulates the release of secretin, which in turn stimulates the exocrine pancreas to release bicarbonate and water so as to raise the pH of the chyle. This is necessary so as to maximize the activity of the digestive enzymes located on the surface of the luminal cell.

As mentioned, starch digestion begins in the mouth with salivary amylase. It pauses in the stomach as the stomach contents are acidified, but resumes when the chyle enters the duodenum and the pH is raised. The amylase of the pancreatic juice is the same as that of the saliva. It attacks the same bonds in the same locations and produces the same products: maltose, maltotriose, and the small polysaccharides (average of 8 glucose molecules) called α-limit dextrins. The limit dextrins are further hydrolyzed by α-glucosidases on the surface of the luminal cells. The hydrolysis of the bonds not attacked by α-amylase or α-glucosidase, or the disaccharidases maltase, lactase, or sucrase, are passed to the lower part of the intestine where they are attacked by the enzymes of the intestinal flora. Most of the products of this digestion are used by the flora themselves; however, the microbial metabolic products may be of use. The flora can produce useful amounts of short-chain fatty acids and lactate as well as methane gas, carbon dioxide, water, and hydrogen gas. The carbohydrates of legumes typify the substrates these flora use. Raffinose, which is an α-galactose $1{\rightarrow}6$ glucose $1{\rightarrow}2$ β-fructose, and trehalose, an α-glucose $1{\rightarrow}1$ α-glucose are the typical substrates from legumes for these flora. The flora will also attack portions of the fibers and celluloses that are the structural elements in fruits and vegetables. Again, some useful products may be produced, but the bulk of these complex polysaccharides having β linkages and perhaps other substituent groups as part of their structure are largely untouched by both intestinal and bacterial enzymes.

These undigested unavailable carbohydrates serve very useful functions:

1. They provide bulk to the diet, which in turn helps to regulate the rate of food passage from mouth to anus.
2. They act as adsorbants of noxious or potentially noxious materials in the food.
3. They assist in the excretion of cholesterol and several minerals, thereby protecting the body from overload.

Populations consuming high-fiber diets seem to have fewer health problems. They have a lower incidence of colon cancer, fewer problems with constipation, and as a general rule, have lower serum cholesterol levels.

The disaccharides in the diet are hydrolyzed to their component monosaccharides by enzymes also located on the surface of the luminal cell. Lactose is hydrolyzed to glucose and galactose by lactase, sucrose is hydrolyzed by sucrose to fructose and glucose, and maltose is hydrolyzed by maltase to two molecules of glucose. Table 6 lists these enzymes together with their substrates and products.

TABLE 6
Enzymes of Importance to Carbohydrate Digestion

Enzyme	Substrate	Products
α-Amylase	Starch, amylopectin, glycogen	Glucose, maltose, maltotriose, α-limit dextrin
α-Glucosidase	α-Limit dextrin	Glucose
Lactase	Lactose	Galactose, glucose
Maltase	Maltose	Glucose
Sucrase/isomaltase	Sucrose/α-limit dextrin	Glucose, fructose

Once the monosaccharides are released through the action of the above enzymes they are absorbed by one of several mechanisms. Glucose and galactose are absorbed by an energy-dependent, sodium-dependent, carrier-mediated mechanism. This mechanism is termed active transport because glucose is transported against a concentration gradient. Because the transport is against a concentration gradient, energy is required to "push" the movement of glucose into the enterocyte. This transport is diagrammed in Figure 7. Glucose and galactose appear to compete for the same active transport system. They also compete for a secondary transporter, a sodium-independent transporter found in the contraluminal membrane. The two transporters differ in molecular weight. The sodium-dependent transporter has a weight of 75 kDa while the sodium-independent transporter weighs 57 kDa. This sodium-independent transporter is a member of a family of transporters called GLUT 1, 2, 3, 4, or 5. Each of these transporters are specific to certain tissues. The mechanism of their action is shown in Figures 7 and 20. Mobile glucose transporter recruitment and action is described in Section VII.C.

Fructose is not absorbed via an active transport system but by facilitated diffusion. This process is independent of the sodium ion and is specific for fructose. In the enterocyte much of the absorbed fructose is metabolized such that little fructose can be found in the portal blood even if the animal is given an intraluminal infusion of this sugar. On the other hand, an infusion of sucrose will sometimes result in measurable blood levels of fructose. The reason why this occurs may be due to the location of sucrase on the enterocyte. Rather than extending out into the lumen as do the other disaccharidases anchored to the enterocyte by a glycoprotein, sucrase is closely attached to the enterocyte membrane and the sucrose molecule is closely embraced by the enzyme. The hydrolysis of sucrose and subsequent transport of its constituent monosaccharides occurs such that both monosaccharides enter the enterocyte simultaneously. If the diet is particularly rich in sucrose the rise in both glucose and fructose in the portal blood will be measurable. This has some interesting consequences as will be discussed in Section VI below.

Of the other monosaccharides present in the lumen, passive diffusion is the means for their entry into the enterocyte. Pentoses, such as those found in plums or cherries, and other minor carbohydrates will find their way into the system only to be passed out of the body via the urine if the carbohydrate cannot be used.

VI. METABOLISM

A. OVERVIEW

Once absorbed by the intestinal cell, glucose passes into the portal blood and circulates first to the liver and then throughout the body. Glucose is the universal and in many cases the preferred fuel for almost all cells. Even though humans consume almost as much energy from carbohydrate as from fat, the body will prefer to oxidize that carbohydrate and store that fat. However, because one is not constantly consuming food, these fuel choices are not always possible. The body can protect itself from a lack of food energy by using stored energy. Some of this store (less than a day's need) can be provided by glycogen, a polymer of glucose. Hence, glucose in excess of immediate oxidative need is used to synthesize glycogen in the

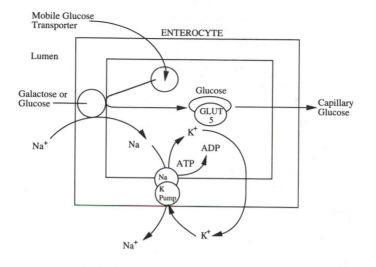

FIGURE 7. Active transport of glucose from the lumen into the enterocyte, showing the role of energy-dependent Na^+K^+ exchange and the mobile glucose transporter (GLUT 5). Once all the glucose has been transported across the enterocyte, the mobile glucose transporter returns to its storage site, only to be recruited once again when more glucose is present in the lumen.

muscle and liver. Once the glycogen stores are filled, surplus glucose from the diet can be converted to fatty acids and stored as triacylglycerols in the adipose tissue. In times of need, this fat can be oxidized as can the stored glycogen. For those cells having an absolute requirement for glucose (certain brain cells) this important fuel can be provided through glycogenolysis or synthesized via gluconeogenesis in the liver and kidney.

All of these processes (see Figure 8), including food intake regulation (see Unit 3), glucose oxidation, lipid oxidation, fatty acid synthesis glycogenesis, glycogenolysis, and gluconeogenesis are under genetic, dietary, and hormonal control. This control is carefully integrated such that normal blood glucose levels are maintained at 100 ± 20 mg/dl. Excursions below or above this range may occur. If the excursion is of short duration (minutes) there is no cause for alarm. However, if these excursions are of more than several minutes or hours, then, depending on the reason for these excursions, medical assistance may be required. Before a discussion of the regulation of glucose homeostasis can be entered, it is first necessary to describe the various pathways involved in this regulation.

B. GLYCOLYSIS

The glycolytic pathway for the anaerobic catabolism of glucose can be found in all cells in the body. The pathway begins with glucose, a 6-carbon unit, and through a series of reactions produces 2 molecules of ATP and 2 molecules of pyruvate. The pathway is shown in Figure 9. The control of glycolysis is vested in several key steps. The first step is the activation of glucose through the formation of glucose-6-phosphate. In the liver and pancreatic β cell this step is catalyzed by the enzyme glucokinase. A molecule of ATP is used and magnesium is required. Glucose-6-phosphate is a key metabolite. It can proceed down the glycolytic pathway, or move through the hexose monophosphate slunt (or "shunt"), or be used to make glycogen. How much glucose-6-phosphate is oxidized directly to pyruvate depends on the nutritional state of the animal, the type of cells, the genetics of the animal, and its hormonal state. Some cell types, the brain cells for example, do not make glycogen. Some people do not have shunt activity in the red cell because the code for glucose-6-phosphate dehydrogenase has mutated such that the enzyme is not functional. Insulin-deficient animals likewise might have little shunt and glycolytic activity due to the lack of insulin's effect on the synthesis of its enzymes. All these factors determine how much glucose-6-phosphate goes in which direction.

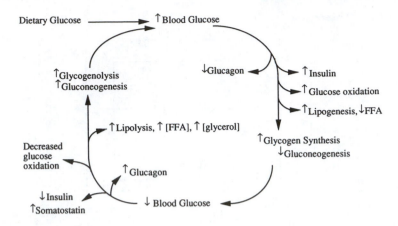

FIGURE 8. Overview of glucose metabolism. As blood glucose levels rise due to influx of dietary glucose, blood insulin levels rise and glucagon levels fall. Glucose oxidation increases as does glycogenesis and lipogenesis. Gluconeogenesis fails. As the blood glucose levels fall these processes reverse. Glucagon levels rise, insulin falls; glycogenolysis and gluconeogenesis rise and peripheral glucose oxidation decreases.

Two enzymes are used for the activation of glucose: glucokinase and hexokinase. In the liver both enzymes are present. While hexokinase activity is product inhibited, glucokinase is not. The hexokinase in the nonhepatic tissues must be product inhibited to prevent the hexokinase from tying up all the Pi in the cells as glucose-6-phosphate. The Km for glucokinase is greater than that for hexokinase so the former is the main enzyme for the conversion of glucose to glucose-6-phosphate in the liver. The other enzyme will phosphorylate not only glucose, but other six-carbon sugars such as fructose. However, the amount of fructose phosphorylated to fructose-6-phosphate is small in comparison to the phosphorylation of fructose at the carbon 1 position catalyzed by fructokinase. The metabolism of fructose is shown in Figure 11.

Glucose-6-phosphate is isomerized to fructose-6-phosphate and then is phosphorylated once again to form fructose-1,6-bisphosphate. Another molecule of ATP is used, and again magnesium is an important cofactor. Both kinase reactions are rate controlling reactions in that their activity determines the rate at which subsequent reactions proceed. The phosphofructokinase reaction is unique to the glycolytic sequence while the glucokinase or hexokinase step is not. Thus, one could argue that the formation of fructose-1,6-bisphosphate is the first *committed* step in glycolysis. Glycolysis is inhibited when phosphofructokinase is inhibited. This occurs when levels of fatty acids in the cytosol rise as in the instance of high rates of lipolysis and fatty acid oxidation. Phosphofructokinase activity is increased when levels of fructose-6-phosphate rise or when cAMP levels rise. Stimulation occurs also when fructose-2,6-bisphosphate levels rise. In any event, glycolysis then proceeds with the splitting of fructose-1,6-bisphosphate to dihydroxyacetone phosphate (DHAP) and glyceraldehyde-3-phosphate. At this point another rate controlling step occurs. This step is one which shuttles reducing equivalents into the mitochondria for use by the respiratory chain. This is the α-glycerophosphate shuttle, shown and discussed in Unit 3. This shuttle carries reducing equivalents from the cytosol to the mitochondria. DHAP picks up reducing equivalents when it is converted to α-glycerol phosphate. These reducing equivalents are produced when glyceraldehyde-3-phosphate is oxidized in the process of being phosphorylated to 1,3-diphosphate glyceraldehyde. The α-glycerophosphate enters the inner mitochondrial membrane, whereupon it is converted back to DHAP and releases its reducing equivalents to FAD that, in turn, transfers the reducing equivalents to the mitochondrial respiratory chain. The reason why this shuttle is rate limiting is due to the need to regenerate NAD+. Without NAD+ the glycolytic pathway ceases. NAD+ itself cannot pass through the mitochondrial membrane so substrate shuttle is necessary.

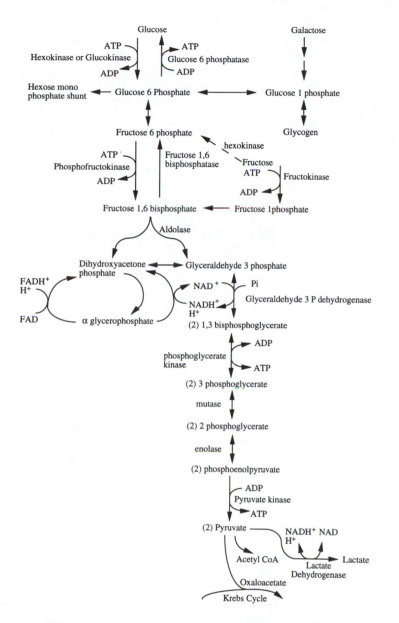

FIGURE 9. The series of reactions which comprise glycolysis.

Another means of producing NAD$^+$ is by converting pyruvate to lactate. This is a nonmitochondrial reaction catalyzed by lactate dehydrogenase. It occurs when an oxygen debt is developed, as happens in exercising muscle. In these muscles more oxygen is consumed than can be provided. Glycolysis is occurring at a rate faster than can be accommodated by the respiratory chain that joins the reducing equivalents transferred to it by the shuttles to molecular oxygen making water. If more reducing equivalents are generated than can be used to make water, the excess are added to pyruvate to make lactate. Thus, rising lactate levels are indicative of oxygen debt.

There are other shuttles which also serve to transfer reducing equivalents into the mitosol. These are the malate-aspartate shuttle and the malate-citrate shuttle. Neither of these are rate limiting with respect to glycolysis. The malate-aspartate shuttle has rate controlling properties with respect to gluconeogenesis while the malate-citrate shuttle is important to lipogenesis.

Once 1,3-bisphosphate glyceraldehyde is formed it is converted to 3-phosphoglyceralde-hyde with the formation of 1 ATP. The 3-phosphoglyceraldehyde then goes to 2-phosphoglyc-eraldehyde and then to phosphoenolpyruvate. These are all bidirectional reactions that are also used in gluconeogenesis. The phosphoenolpyruvate is dephosphorylated to pyruvate with the formation of another ATP. Because of the great energy loss to ATP formation at this step this reaction is not reversible. Gluconeogenesis uses another enzyme, phosphoenolpyruvate carboxykinase, to reverse this step. Glycolysis uses pyruvate kinase to catalyze the reaction. At any rate, pyruvate can now be activated to acetyl CoA which can enter the Krebs citric acid cycle.

The glycolytic pathway is dependent on both ATP for the initial steps of the pathway, the formation of glucose-6-phosphate and fructose-1,6-bisphosphate, and on the ratio of ATP to ADP and inorganic phosphate, Pi. In working muscle the continuance of work and the continuance of glycolysis depends on the cycling of the adenine nucleotides and the export of lactate. ATP must be provided at the beginning of the pathway and ADP as well as Pi must be provided in the latter steps. If the tissue runs out of ATP or ADP or Pi, or accumulates lactate and H^+, glycolysis will come to a halt, and work cannot continue. This is what happens to the working skeletal muscle. Exhaustion sets in when glycolytic rate is down-regulated by an accumulation of lactate.

An interesting clinical condition arises in some humans and in pigs which have a genetic error in the regulation of their lactate export and adenine nucleotide cycling. This error is unnoticed unless the individual is anesthetized with an anesthesia such as halothane. When anesthetized, body temperature rises precipitously, muscle rigor and acidosis quickly follow. This condition is known as malignant hyperthermia and occurs in 1 child in 15,000 and 1 adult in 50,000 to 100,000. Unless quickly recognized and measures taken to reduce the body temperature and combat the acidosis, death will result. The biochemical explanation has to do with ATP, ADP, and Pi cycling and the export of lactate from the muscle cell. Apparently, the anesthesia affects several exchange mechanisms in the membranes within and around the muscle cell. Affected is the coupling of respiration to ATP synthesis by the mitochondria, and the energy normally trapped in the high-energy bond of the ATP molecule is released as heat. Probably the ADP generated in the early ATP-dependent steps of glycolysis is not sent into the mitochondria for rephosphorylation into ATP and, instead, is recycled through substrate phosphorylation. Since ADP is exchanged (via several different exchange mechanisms) for ATP, the cell must make some adjustments in its metabolism. Muscle tends to use the glycolytic pathway with the excess product, pyruvate, sent back to the liver as lactate. While muscle does not lack mitochondria, its mitochondrial activity cannot keep pace with its glycolytic flux when the muscle is working hard and long, or in this instance, when the person with the genetic disease of malignant hyperthermia is anesthetized with halothane. Hence, the pyruvate/lactate spillover. The lactate must exit the cell via a lactate/H^+ symport. This requires a normal or accelerated blood flow. If the lactate and H^+ are not carried away by the blood, they accumulate. H^+ inhibits the activity of phosphofructokinase and lactate acts as a feedback inhibitor of glycolysis.

When an anesthesia such as halothane is used on susceptible individuals there is a further disruption in the control of glycolysis. There is an accelerated futile cycling between fructose-6-phosphate and fructose-1,6-phosphatase, as well as a dramatic decrease in glycolytic flux. The decrease in flux is secondary to the lactate and H^+ accumulation. In halothane anesthesia blood flow is reduced. This, coupled with the genetic error(s) in the membrane(s), results in the phenotypic expression of the malignant hyperthermic genotype.

C. HEXOSE MONOPHOSPHATE SHUNT

The shunt provides an alternate pathway for the use of glucose-6-phosphate. It is an important pathway because it generates reducing equivalents carried by NADP and because it generates a phosphorylated ribose for use in nucleotide synthesis. It is estimated that approximately 10% of the glucose-6-phosphate generated from glucose is metabolized by the shunt.

As can be seen in Figure 10, the shunt contains two NADP-linked dehydrogenases, glucose-6-phosphate dehydrogenase and 6-phosphogluconate dehydrogenase. These two enzymes comprise the rate limiting steps in the reaction sequence. In the instance where there is an active lipogenic state, these reactions provide about 50% of the reducing equivalents needed by the lipogenic process (see Unit 6). In fact, if one wanted a quick assessment of the lipogenic response to a variety of treatments one could measure the activity of these enzymes using an aliquot of a tissue homogenate plus enough substrate and magnesium to optimize the conditions of the assay. There is an excellent correlation between this dehydrogenase activity and lipogenesis.

Lipogenesis is not the only process that requires reducing equivalents carried by NADP. The microsomal P450 enzymes need them as does the maintenance of glutathione in the reduced state. The glutathione system in the red cell maintains the redox state and integrity of the cell membrane. If sufficient reducing equivalents are not produced by the shunt dehydrogenase reactions to reduce glutathione, the red cell membrane integrity is lost and hemolytic anemia results. This is important to the red blood cell function of carrying oxygen and exchanging it for carbon dioxide.

There are a number of genetic mutations in the code for red cell glucose-6-phosphate dehydrogenase. The code is carried as a recessive trait on the X chromosome and thus only males are affected. These mutations are usually silent. That is, the male, having a defective red cell glucose-6-phosphate dehydrogenase, does not know he has the problem unless his cells are tested *or* unless he is given a drug such as quinine or one of the sulfur antibiotics that increases the oxidation of NADPH+H⁺. When this happens NADPH+H⁺ is depleted and is not available to reduce oxidized glutathione. In turn, the red cell ruptures. In almost all cases the affected male has sufficient enzyme activity to meet the normal demands for NADPH+H⁺. It is only when stressed by these drugs that a problem develops.

In any event, as shown in Figure 10, glucose-6-phosphate proceeds to 6-phospho-glucolactone, a very unstable metabolite which is in turn reduced to 6-phosphogluconate. 6-Phosphogluconate is decarboxylated and dehydrogenated to form ribulose-5-phosphate with an unstable intermediate (keto-6-phosphogluconate) forming between the 6-phosphogluconate and ribulose-5-phosphate. Ribulose-5-phosphate can be isomerized to ribose-5-phosphate or epimerized to xylulose-5-phosphate. Xylulose and ribose-5-phosphate can reversibly form sedoheptulose-7-phosphate with release of glyceraldehyde-3-phosphate. This, of course, will be recognized as a component of the glycolytic sequence (see Figure 10).

D. INTERCONVERSION OF DIETARY SUGARS
1. Fructose

In the course of digestion, the simple sugars fructose and galactose are released from sucrose and lactose, respectively. These sugars are usable by most cells after they are converted to glucose. There are specific cells that have specific needs for these monosaccharides. The testes need fructose for sperm production and the mammary cells need galactose for lactose production. In each instance there are reactions that are of interest to the nutrition scientist. Shown in Figure 11 is the metabolism of fructose.

Although two enzymes are available for the phosphorylation of fructose, one of these, the fructokinase, is present only in the liver. Just as hexokinase has a lower Km for glucose than glucokinase for the substrate glucose, so too does hexokinase with respect to fructose and fructokinase. The Km for fructokinase is so high that in fact most of the dietary fructose, whether as the free sugar *or* as a component of sucrose, is metabolized in the liver. This is in contrast to glucose which is metabolized by all the cells in the body. As a result, fructose- or sucrose-rich diets fed to rats or mice will result in a fatty liver. This occurs because the dietary overload of fructose or sucrose exceeds the capacity of the liver to oxidize it so it uses the sugar

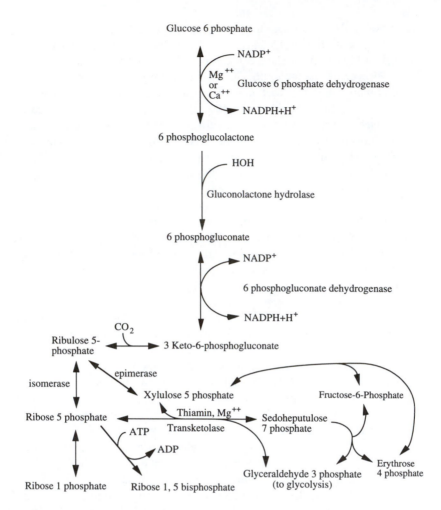

FIGURE 10.   Reaction sequence of the hexose monophosphate shunt commonly referred to as the "shunt".

metabolites as substrate for fatty acid and triacylglyceride synthesis. Until the hepatic lipid export system increases sufficiently to transport this lipid to the storage depots, the lipid accumulates, hence, the fatty liver. Normal rodents adjust to this fructose intake such that after a few weeks the liver returns to its normal (~4%) fat content. Those rodents with diabetic tendencies do not adapt and the fatty liver persists throughout their life. Humans rarely consume high-fructose diets that compare to those offered to laboratory rats. Nonetheless, when the consumption of beverages and foods containing the high-fructose syrups began to climb, nutrition scientists began to question whether this dietary change might have untoward effects. Given the length of the human life span, it is too soon to predict whether this concern was well placed.

The pathway for fructose metabolism shows three enzymes, any one of which if mutated results in a condition known as fructosemia. The first is relatively harmless; it involves a mutation in the gene for fructokinase. As discussed above, hexokinase will phosphorylate fructose and, if the dietary burden is light, the disease of fructosemia will be harmless. Its characteristics of elevated blood and urine levels of fructose are harmless. A second mutation has been identified in the gene for aldolase B. This is the enzyme which catalyzes the splitting of fructose-1-phosphate to glyceraldehyde phosphate and dihydroxyacetone phosphate. Recall that aldolase A catalyzes the splitting of fructose-1,6-bisphosphate. Aldolase A is found in all tissues whereas aldolase B is located in the liver only. The mutation is such that the enzyme

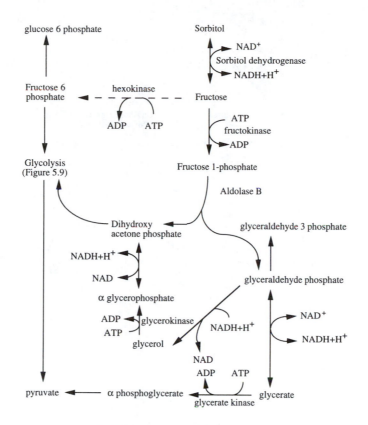

FIGURE 11. Metabolism of fructose.

has a reduced affinity for its substrate, fructose-1-phosphate. The results of this reduced affinity include hypoglycemia due to an inhibition of glycogenolysis by fructose-1-phosphate. This hypoglycemia is not responsive to glucagon stimulation. Prior to the identification of the aldolase B gene mutation, this form of fructosemia was misdiagnosed as one of the glycogen storage diseases because of the presence of hypoglycemia in the face of ample liver glycogen stores. In addition to the disturbance in glycogenolysis, patients with this disorder vomit after a fructose load, have elevated levels of urine and blood fructose, grow poorly with evidence of jaundice, have hyperbilirubinemia (high levels of bilirubin in the blood), albuminuria (albumin in the urine), and amino aciduria (amino acids in the urine) and some patients may have damaged renal proximal convoluted tubules.

The third mutation involves only the liver enzyme, fructose-1,6-bisphosphatase. The muscle enzyme is normal in activity. This enzyme is a key enzyme in the hepatic gluconeogenic pathway so, as one might expect, hypoglycemia is one of the characteristics of a mutation in this enzyme. Other characteristics include an enlarged liver, poor muscle tone, and increased blood lactate levels. All of these mutations are uncommon and all are autosomal recessive traits. Heterozygotes are not detectable.

2. Galactose

Another monosaccharide of importance, especially to infants and children, is galactose which is a component of the milk sugar, lactose. In the intestine, lactose is hydrolyzed to its component monosaccharides, glucose and galactose. Galactose is converted to glucose and eventually enters the glycolytic sequence as glucose-6-phosphate. The entire pathway is shown in Figure 12. Galactose is phosphorylated at carbon 1 in the first step of its conversion to glucose. It can be isomerized to glucose-1-phosphate or converted to UDP-galactose by exchanging its phosphate group for a UDP group. This UDP-galactose can be joined with

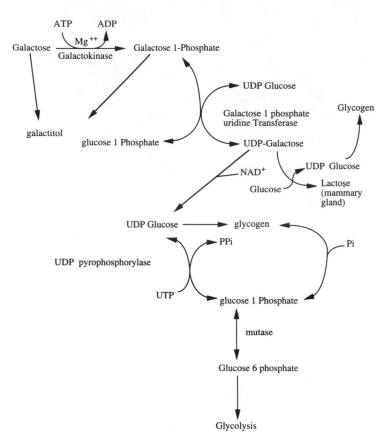

FIGURE 12.   Conversion of galactose to glucose.

glucose to form lactose in the adult mammary tissue under the influence of the hormone prolactin. However, usually the UDP-galactose is converted to UDP-glucose and thence used to form glycogen. When glycogen is degraded, glucose-1-phosphate is released, which in turn is isomerized to glucose-6-phosphate and enters the glycolytic sequence.

Three autosomal recessive mutations in the genes for enzymes involved in galactose conversion to glucose have been described. Galactosemia results in each instance. Two of these mutations involve the gene for galactose-1-phosphate uridyl transferase. Two variants have been described. One is fairly innocuous in that the mutation occurs only in the enzymes found in the red cell. This variant is called the Duarte variant and affected individuals have 50% less red cell galactose-1-phosphate uridyl transferase activity than normal individuals. These people have no other discernible characteristics. The second variant is far more severe in its effects on the patient. The enzyme in the liver is abnormal and does not function to convert galactose-1-phosphate to UDP galactose. As a result, galactose-1-phosphate accumulates, and some is converted to the sugar alcohol, galactitol, via NADH aldose reductase action. Cataracts in the eye form in this disease, accompanied by mental retardation and increased tissue levels of galactose-1-phosphate, galactitol, and galactonic acid. These last metabolites are excreted in the urine. Also characteristic of this mutation in galactose-1-phosphate uridyl transferase are decreased blood glucose levels, decreased glycogenesis, decreased mutase activity, and decreased pyrophosphorylase activity.

Since UDP-galactose is necessary for the formation of the galactoyl lipids, chondroitin sulfate formation is decreased. A mutation in the gene for galactokinase also results in accumulations of galactose and galactitol and cataracts. The galactitol accumulation was found to be the causative agent in the formation of cataracts. Except for cataract formation due to galactitol accumulation, no other symptoms have been described for this form of galactosemia.

3. Mannose

Although the main monosaccharides are glucose, fructose, and galactose, occasionally the diet provides other sugars. These are the pentoses, xylose and xylulose, found in plums, cherries, and grapes. Usually, they are converted to the sugar alcohol xylitol through the action of the NADP-linked enzyme xylose/xylulose dehydrogenase and the xylitol is excreted in the urine. However, a mutation in the gene for this enzyme has been detected and characterized by the presence of xylose or xylulose in the urine instead of xylitol. This has no clinical significance except if the urine is screened for reducing sugars without discriminating for glucose just after such a person has consumed the fruits containing these sugars. If the person is not studied more carefully, there is the off chance of a misdiagnosis of diabetes based on the presence of these reducing sugars in the urine. This is not a very likely occurrence.

Lastly, mannose, another sugar found in food, is converted to fructose via phosphorylation and isomerization:

$$Mannose \rightarrow Mannose\text{-}6\text{-}phosphate \rightarrow Fructose\text{-}6\text{-}phosphate \rightarrow Glycolysis$$

$$\downarrow$$

$$Glycolysis$$

To date, no genetic errors have been described with respect to this sugar.

E. GLYCOGENESIS AND GLYCOGENOLYSIS

Glucose is an essential fuel for working muscle as well as for the brain. In order to ensure a steady supply of this fuel, some glucose is stored in the liver and muscle in the form of glycogen. This is a ready supply of glucose accessed when stimulated to release its glucose by the catabolic hormones glucagon, epinephrine, the glucocorticoids, and thyroxine and/or by the absence of food in the digestive tract. Because the glycogen molecule has molecules of water as part of its structure, this is a very large molecule and cumbersome to store in large amounts. In fact, detailed studies of the nature of the body's fuel stores have shown that the average 70-kg man has only an 18-hour fuel supply stored as glycogen, while that same individual might have up to a 2-month supply of fuel stored as fat. Nonetheless, the synthesis of glycogen and its release of glucose in time of need is an important aspect of carbohydrate nutrition.

Shown in Figure 13 is an overview of glycogenesis and glycogenolysis. Figure 14 gives details of the glycogenolytic cascade. Muscle and liver glycogen stores have very different functions. Muscle glycogen is used to synthesize ATP for muscle contraction, whereas hepatic glycogen is the glucose reserve for the entire body particularly the central nervous system. The amount of glycogen in the muscle is dependent on the physical activity of the individual. After bouts of strenuous exercise, the glycogen store will be depleted, only to be rebuilt during the resting period following exercise. One aspect of physical training is concerned with the expansion of the muscle glycogen store. Through repeated depletion-repletion routines, athletes hope to increase the size of this store so as to increase their endurance. Athletes follow an exercise/recovery routine as well as a dietary carbohydrate routine (a normal carbohydrate diet followed by a carbohydrate-rich diet just prior to competition) that they hope will improve their performance through increasing their muscle glycogen store.

The different types of muscle store and use glycogen for glucose and ATP generation differently. Overall, about 8% of muscle glycogen is converted to glucose and some of

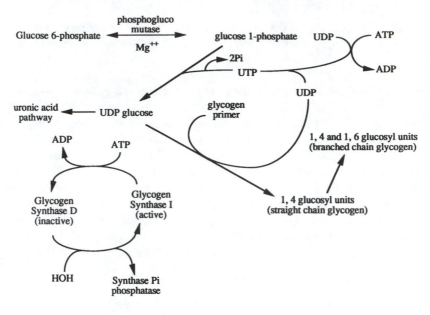

FIGURE 13.   Glycogen synthesis (glycogenesis).

this is released into the bloodstream. The remainder is oxidized via the glycolytic pathway. Myocytes lack glucose-6-phosphatase so glucose release from gluconeogenesis is not possible. Exercise or "work" by "red" muscle fibers that are richly endowed with mitochondria can oxidize glucose fully to provide ATP and result in water and carbon dioxide. These fiber types are found in the heart muscle and the long muscles of legs and arms. White muscle, in contrast, has tremendous capacity for glycogenesis, glycogenolysis, and glycolysis, but has far fewer mitochondria than does the red muscle. Hence, work by white muscle results in an accumulation of lactate released to the bloodstream since the glucose being used cannot be completely oxidized to CO_2 and water. While red muscle can continue to work indefinitely given its generous blood supply and mitochondrial complement, white muscle cannot. It can provide the sudden burst of activity needed for sprinting, for example, but its endurance is limited. Most muscle groups in the human body are mixtures of red and white fibers and, as such, physical training will capitalize on the fiber type best used for the type of competition (i.e., sprinting vs. marathon running) anticipated.

Hepatic glycogen stores are dependent on nutritional status. They are virtually absent in the 24-hour starved animal while being replenished within hours of *ad libitum* feeding. Clusters of glycogen molecules with an average molecular weight of 2×10^7 form quickly when an abundance of glucose is provided to the liver. As noted, the amount of glycogen in the liver is diet dependent. In fact, there is a 24-hour rhythmic change in hepatic glycogen that corresponds to the feeding pattern of the animal. In nocturnal animals such as the rat, the peak hepatic glycogen store will be found in the early morning hours while the nadir will be found in the evening hours just before the nocturnal feeding begins. In humans accustomed to eating during the day, the reverse pattern will be observed.

Glycogen synthesis begins with glucose-1-phosphate formation from glucose-6-phosphate through the action of phosphoglucomutase. Glucose-1-phosphate then is converted to uridine diphosphate glucose (UDP-glucose) which can then be added to the glycogen already in storage (the glycogen primer). UDP-glucose can be added through a 1,6 linkage or a 1,4 linkage. Two high-energy bonds are used to incorporate each molecule of glucose into the glycogen. The straight chain glucose polymer is comprised of glucoses joined through the 1,4 linkage and is less compact than the branched chain glycogen which has both 1,4 and 1,6 linkages as shown in Figure 15. The addition of glucose to the primer glycogen with a 1,4

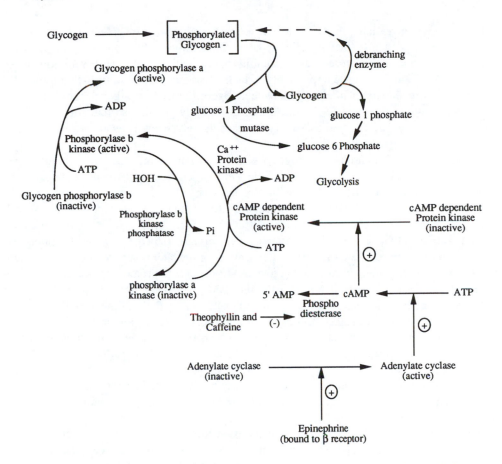

FIGURE 14. Stepwise release of glucose molecules from the glycogen molecule (glycogenolysis).

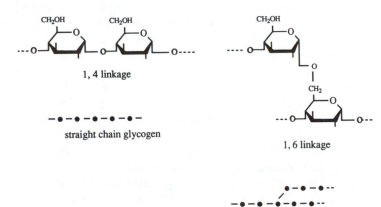

FIGURE 15. Glycogen structures.

linkage is catalyzed by the glycogen synthase enzyme while the 1,6 addition is catalyzed by the so-called glycogen branching enzyme (amylo 1→4, 1→6 transglucosidase). Once the liver and muscle cell achieve their full storage capacity, these enzymes are product inhibited and glycogenesis is "turned off". Glycogen synthase is inactivated by a cAMP-dependent kinase and activated by a synthase phosphatase enzyme that is stimulated by changes in the ratio of ATP to ADP. Glycogen synthesis is stimulated by the hormone insulin and suppressed by the catabolic hormones. The process does not fully cease, but operates at a very low level. Glycogen does not accumulate appreciably in cells other than liver and muscle although all cells contain a small amount of glycogen. Note in Figure 13 that a glycogen primer is required for glycogen synthesis to proceed. This primer is carefully guarded so that some is *always* available when glycogen is synthesized. This means that glycogenolysis *never* fully depletes the cell of its glycogen content.

Glycogenolysis is a carefully controlled series of reactions referred to as the glycogen cascade. It is called a cascade because of the stepwise changes in activation states of the enzymes involved. To release glucose for oxidation by the glycogenolytic pathway, the glycogen must be phosphorylated. This is accomplished by the enzyme glycogen phosphorylase. Glycogen phosphorylase exists in the cell in an inactive form (glycogen phosphorylase b) and is activated to its active form (glycogen phosphorylase a) by the enzyme phosphorylase b kinase. In turn, this kinase also exists in an inactive form which is activated by the calcium-dependent enzyme, protein kinase, and active cAMP-dependent protein kinase. These activations each require a molecule of ATP. Lastly, the cAMP-dependent protein kinase must have cAMP for its activation. This cAMP is generated from ATP by the enzyme adenylate cyclase which, in itself, is inactive unless stimulated by a hormone such as epinephrine, thyroxine, or glucagon. As can be seen, this cascade of activation is energy dependent, with three molecules of ATP needed to get the process started. Once started, the glycolytic pathway will replenish the ATP needed initially as well as provide a further supply of ATP to provide needed energy. As mentioned, the liver and muscle differ in the use of glycogen. This also affects how ATP is generated within the glycogen-containing cell and how much is generated by cells that do not store glycogen.

In part, our understanding of how glycogen is used or how glycogenolysis occurs has come about because of some spontaneous mutations in the genes coding for the enzymes involved. While these mutations in several instances are devastating to the affected person, they have shed light on the control of the overall balance of glycogenesis and glycogenolysis.

One very rare autosomal recessive disease is due to a mutation in the gene for the branching enzyme. This results in an accumulation of straight chain glycogen which, because it is less compact than the normal branched chain glycogen, results in an enlarged liver. This disorder is called amylopectinosis and is usually grouped with the other disorders characterized by enlarged glycogen stores. However, this disorder affects synthesis rather than degradation (which is normal) and there is not an excess in glycogen. People with this disorder have a problem with the synthesis of branched glycogen in the muscle and have poor muscle tone. They are exercise intolerant. Poor weight gain and early death are also characteristic of the disorder.

Five mutations in the genes which code for the enzymes of glycogenolysis have been described. These include a mutation in the lysomal α-1,4-glucosidase (also called acid maltase) which results in a generalized excess of glycogen not only in the liver and muscle but also in the viscera and central nervous system. This disorder is called Pompe's disease and is characterized by an enlarged liver and heart and extreme muscular weakness.

A mutation in the gene for the debranching enzyme (amylo-1,6-glucosidase) results in the accumulation of highly branched short-chain glycogen in the muscles and liver. The usual glycogen has a branch point at every fourth glucosyl residue in the interior of the molecule and further apart on the outer regions. The glycogen stored in people lacking the debranching enzyme have their branch points very close together. This occurs when glucose is mobilized from glycogen and only the outer limbs of the molecule are used. Without a functioning debranching enzyme, the remaining inner core is untouched. These cores accumulate and are responsible for the enlarged liver and heart. Because the glycogen gives up only a small amount of its glucose, the muscle which needs it for ATP synthesis is very weak. This condition is called Forbes disease.

McArdle's disease affects only the muscle, and the enzyme lacking is the muscle phosphorylase. Patients with this disorder are intolerant to exercise and accumulate glycogen in the muscle but not the liver. This disorder was discovered in military recruits during World War II, when in a few isolated instances, young men were found who could not endure the rigorous physical training of boot camp. Unfortunately, the first few were thought to be malingerers and were forced to exercise to death by their drill instructors. When their deaths were investigated, the reason for their exercise intolerance was understood. The mutation in the muscle phosphorylase gene might not have been discovered otherwise.

In the liver, a mutation in phosphorylase is far more serious. This disorder, known as Her's disease, results in growth retardation, an enlarged liver due to glycogen accumulation, and elevated serum lipids. In both McArdle's disease and Her's disease, glycogen is not phosphorylated because of a mutation in the enzyme which catalyzes the initial step in glycogenolysis. This is also the case for another glycogen storage disease, but instead of a mutation in the gene for phosphorylase, the mutation is in the gene for the phosphorylase kinase, the enzyme that is responsible for the activation of glycogen phosphorylase b to glycogen phosphorylase a. Without the addition of energy through the hydrolysis of ATP, the glycogen phosphorylase cannot transfer this phosphate to the glycogen molecule and produce a molecule of glucose-1-phosphate. People with this disorder have the same symptoms as those with Her's disease and, in addition, have increased rates of gluconeogenesis and hypoglycemia when without food for long periods of time. They also have decreased phosphorylase activity in hepatocytes and leukocytes.

All of these disorders in glycogen synthesis and degradation are rare and all appear as autosomal recessive traits. They are listed in Table 7. Their long-term outlook is not very good. Nutritional manipulations include a continual nasogastric drip of a starch suspension which is directed towards reducing hypoglycemia episodes. Because the hypoglycemia is due to an inability to normally mobilize the glycogen-glucose, care must be given to avoid prolonged periods without food. The glucose that is needed by all the body's cells must be provided either by the diet or through an active gluconeogenic process.

F. GLUCONEOGENESIS

The provision and maintenance of normal blood glucose levels in the absence of food involves not only glycogenolysis but the synthesis of glucose from noncarbohydrate precursors. This process is called gluconeogenesis and is shown in Figure 16. Gluconeogenesis occurs primarily in the liver and kidney. Most tissues lack the full complement of enzymes needed to run this pathway. In particular, the enzyme phosphoenolpyruvate carboxykinase is not found. Shown in Figure 16 are the enzymes that are unique to gluconeogenesis. The other reactions shown use the same enzymes as glycolysis (see Figure 9) and do not have control properties with respect to gluconeogenesis. The rate limiting enzymes of interest are glucose-6-phosphatase, fructose-1,6 biphosphatase, and phosphoenolpyruvate carboxykinase (PEPCK). Pyruvate kinase and pyruvate carboxylase are also of interest because their control is a coordinated one with respect to the regulation of PEPCK.

The capacity to synthesize glucose in times of need is absolutely essential to survival. Blood glucose must be maintained so that those tissues, i.e., brain, that have an absolute requirement for this fuel can continue to function. While gluconeogenesis is essential, it must be carefully controlled so that excess glucose is not produced. The process is energetically very expensive. Because it uses as substrates the carbon chains of deaminated amino acids, if it were not closely regulated, undue protein catabolism with its associated ammonia load could be devastating. Fortunately, there are a number of fail-safe controls in place that do not allow this to occur.

TABLE 7
Amino Acid That Contribute
Carbon Chain for the Synthesis
of Glucose

Amino acid	Enters as
Alanine	Pyruvate
Tryptophan→Alanine	Pyruvate
Hydroxyproline	Pyruvate
Serine	Pyruvate
Cysteine	Pyruvate
Threonine	Pyruvate
Glycine	Pyruvate
Tyrosine	Fumarate
Isoleucine	Succinyl CoA
Methionine	Succinyl CoA
Valine	Succinyl CoA
Histidine→Glutamate	α-Ketoglutarate
Proline→Glutamate	α-Ketoglutarate
Glutamine→Glutamate	α-Ketoglutarate
Arginine→Glutamate	α-Ketoglutarate

1. Cori and Alanine Cycles

The pathway shown in Figure 16 provides glucose to all cells in the body. Under normal dietary conditions the glucose synthesized in the kidney is used by the kidney as fuel to run the kidney's metabolism. Only under conditions of prolonged starvation (more than 48 hours) will the kidney contribute significant amounts of glucose to the circulation. Thus, circulating glucose produced by gluconeogenesis comes from the liver. There are two important metabolite or substrate cycles that are crucial to the effective regulation of blood glucose levels. One is the Cori cycle shown in Figure 17 and the other is the alanine cycle shown in Figure 18.

The Cori cycle involves the use of glucose by muscle and the red blood cell. Glucose is oxidized via glycolysis to two molecules of lactate. The lactate is delivered to the liver which converts it back to glucose via gluconeogenesis. The red cell produces 2 ATPs through the glycolytic process while the liver uses 6 ATPs to resynthesize the glucose. The alanine cycle differs in that the exchange is between muscle and the liver and uses alanine. Since the muscle cell has mitochondria, it can use the reducing equivalents generated by the glycolytic sequence to generate 4 to 6 moles of ATP. Rather than lactate, the muscle cell sends pyruvate (as alanine) to the liver if the pyruvate cannot be fully oxidized in the muscle cell. Actually, it is not pyruvate but its transaminated product, alanine, that is sent to the liver. Once in the hepatocyte this alanine is deaminated (the amino group used for urea synthesis) and the resultant pyruvate used to resynthesize glucose via gluconeogenesis.

These cycles are important in glucose homeostasis because they provide the means for supplying glucose to tissues that need it and which cannot *complete* its oxidation. In order to participate in these cycles, the peripheral cells must release either lactate or pyruvate or alanine as their metabolic end product of glycolysis. Further, the use of the NADH generated by the glycolytic sequence differentiates whether the Cori cycle or the alanine cycle is used. If the former, the $NADH+H^+$ is used to reduce pyruvate to lactate. In the latter, the $NADH+H^+$ is used as part of a shuttle system for the entry of reducing equivalents into the mitochondrial respiratory chain. This $NADH+H^+$ is *not* available for pyruvate reduction. Pyruvate is thus available for transamination and is converted to alanine which, in turn, is used by the liver for glucose synthesis. Although the alanine cycle is an important mechanism in the regulation of the blood glucose level, other amino acids can also serve as glucose precursors. Listed in Table 7 are amino acids that can be used in this way.

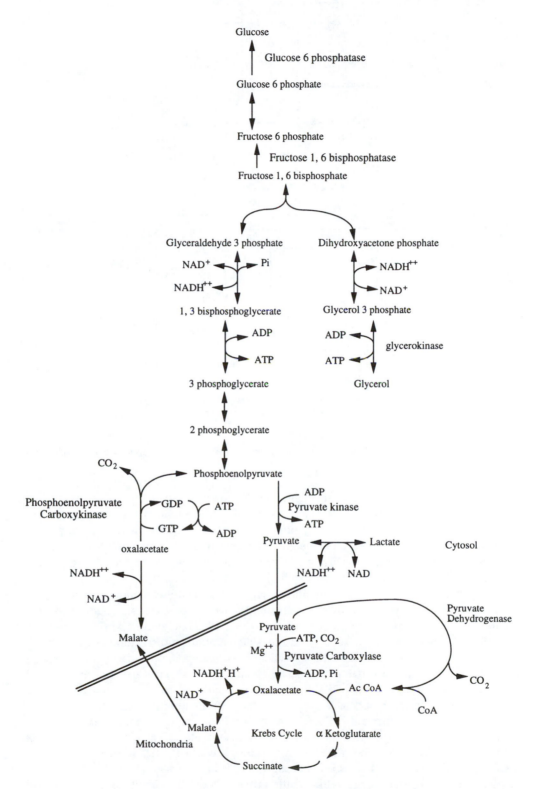

FIGURE 16. Pathway for gluconeogenesis.

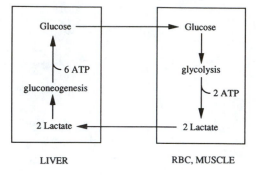

FIGURE 17.   The Cori cycle.

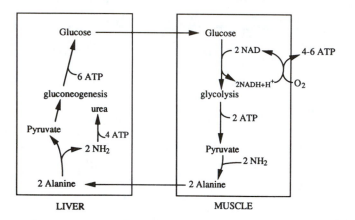

FIGURE 18.   The alanine cycle. Both the Cori cycle and the alanine cycle serve to ensure a supply of glucose to cells requiring it.

People who consume high-protein, high-fat diets frequently use their excess protein intake to provide the carbon skeletons for glucose synthesis. In addition, when people have been without food for several days, the body proteins are catabolized for energy and to provide glucose precursors. As can be seen in the gluconeogenic pathway shown in Figure 16 as well as in the Cori and alanine cycles (Figure 18), gluconeogenesis uses more ATP than glycolysis produces. This is a costly process but one that is essential to survival.

The difference in ATPs used and produced implies that the mitochondria are important to the regulation of the pathway. Indeed, one shuttle, the malate-aspartate shuttle shown in Figure 19, has rate controlling properties. The malate-aspartate shuttle works to transport reducing equivalents into the mitochondria and ATP out of the mitochondria in exchange for ADP. Malate is transported into the mitochondria whereupon it gives up two reducing equivalents and is transformed into oxalacetate. Oxalacetate cannot traverse the mitochondrial membrane so it is converted to α-ketoglutarate in a coupled reaction that also converts glutamate to aspartate. Aspartate travels out of the mitochondria (along with ATP) in exchange for glutamate. Once out in the cytosol, the reactions are reversed: aspartate is reconverted to glutamate, α-ketoglutarate is reconverted to oxalacetate, which in turn can be reduced to malate or decarboxylated to form phosphoenolpyruvate. Measurement of the activity of this shuttle has revealed that the more active the shuttle, the more active is gluconeogenesis. This is because the shuttle provides a steady supply of oxalacetate via α-ketoglutarate in the cytosol. This oxalacetate cannot get there any other way. As mentioned, it is generated by the Krebs cycle in the mitochondria but cannot leave this compartment.

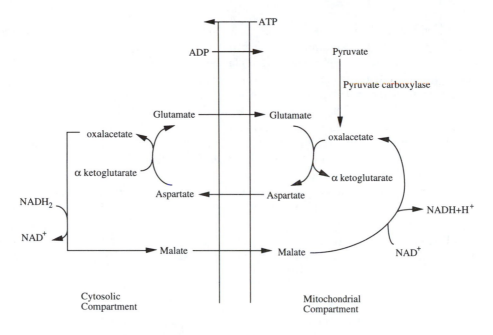

FIGURE 19. Malate-aspartate shuttle.

Oxalacetate is essential to gluconeogenesis because it is the substrate for PEPCK which catalyzes its conversion to phosphoenolpyruvate (PEP). This is an energy-dependent conversion which overcomes the irreversible final glycolytic reaction catalyzed by pyruvate kinase. The activity of PEPCK is closely coupled with that of pyruvate carboxylase. Whereas the pyruvate kinase reaction produces 1 ATP, the formation of PEP uses 2 ATPs: one in the mitochondria for the pyruvate carboxylase reaction and one in the cytosol for the PEPCK reaction. PEPCK requires GTP provided via the nucleoside diphosphate kinase reaction which uses ATP. ATP transfers one high-energy bond to GDP to form ADP and GTP.

The enzyme PEPCK has been studied extensively as scientists have tried to understand the gluconeogenic process. In starvation or uncontrolled diabetes, PEPCK activity is elevated as is gluconeogenesis. Starvation elicits a number of catabolic hormones that serve to mobilize tissue energy stores as well as precursors for glucose synthesis. Uncontrolled diabetes elicits similar hormonal responses. In both instances, the synthesis of the PEPCK enzyme protein is increased. Unlike other rate limiting enzymes, PEPCK is not regulated allosterically or by phosphorylation-dephosphorylation mechanisms. Instead, it is regulated by changes in gene transcription of its single-copy gene from a single promoter site. This regulation is unique because all of the known factors (hormones, vitamins, metabolites) act all in the same place. They either turn on the synthesis of the messenger RNA for PEPCK or they turn it off. What is also unique is the fact that only liver and kidney cells translate this message into active enzyme protein which catalyzes PEP formation. Other cells and tissues have the code for PEPCK in their nuclear DNA but do not synthesize the enzyme. Instead, these cell types synthesize the enzyme which catalyzes glycerol synthesis. In effect, then, only the kidney and liver have active gluconeogenic processes.

The next few steps in gluconeogenesis are identical to those of glycolysis but are in the reverse direction. When the step for the dephosphorylation of fructose-1,6-bisphosphate occurs there is another energy barrier, and instead of a bidirectional reaction catalyzed by a single enzyme, there are separate forward and reverse reactions. In the synthesis of glucose, this reaction is catalyzed by fructose-1,6-bisphosphatase and yields fructose-6-phosphate. No ATP is involved but a molecule of water and an inorganic phosphate are produced. Rising levels of fructose-2,6-bisphosphatase allosterically inhibits gluconeogenesis while it stimulates glycolysis. AMP likewise inhibits gluconeogenesis at this step.

Lastly, the removal of the phosphate from glucose-6-phosphate via the enzyme complex glucose-6-phosphatase completes the pathway to yield free glucose. Again, this is an irreversible reaction which does not involve ATP. The glucose-6-phosphate moves to the endoplasmic reticulum where the phosphatase is located. Should there be a mutation in the gene for the translocation of glucose-6-phosphate to the endoplasmic reticulum or in its phosphatase, glucose cannot be released and hypoglycemia will result. This reaction is also used when glycogenolysis provides the phosphorylated glucose. In either instance, free glucose is not released to the circulation. The resultant disease is called Von Gierke's disease. In addition to hypoglycemia, this rare, autosomally recessive disease is characterized by an enlarged liver due to excess glycogen stores, elevated blood lipids, decreased sensitivity to insulin, brain damage, and a shortened life span. About 25% of all patients with some form of glycogen storage disease have Von Gierke's disease. Aside from providing many small meals throughout the day and night to prevent the hypoglycemia, there is little else that dietary maneuvers can achieve.

G. GLUCOSE HOMEOSTASIS

In the foregoing sections, each of the metabolic pathways involved in the use and production of glucose was discussed with the goal of providing a framework for understanding how the blood glucose level is maintained within very close limits. Soon after food is consumed, digested, and absorbed, the blood glucose levels rise. Glucose is a hydrophillic compound and can circulate freely in the bloodstream without the need for a special carrier. However, as a hydrophilic compound, it cannot penetrate the plasma membrane surrounding the cells of the body without help. The mechanism for glucose entry is dependent on the hormone insulin and on a special protein called the mobile glucose transporter. There are five different glucose transporters, called GLUT 1, 2, 3, 4, and 5. Some cell types have only one of these while others have more than one.

The transporters differ slightly in their structure and function with respect to the function of the tissues which contain them. Table 8 lists the transporters and their location. The glucose transporter is referred to as a mobile transporter because when it is not in use it is sequestered in an intracellular pool. When needed, it leaves its storage site, moves to the interior aspect of the plasma membrane, forms a loose bond with the membrane, picks up the glucose molecule, and moves it through the membrane into the cytosol whereupon the glucose can be phosphorylated and metabolized. Figure 20 illustrates how these transporters work when the recruitment of the transporter is responsive to insulin signaling.

The action of insulin is initiated when it binds to the plasma receptor. In the binding process, the transport form of insulin, proinsulin, is cleaved with the release of the C-peptide. The insulin receptor extends through the plasma membrane and has an intrinsic protein kinase as part of its structure. When insulin binds to the receptor, almost instantly autophosphorylation of the receptor occurs with phosphate groups from ATP attached to the exposed tyrosine residues. Phosphorylation of the tyrosine residues requires the movement of the calcium ion from its storage site on the endoplasmic reticulum. This mobilization of calcium occurs when phosphatidyl inositol triphosphate and diacylglycerol are produced from the membrane phospholipid, phosphatidylinositol. In turn, the diacylglycerol stimulates the temporary binding of Ca^{++} to the kinase to facilitate the phosphorylation of the tyrosine residues. All of these reactions result in a change in the phosphorylation state of the transporter in its storage site, facilitating its release and migration to the cell surface. This then, accomplishes the goal of moving the glucose from the bloodstream into the cell for its appropriate disposal.

Not all cells mobilize their glucose transporters under the influence of insulin. Some use a different mechanism. Brain cells are an example, as are the β cells in the islets of Langerhans in the pancreas. These cell types have stringent requirements for glucose as their principle

TABLE 8
Location of the Mobile Glucose Transporters

Transporter	Location
GLUT 1	Ubiquitous but found mainly in brain, placenta, and cultured cells. Is not particularly responsive to insulin regulation
GLUT 2	Liver, β cells of pancreas, kidney
GLUT 3	Ubiquitous in human tissue
GLUT 4	Adipose tissue, heart, skeletal muscle
GLUT 5	Small intestine

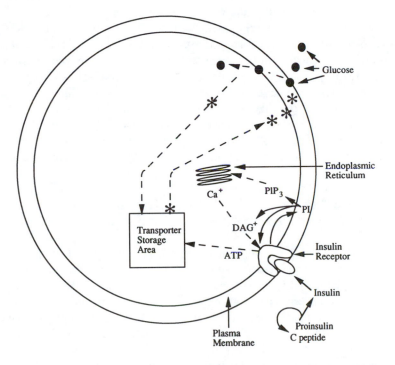

FIGURE 20. As blood glucose levels rise, the β cell of the pancreas releases insulin. Insulin binds to its receptor on the surface of the target cell and signals the release of the mobile glucose transporter from its storage site. The transporter migrates to the plasma membrane, picks up the glucose and transports it to the cytosol, whereupon it releases it.

metabolic fuel yet their use and transport of glucose is independent of insulin bound to a plasma membrane receptor. The presence of mobile glucose transporters has been ascertained by a number of scientists, yet their recruitment and the signals necessary for this recruitment are largely unknown.

As mentioned, insulin bound to its receptor on the plasma membrane is essential to the entry of glucose into insulin-dependent cells. When a person (or animal) consumes a glucose-rich food and that glucose appears in the bloodstream, the glucose stimulates the pancreatic β cells in the islets of Langerhans to release insulin. How the glucose transporter is recruited is not specifically known, but nonetheless, glucose enters the cytosol of the β cell via GLUT 2 and is phosphorylated to glucose-6-phosphate by the enzyme glucokinase. It is thought that this phosphorylation step provides the signal to the β cell to release insulin from its insulin store. Aberrations in pancreatic glucokinase result in impaired insulin release and subsequent impairment in the use of glucose. Again, exactly how this signal is generated is not known.

The PIP cycle is involved as is the tyrosine kinase and the calcium ion, but information is lacking on the specifics of the mechanism. The transport of glucose and subsequent release of insulin via the Golgi complex also involves the sodium and potassium ions and ATP.

As the blood glucose levels fall because of the insulin-stimulated use of this glucose, less glucose is transported into the β cell and thus less insulin is released. In turn, all of the various cells which use glucose will have less glucose to use as well as less insulin bound to its receptor signaling glucose use. In the fully fed state, insulin is the key to normal glucose oxidation or conversion to glycogen or fatty acids. However, in the absence of continuous feeding, the body must adjust its metabolism to ensure a continuous fuel supply. Other hormones now play key roles as the blood glucose falls. These hormones switch metabolism from glucose disposal to blood glucose maintenance. First they exert an anti-insulin action at insulin target cells. They interfere with the insulin-stimulated glucose uptake. In so doing, they promote insulin resistance. That is, the cells are resisting the positive effects of insulin on glucose uptake and oxidation via glycolysis. Second, these hormones provide signals that enhance glycogenolysis and gluconeogenesis to provide glucose to those cells that need it. The enhancement of glycogenolysis in the liver precedes that of gluconeogenesis since glycogen is more readily available than are the substrates for gluconeogenesis. In addition, glycogenolysis is energetically less expensive than is gluconeogenesis. Third, lipolysis and fatty acid oxidation are enhanced to provide energy and glycerol for glucose synthesis. All of these inhibitions and enhancements are coordinated so that the blood glucose level remains within the normal range of 80 to 120 mg/dl. Excursions above and below might occur briefly, but as soon as they appear, compensatory mechanisms are put into place to maintain overall glucose homeostasis.

VII. ABNORMALITIES IN THE REGULATION OF GLUCOSE HOMEOSTASIS: DIABETES MELLITUS

Just as we have learned about the details of glycogen synthesis and use through the study of genetic anomalies in this process, so too have we learned about the regulation of glucose homeostasis through the study of a large number of genetic errors which result in the disease, diabetes mellitus. Current estimates of the number of genetic mutations thought to be responsible for the development of this disease range from 20 to 100, depending on the definitions used for the disease. Approximately 5% of the total population in the U.S. carry one of these mutations and will at some time in their life span develop the disease.

Of the total population with diabetes mellitus, about 10% have the disease as a result of pancreatic insulin production failure while 90% develop the disease as a response to one or more failures in the target tissues: liver, muscle, or adipose tissue. This population difference is the basis for the division of the diseases into two broad types. Type I disease comprises the group of diseases that relate to the failure of the pancreas to produce sufficient insulin. This group is referred to as the insulin-dependent type of diabetes mellitus (IDDM). Type II disease refers to that group of diseases that develop in response to abnormalities in the target tissues. The latter group of diseases is called noninsulin-dependent diabetes mellitus (NIDDM).

Diabetes mellitus is characterized by defective glucose utilization. In its most severe form, the symptoms of excessive thirst, excessive urination, rapid weight loss and, perhaps, coma and death are observed. It is a disease that has been known for centuries, having been described in the medical writings of the ancient Greeks and Egyptians. Even then it was recognized that diet was an important factor in its development as was obesity.

Although diabetes is a collection of diseases arising for a variety of reasons, its diagnosis is based on the results of a glucose tolerance test. Examples of the results of this test are shown in Figure 21. Glucose tolerance in persons suspected of having diabetes mellitus is tested by giving the person a large dose (usually 1 g/kg body weight) of glucose and monitoring the blood glucose level before and at 30-minute intervals after the glucose. Variations on the procedure have been developed for screening purposes. A single fasting blood sample may be examined for its glucose content, or a fasting plus a 2-hour post-meal blood sample may be examined, or the test may be 5 hours in duration rather than the usual 2 hours. The type of test for the presence of the disease is usually determined by the patient's symptoms and the family history. In normal nondiabetic fasted individuals, administration of a bolus of glucose elicits a typical rise then fall in blood glucose levels, as shown in Figure 21. In contrast, diabetic individuals may have an elevated fasting blood glucose level and may have a failure to appropriately reduce the glucose level after the test dose. Abnormal glucose tolerance is defined in several ways: there may be a departure from the normal fasting blood glucose level (80 to 120 mg/dl) and/or post-challenge values may be excessively high (exceeding 250 mg/dl) and/or fail to return to the pre-challenge blood glucose level by 120 minutes after the challenge. Blood insulin values may exceed normal in some individuals and this is interpreted as a sign of target tissue insulin resistance. These individuals are referred to as hyperinsulinemic. They may be hyperinsulinemic yet have normal blood glucose levels and normal glucose tolerance.

There are several variations in response to a glucose challenge and these will be discussed subsequently. However, because the use of glucose is critical to almost every cell in the body, any deviation in any of the many metabolic steps involved in its use must be included in the definition for diabetes mellitus. Table 9 lists the general categories of spontaneous mutations that have been identified as causes of diabetes mellitus.

A. IDDM: CONSEQUENCES OF INSULIN DEFICIENCY

Much of what has been learned about the consequences of IDDM has been due to the use in experimental animals of β islet cell cytotoxic agents. These agents destroy the insulin-producing islet cells, making it possible to study the acute and chronic responses to insulin deficiency. The literature on this aspect of diabetes research is voluminous. From it we have learned how insulin functions in the body.

Insulin deficiency characterized by high blood glucose levels results in the excessive thirst, urinary loss, and rapid body wastage so typical of severe IDDM. The body fat stores are raided, but because insulin is needed to complete fatty acid oxidation, this oxidation is incomplete. As a result, acetone, β-hydroxybutyrate, and acetoacetate, products of incomplete fatty acid oxidation, accumulate. These are the ketone bodies. Elevated blood levels of these ketones (ketonemia) are observed as is an elevated urinary excretion (ketonuria). Rising levels of ketones increase the need for buffering power since they tend to lower pH. Acidosis is a characteristic feature of diabetes. Not only are the fat stores raided, but so too is the body protein. Proteolysis (body protein breakdown) is enhanced and amino acids thus liberated are used for energy or as substrates for intracellular glucose synthesis. The ammonia released as a product of the deamination of these amino acids assists in the buffering of the accumulating ketones. However, this ammonia is in itself cytotoxic, so the body must increase its capacity to convert it to urea. Humans with uncontrolled diabetes thus are characterized by a loss in body protein, an increase in blood and urine levels of ammonia, an increase in urea synthesis, a negative nitrogen balance, a loss in fat store, elevated blood and urine levels of glucose, and elevated levels of fatty acid oxidation products. Some of these metabolic products are also excreted via the lungs in the expired air. The breath of an uncontrolled diabetic has the aroma of the ketones — somewhat like the aroma of fingernail polish remover.

1. Pancreatic β Islet Cell Failure

Several explanations for pancreatic insulin production failure have been offered. The two most generally accepted are (1) failure due to autoimmune disease, and (2) failure due to viral destruction of the islet β cells. In each of these instances, the genetic heritage of the individual plays a role. In both, the immune system is involved. In the former, the autoimmune disease, the insulin-producing pancreatic islet cell is destroyed because the immune system has sensed

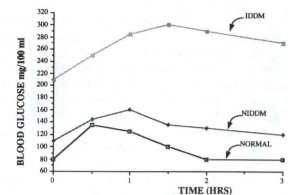

FIGURE 21. Typical glucose tolerance values for normal people and for people with either NIDDM or IDDM. Note that the normal response to a glucose challenge includes a rise followed by a fall in the blood glucose. The NIDDM patient may have a normal fasting blood glucose, but the rise following the challenge is greater than normal and the fall is barely perceptible. The patient with IDDM may have higher values at all time points. Within each group of subjects, however, there may be considerable variation.

TABLE 9
Abnormalities in Cells, Tissues, or Systems that are Associated with Diabetes Mellitus

Abnormality[a]	Result
T cell receptor (recognizes self antigen)	Autoimmune destruction of β cells
Inability to repel certain viruses	Viral destruction of β cells
Amino acid substitution in A or B chains of insulin	Major, minor or no effect on insulin activity
Amino acid substitution in C chain of proinsulin	No C chain cleavage to produce insulin
β Cell glucokinase	Inability to recognize the glucose signal for insulin release
Obesity	Distortion of fat cell membrane insulin receptor; tissue insensitivity to insulin
Insulin receptor protein	Defective structure fails to fully bind insulin to the target cell membrane and/or fails to send send signal to mobilize glucose transporters; tissue insensitivity to insulin
Mobile glucose transporters	Failure to move glucose into target cell
Intracellular enzymes	Failure to process glucose

[a] Within each of these disorders, several different mutations causing the same clinical state have been found.

the presence of an antigen which it recognizes not as a self-made protein but as a foreign protein. What this self antigen might be is not known, but as a result of the antigen-antibody reaction the insulin-producing β cells of the pancreatic islets are destroyed, and with this destruction the clinical symptoms of severe diabetes of the insulin-dependent type develop.

Epidemiologists have noted that, following epidemics of diseases such as flu (influenza), there are upsurges in the number of newly diagnosed people with diabetes. Not all people who contract flu develop IDDM nor have all people who develop IDDM had their disease preceded by flu. In some people, certain types of viral infections are followed by the development of IDDM. Laboratory studies using susceptible and nonsusceptible strains of mice and rats have likewise shown this series of events. It would appear that certain genes for the immune system have mutated such that the body is unable to repel certain of the viruses, and that these viruses in turn target the insulin-producing β cells of the pancreatic islets. Whereas most people have immunocompetent systems that protect their pancreas from such viral attack, some do not. In these people, if they are exposed to these viruses, IDDM results. If unexposed, they do not develop IDDM.

2. Autoimmune Disease

IDDM may be the result of autoimmune disease. Autoimmunity is characterized by an increase in the number of T cells. T cells, originating in the thymus, are a type of cell which is an essential component of the immune system. It recognizes internal antigens (self antigens) and produces antibodies to these antigens. In some instances, the recognition is nonspecific. That is, antibodies are raised to a group of related antigens. Serial evaluations of human, rat, and mouse pancreatic tissue have shown progressive autoimmunologically mediated destruction of the islet cells. Humans, if treated with the immunosuppressive drug, cyclosporin, early in the course of IDDM, will have their disease suppressed. Cyclosporin blocks the calcium-dependent pathways of T cell gene expression. T cell activation is initiated by the T cell receptor which recognizes an antigen on the correct histocompatibility complex on the surface of the antigen presenting cell. Transmission of this signal to the nucleus of the cell involves the calcium ion, a complex of related proteins, and the phosphatidylinositol cycle which is responsible for the movement of the calcium ion from the intracellular store to where it is needed. Cyclosporin blocks this calcium-mediated signaling system and in so doing blocks the T cell recognition of self antigens. This response to immunosuppression by cyclosporin gives clear indication of the involvement of the immune system in the pathophysiology of IDDM. Further evidence of the involvement of the immune system has included studies of the inheritance of the diabetic tendency and the inheritance of human leukocyte antigens (HLA) encoded by genes on the short arm of chromosome 6.

The HLA, A, B, and C genes are termed class 1 genes and encode antigens present in most cells. These antigens are important in T-cell recognition and in the rejection of aberrant cells. Aberrant cells can include cancerous cells, viral infected cells, or cells from allografts. It can also include certain self-cell types. Of interest is the fact that some years ago, scientists at the Jackson Laboratory, using traditional gene mapping techniques to identify the inheritance of the diabetic trait in the db/db mouse, reported that the diabetic trait in this mouse was carried on chromosome 6, the same chromosome that carries the codes for antigen recognition.

3. Diabetes Secondary to Viral Infections

Studies of the incidence of IDDM in human populations indicate that major increases in new cases have followed outbreaks of communicable viral diseases. Certain strains of mice likewise have been found to develop IDDM following exposure to two closely related viruses, the encephalomyocarditis virus and the Coxsackie B virus. Not all rodents, however, will respond to these viruses by developing IDDM. Some strains are responsive while others are not. This suggests a genetic determination of susceptibility to these infections that probably involves genes that code for the various components of the immune system. Such variability in the human population is also likely and explains why some humans may develop IDDM secondary to a viral infection while others do not. Notkins and co-workers have demonstrated that susceptibility is genetically determined. Viruses work by inserting their DNA into normal cells, thus converting them to an abnormal cell or causing the normal cell to destroy itself. If the person was susceptible, he/she would not be able to repel the virus and prevent its entry into the β cell. Fluorescein labeling of viral antibody has confirmed the entry of such viruses into the β cell. Evidence of virus-induced IDDM in man has been gathered through post-mortem studies of pancreatic tissue excised from children with fatal viral infections caused by a variety of viruses. Of 250 children studied, only 7 had a Coxsackie B infection and, of these, 4 had significant β cell destruction and evidence of acute or chronic inflammation in the islet tissue.

4. Genetic Errors in Insulin Structure

In addition to islet cell failure, the possibility exists that the islet cell may not be producing insulin in the appropriate amino acid sequence to have full biological activity. Insulin gene mutations have been documented in both humans and the mouse which result in a variety of amino acid substitutions and have a variety of effects on insulin action. Steiner et al., for example, studied a number of families with aberrant insulin genes. Ten families were studied that had single-point gene mutations that resulted in amino acid substitutions in the proinsulin molecule. Six of these substitutions resulted in the secretion of defective insulin molecules due to changes within the A or B chains. These changes resulted in molecules that were immunoreactive but did not bind to the plasma membrane insulin receptor site on the adipocyte. Four additional families were found to have insulin gene mutations which prevented the recognition of the C-peptide A chain dibasic cleavage site and its removal. These families had high levels of proinsulin in the blood because the C-peptide was not removed upon binding of the insulin to the receptor site. Proinsulin is the large insulin molecule released by the pancreas. When insulin reaches its target tissue, a fraction of this large molecule is split off. This fraction is called the C-chain or C-peptide. Proinsulin is 1/40th to 1/60th as active as insulin. The aberrant proinsulin molecule may have the appropriate β cell processing protease but not the appropriate C-peptide recognition site.

The variability of the insulin gene in a group of phenotypically normal individuals has been studied. Although several variants have been found, none were considered mutants. That is, the base pair substitutions that coded for specific amino acids in the insulin molecules were in places that did not affect the conformation of the molecule or the active site in the insulin molecule, nor did they affect the cleavage of proinsulin to active insulin. The variety of base pair substitutions and subsequent amino acid substitutions in the insulin molecule appears to be large, yet the impact of these aberrations (if they can be called aberrations) is very small or nonexistent. However, should substitutions occur that affect proinsulin cleavage or reactive sites in the insulin molecule, then diabetes would develop. Whether the diabetes is insulin-dependent or noninsulin-dependent would, as mentioned, depend on the nature of the defect.

Recently there has developed an hypothesis that islet cell failure is due to a mutation in the gene for glucokinase. Glucokinase is the enzyme that converts glucose to glucose-6-phosphate and this conversion is thought to signal insulin release. Aberrant glucokinase gene expression would mean that glucose as a potent stimulator for insulin release would not have this function. Several mutations in the glucokinase gene in the β cell have been found in humans. These mutations appear to be tightly linked to the development of NIDDM and result in a decrease in glucose phosphorylation. NIDDM rather than IDDM develops because nutrients other than glucose can act as secretogogues and the action of these nutrients on insulin release is independent of glucokinase activity. Several amino acids as well as several three-carbon metabolites can stimulate insulin release.

B. NIDDM: TARGET TISSUE DISEASE

The range of disorders in humans and laboratory animals that fit the description for NIDDM is far greater than that for IDDM. For most of the NIDDM disorders, obesity is a concurrent feature. This obesity either precedes or accompanies the development of abnormal glucose tolerance. The animals that are genetically obese usually overeat, and studies of the neuroendocrine influence on food intake have suggested that, in part, the genetic error in these animals may reside in the satiety signaling system in the brain. One feature of obesity that is common to NIDDM is the resistance of the peripheral fat cell to the effects of insulin. The plasma membrane receptor on the fat cell may be aberrant in structure or number. If abnormal in structure, insulin may not bind to it. This may occur either because the receptor protein is abnormal or because the fat cell is enlarged by its stored fat and the receptor structure is distorted. When the fat cell shrinks, i.e., when the obese person loses a large percentage of excess stored fat, insulin binding is normalized. Insulin binding, in this instance, is directly related to fat cell size, which in turn is directly related to the size of its fat store. The insulin resistance, thus observed, refers to the particular abnormality of the fat cell insulin receptor conferred upon it by its excess fat store.

Insulin resistance can, however, occur for other reasons, and it can occur in other cell types as well. By definition, insulin resistance means that it takes abnormally large amounts of insulin to regulate or control blood glucose within normal limits. A person with insulin resistance may not develop abnormal glucose tolerance *if* the pancreas is able to sustain an abnormally high insulin output. In this circumstance, the individual may be insulin resistant and hyperinsulinemic, but not hyperglycemic or have abnormal glucose tolerance. Eventually, the islet β cells may not be able to sustain this high insulin output and the insulin resistance will then progress to abnormal glucose tolerance and subsequently to the diabetic hyperglycemic state. Insulin resistance may be a feature of the fat cell, and/or the muscle cell, and/or the liver cell, and in each instance genetic errors in the DNA which code for this particular plasma membrane structure have been found. Insulin receptors have been isolated and their structures analyzed and sequenced. The part of the DNA that codes for these structures has been cloned. Making a cDNA clone allows the scientist to study the way the gene works and what happens if it mutates. It is generally agreed that the receptor is synthesized as a single polypeptide precursor of 1382 amino acids which contains a signal peptide of 27 amino acids, the α subunit of 735 amino acids (including four basic amino acids of the processing site), and the β subunit of 620 amino acids. After glycosylation, processing, and disulfide bonding, it is expressed as a heterotetramer composed of two α subunits with a molecular weight of 95,000. The α subunit is entirely located on the exterior aspect of the plasma membrane while the β subunit extends through the plasma membrane into the cytoplasm. The human insulin receptor gene is located on chromosome 19. It consists of 22 exons which span 120 kb. The α subunit is encoded by the first 120 kb and includes a signal peptide, an insulin binding region, and a cysteine-rich region. The β subunit is encoded by the last 30 kb. As mentioned, this subunit is the portion of the receptor molecule that crosses the plasma membrane. It has a proreceptor processing site and the final portion of the unit of the receptor molecule consists of tyrosine kinase. When insulin binds to the α subunit, autophosphorylation occurs, resulting in activation of tyrosine kinase. If the DNA coding for the receptor protein has mutated such that lysine, an important amino acid for ATP binding and receptor activity, is replaced by arginine, alanine, or methionine, the receptor is no longer able to mediate insulin action. Thus, lysine is a critical component of the 1030 ATP binding site. Clusters of tyrosine residues are also critical to the autophosphorylation process. If tyrosine is replaced by phenylalanine, again, receptor activity is compromised. Other mutations in the code for the receptor protein which affect its amino acid sequence have been reported. These mutations (depending on their location) likewise can affect the activity of the receptor and, in turn, can explain insulin resistance.

C. MOBILE GLUCOSE TRANSPORTERS

Insulin resistance can also be attributed to post-receptor defects. Errors in the codes for the mobile glucose transporter (called GLUT 1,2,3,4 and 5) have received considerable attention, especially as these errors may relate to the development of obesity. These are summarized in Table 10. Peripheral glucose uptake may be impaired if the mobile glucose transporter (GLUT 4) in the adipocyte is aberrant. An aberrant adipocyte transporter would result in less insulin-stimulated glucose uptake by these cells with the result of increased levels of circulating glucose, which in turn would lead to hyperglycemia and hyperinsulinemia. Note the similarity of clinical features between this genetic error and the error described above that involves the gene for the insulin molecule. In both instances, one observes peripheral fat cell resistance together with compensatory increases in hepatic glycolysis, pentose shunt, glycogenesis, lipogenesis, hepatic lipid output, and adipocyte lipid uptake and storage. The compensatory increases in hepatic metabolism are probably driven by both the hyperinsulinemia,

TABLE 10
Aberrant Mobile Glucose Transports and Their Consequences

Protein	Consequences of an error
GLUT 1	Minimal changes in glucose uptake by all tissues that use glucose
GLUT 2	Liver — glucose metabolic pathways suppressed; increased gluconeogenic activity
	β Cell — pancreas unresponsive to glucose stimulation; kidney - increased gluconeogenic activity
GLUT 3	Minimal changes in glucose uptake and metabolism
GLUT 4	Adipose tissue — decrease in glucose use by fat cell; compensatory increase in hepatic glucose use; increase in hepatic lipogenesis and lipid output; increase in hepatic glycogen store
	Heart, muscle — decrease in glucose use by muscle could be lethal if compensatory use of fatty acids and ketones is insufficient
GLUT 5	Small intestine — glucose uptake by intestinal cells is impaired. If diet is high in carbohydrates, osmotic diarrhea might result

with its effects on anabolic processes, and the hyperglycemia, which provides a continuous high level of substrate for these anabolic pathways.

Studies of obese diabetic Zucker (ZDF/drt) rats and obese diabetic A^{vy}/a mice have suggested that the substrate glucose may have regulatory properties with respect to the expression of the gene for the mobile glucose transporters in liver, muscle, and fat cells. This suggestion was based on the observation that alterations in GLUT 2 and/or GLUT 4 proteins were not associated with the obesity per se, but were secondary to severe hyperglycemia that was the result of the diabetic state. Incidentally, studies of GLUT 1 and GLUT 4 in adipocytes from normal rats showed that feeding a high-glucose diet increases GLUT 4 activity while feeding a high-fat diet isocalorically decreased GLUT 4 activity and increased GLUT 1 activity. These results indicated that the two transporters differed in their response to insulin and glucose. In normal nondiabetic rats, GLUT 1 activity is probably responsible for basal glucose uptake while GLUT 4 is under the control of insulin. When insulin levels are high, GLUT 4 activity is high, whereas GLUT 1 seems to be independent of the hormone but responsive to the nutritional state of the body. It also appears from studies of normal and genetically obese and/or diabetic animals that the multiplicity of glucose transporters, while seemingly redundant, comprise a "fail-safe" mechanism to ensure glucose disposal. Should one of the isoforms be aberrant because of a genetic error, there would be a backup transporter that could increase in activity to compensate for the genetically determined loss.

The study of dietary factors which affected GLUT 1 and GLUT 4 activity also provides some insight into the nature of nutrient-gene interactions that may explain NIDDM. As mentioned in the introduction, economic constraints, food rationing, and lifestyle choices can affect the time course and severity of NIDDM. Lifestyle choices include decisions about the quantity and composition of the food consumed as well as the level of physical activity. As indicated above, the diet composition can affect the recruitment of GLUT 1 and GLUT 4 transporters. If the NIDDM patient had an error in one or the other of these transporters, clearly, the choice of the diet would be critical in the disposal of glucose by the adipocyte and, in turn, critical to the regulation of glucose homeostasis. In addition, exercise has been shown to affect the regulation of glucose transport in skeletal muscle.

With exercise, the number of GLUT 4 transporters increases, independent of insulin status. This explains the decrease in insulin need by diabetic athletes, an observation frequently made but poorly understood in practical terms. With exercise, the muscle uses glucose without the need for insulin bound to the receptor. Insulin is thus not needed for the recruitment and translocation of GLUT 4 transporters. With this in mind, if NIDDM develops as a result of an error in the insulin receptor, then exercise will promote glucose use and facilitate the reduction in blood glucose. If the person thus includes daily exercise and avoids high energy and/or high carbohydrate diets, then the phenotypic expression of the genotype for either a receptor or transporter error might be postponed or avoided. In turn, one can understand why the incidence of NIDDM decreases with restricted food supplies and increases in physical activity as happens during times of economic duress or war.

While all of the above-described mutations can lead to abnormal glucose tolerance and, in some people, many of the secondary problems associated with diabetes, diabetes mellitus itself can be a secondary problem as a result of other diseases. While these diseases have not been discussed in detail, the reader should be aware of their occurrence. Lead toxicity, for example, results in damage to the pancreas and, subsequently, to glucose intolerance. Other toxicities can have similar effects. Diseases of other endocrine organs, especially those producing counter-insulin hormones, likewise will result in characteristic changes in glucose tolerance. In this category are diseases of the adrenal cortex (Cushing's disease or excess cortisol release), or tumors in the brain which result in excess ACTH production, or diseases which result in excess growth hormone release or excess glucagon release, or diseases of the thyroid gland which impair thyroxin release. All of these diseases result in hormonal imbalance, peripheral insulin resistance, and subsequently affect insulin action. When these diseases are treated successfully, frequently the diabetic characteristic disappears. Sometimes, if the primary disease goes too long without treatment, irreversible changes in the pancreas and target tissues occur. Whether there are genetically determined reasons for these other endocrine diseases is not known. Generally speaking, relative to the incidence of diabetes mellitus, these other endocrine diseases are rare. So too are the instances of heavy metal intoxication. Nonetheless, no discussion of diabetes mellitus in its many forms would be complete without their mention.

VIII. OTHER HEALTH CONCERNS IN CARBOHYDRATE NUTRITION

Already discussed are the genetic errors in glycolysis, shunt activity gluconeogenesis, and glycogen turnover. These are summarized in Table 11. Few of these affect large numbers of people and few can be managed successfully to normalize health and life span. In addition, the dietary and nondietary aspects of the many forms of diabetes mellitus have been presented. In the present section, attention to other issues of importance to carbohydrate nutrition will be given. These are related to the intake of nondigestible fiber, lactose, and alcohol.

A. FIBER

A number of years ago, several scientists noticed that populations whose traditional diets were rich in fibrous food had low incidences of colon cancer as well as heart disease and diabetes mellitus. They compared these diets to those typically consumed by people in the U.S. and Europe and suggested that the health status of these populations was related to their high-fiber diets. With the consumption of high-fiber diets, the feces were bulkier, more moist, and more frequent than when low-fiber diets were consumed. These reports attracted a lot of attention and a plethora of high-fiber foods appeared in the market place. People began to consume these products in the hopes of having similar benefits conferred. Just as a single prescription from the drugstore cannot cure all diseases, the same can be said about a dietary change with respect to colon cancer, heart disease, and diabetes mellitus.

Dietary fiber refers to those carbohydrates that are indigestible and unabsorbed. The component glucose moieties are joined by β linkages rather than α linkages. They may also contain additional substituents, but their chief characteristic is that of nondigestibility by the α-amylases of the mammalian gastrointestinal system. These nondigestible carbohydrates are plant products and fall into five major categories: celluloses, hemicelluloses, lignins, pectins, and gums. The celluloses, hemicelluloses, and lignin provide bulk to the gastrointestinal contents due to their property of absorbing water. The increased bulkiness of the gut contents

TABLE 11
Inherited Disorders of Carbohydrate Metabolism

Process	Disease	Enzyme	Symptoms
Digestion	Lactose intolerance	Lactase	Chronic or intermittent diarrhea, flatulence, nausea, vomiting, growth failure in young children
	Sucrose intolerance	Sucrase	Diarrhea, flatulence, nausea, poor growth in infants
Intestinal transport	Glucose-galactose intolerance	Glucose-galactose carrier	Diarrhea, growth failure in infants, stools contain large quantities of glucose and lactic acid
Interconversion of sugars	Galactosemia	Galactose-1-P-uridyl	Increased cellular content of galactose-1-phosphate, eye cataracts, mental retardation, increased cellular levels of galactitol
		Galactokinase	Cataracts, cellular accumulation of galactose and galactitrol
		Galactoepimerase	No severe symptoms
	Fructosemia	Fructokinase	Fructosuria, fructosemia
		Fructose-1-P-aldolase	Hypoglycemia, vomiting after fructose load, fructosemia, fructosuria; in children: poor growth, jaundice, hyperbilirubinemia, albuminuria, amino-aciduria
		Fructose-1,6-diphosphatase	Hypoglycemia, hepatomegaly, poor muscle tone, increased blood lactate levels
	Pentosuria	NADP-lined xylitol dehydrogenase	Elevated levels of xylose in urine
Glucose catabolism	Hemolytic anemia	Glucose-6-phosphate dehydrogenase	Low erythrocyte levels of NADPH, hemolysis of the erythrocyte
		Pyruvate kinase	Nonspherocytic anemia, accumulation of phosphorylated glucose metabolites in the cell, jaundice in newborn
	Type VII glycogenosis	Phosphofructokinase	Intolerance to exercise, elevated muscle glycogen levels, accumulation of hexose monophosphates in muscle
Gluconeogenesis	Von Gierke's disease (Type I glycogenosis)	Glucose-6-phosphatase	Hypoglycemia, hyperlipemia, brain damage in some patients, excess liver glycogen levels, shortened life span, increased glycerol utilization
Glycogen synthesis	Amylopectinosis (Type IV glycogenosis)	Branching enzyme Liver amylot (1,4→1,6)-trans-glucosidase	Tissue accumulation of long-chain glycogen that is poorly branched, intolerance to exercise
Glycogenolysis	Pompe's disease (Type II glycogenosis)	Lysosomal α-1,4-glucosidase (acid matase) Amylo-1,6-glucosidase (debranching enzyme)	Generalized glycogen excess in viscera, muscles, and nervous system, extreme muscular weakness, hepatomegaly, enlarged heart
	Forbe's disease (Type III glycogenosis)	Muscle phosphorylase	Tissue accumulation of highly branched, short-chain glycogen, hyperglycemia, acidosis, muscular weakness, enlarged heart
	McArdle's disease (Type V glycogenosis)	Liver phosphorylase Phosphorylase kinase	Intolerance to exercise
	Her's disease (Type VI glycogenosis)		Hepatomegaly, increased liver glycogen content, elevated serum lipids, growth retardation
	Type IX glycogenosis		Hepatomegaly, increased liver glycogen levels, decreased phosphorylase activity in hepatocytes and leukocytes, elevated blood lipids, hypoglycemia after prolonged fasting, increased gluconeogenesis

stimulates peristalsis and results in shorter passage time and more frequent defecation. In addition to its water-holding property, fibers of the lignin type adsorb cholesterol, aiding in its excretion in the feces. Pectins and gums also influence gastric emptying, but in the opposite direction. These fiber types form gels that slow gastric emptying and slow the digestion and absorption of sugars, starches, and also fats. As a result of these actions, the fibers collectively help to lower the level of serum cholesterol while increasing its excretion. It is for these reasons nutritionists encourage the consumption of fiber-rich plant foods. Fruits are good sources of pectin, while cereal grains and the woody parts of vegetables are good sources of the celluloses, hemicelluloses, and lignins. Dried beans and oats are good sources of gums. The inclusion of foods containing all of these fiber types will no doubt be of benefit with respect to intestinal transit time and may also result in a small decrease in cholesterol absorption. This may have some impact on cholesterol balance. If fiber increases cholesterol excretion and reduces cholesterol recirculation, a small decrease in serum cholesterol level may occur. However, since cholesterol synthesis may rise to compensate for decreased absorption and reabsorption, the net effect with respect to cardiovascular disease development may be minor.

The increased transit speed of high-fiber diets may be of benefit to those people susceptible to colon cancer. The fiber not only adsorbs cholesterol and hastens its excretion, but also adsorbs potentially noxious components of the ingesta, hastening their excretion as well. Thus, carcinogenic compounds have less time for exposure to colon cells and thus less opportunity to convert a normal cell to a cancer cell.

Lastly, as with all comparisons of population groups, one must be careful in the interpretation of the data. Yes, a certain primitive group has less degenerative disease than we do in the U.S. and yes, the diet contains more fiber. Is this a cause and effect scenario? No, it is not. The picture is incomplete without observations on the incidence of other diseases, the average life span, the availability of clean water, immunizations, medical care, and observations on other aspects of life style that can affect disease development.

B. LACTOSE

Lactose, the primary carbohydrate in milk, provides about 40% of the total energy consumed by the newborn infant. The utilization of lactose to provide energy or to provide galactose for the formation of important neural tissue components involves the enzyme lactase. In its absence, lactose is not digested and acts as an osmotic agent, stimulating peristalsis with the clinical symptoms of flatulence, bloating, cramps, malaise, and diarrhea.

Whether lactase deficiency is a congenital error or not is subject to much discussion. In populations that traditionally consume large quantities of milk and milk products, the incidence of lactose intolerance is low. However, when diets contain little milk, lactase deficiency is prevalent. Lactase deficiency has been assessed by a lactose tolerance test or by jejunal biopsies or by both techniques. Lactose intolerance, when assessed by the lactose tolerance test alone, may also include individuals with genetic errors in galactose metabolism.

Lactase deficiency has been reported in 55% of Mexican-American males, 73.8% of adult Mexicans from rural Mexico, 44.7% of Greeks, 56% of Cretans, and 66% of Greek Cypriots, 68.8% of North American Jews, 50% of Indian adults and 20% of Indian children, 45% of Negro children in the U.S., 80% of Alaskan Eskimos, and is greater in Oriental adults compared with Caucasian adults. Current evidence indicates that lactose intolerance is more common than lactose tolerance. Notable exceptions to these observations are Caucasians of Scandinavian or Northern European background. These populations have less than 5% with lactose intolerance and traditionally consume diets containing large amounts of milk and milk products.

Lactose intolerance appears to be age related. Prevalence of lactose intolerance is greater in adult populations than in populations of children, suggesting that if there is a genetic tendency toward lactase deficiency, this tendency may be modified by such environmental factors as milk availability, sanitation, adequacy of diet with respect to essential nutrients, and the presence of parasites. That lactose intolerance does not appear until after weaning and is related to milk drinking or avoidance, suggests that high milk consumption may be a stimulus for prolonging lactase activity in the mucosal brush border during the postweaning period. Genetic studies of lactose intolerant families suggest that true lactase deficiency is an autosomal recessive trait.

Therapy for lactose intolerant individuals consists simply of restricting lactose intakes. Some individuals tolerate fermented products such as yogurt and cheese fairly well, while varying amounts of milk or ice cream induce the typical symptoms of diarrhea and flatulence.

C. ETHANOL

Alcoholic beverages have been consumed by humans since the dawn of history. They have been used to ease anxiety, promote social interaction, and as a vehicle to dominate others. Ethanol, the alcohol in beverages, is the quantitative end product of yeast glycolysis. Small amounts can be synthesized in mammalian cells. Thus, ethanol is a drug, a food, and a metabolite. It has been estimated that upward to 90 million Americans consume alcoholic beverages every day and that about 10% of these people are addicted to its consumption. This affliction is called alcoholism.

Alcoholism is truly a disease that is a result of a nutrient-gene interaction. The nutrient in this instance is alcohol; the gene is as yet unidentified. Although unidentified, there is ample evidence in the literature that supports the concept that the tendency toward alcoholism is inherited. Studies of twins reared by adoptive parents as well as studies of multigeneration families give support to this idea. An alcoholic is more likely than a nonalcoholic to have an alcoholic relative. At least 33% of alcoholics have an alcoholic parent. This has been observed in adopted individuals where the biological parent was unknown to the alcoholic and so the parent's proclivities were not taught. Studies of monozygotic (identical) twins and dizygotic (fraternal) twins indicated a high degree of concordance for alcoholism. If one twin became an alcoholic, the other twin also became one if that twin chose to consume alcohol. The concordance was greater in the identical twins than in the fraternal twins. While scientists agree on the heritable nature of alcoholism, no one gene or group of genes has been identified and found culpable for the disorder.

Ethanol, once consumed, is rapidly absorbed by simple diffusion. The diffusion is affected by the amount of alcohol consumed, the regional blood flow, the surface area, and the presence of other foods. The different segments of the gastrointestinal tract absorb ethanol at different rates. Absorption is fastest in the duodenum and jejunum, slower in the stomach, ileum, and colon, and slowest in the mouth and esophagus. The rate of absorption by the duodenum depends on gastric emptying time, which in turn depends on the kinds and amounts of foods consumed with the ethanol. Certain drugs may also influence gastric emptying time and thus influence absorption. Complete absorption may vary from two to six hours. The type of beverage can influence ethanol absorption. Ethanol from beer is absorbed slower than that found in whisky, which is slower than gin and red wine, and of course pure ethanol is absorbed the fastest of all.

Once absorbed, ethanol is rapidly distributed between the intracellular and extracellular compartments. This is because ethanol is completely miscible in water and thus freely travels anyplace water travels. The uptake of ethanol by the fat depots is minimal. Ethanol crosses the plasma membranes, but in so doing, changes them. When ethanol is in contact with a protein, it denatures it. Thus, large and frequent ethanol exposures results in damage to proteins both within and around the cells. The most damaged tissue is the liver since ethanol is carried directly to this tissue via the portal blood. While gut cells are also damaged, these cells have such a rapid turnover time (less than seven days) that such damage due to intermittent ethanol consumption is not as long-lasting as happens in the liver. Liver cells, in

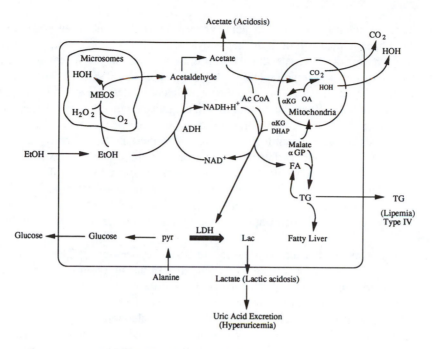

FIGURE 22.   Metabolism of ethanol by the hepatocyte.

contrast, have a longer half-life and once damaged do not repair as readily. Alcoholic liver disease is a major cause of death among those who drink heavily.

Ethanol diffuses from the blood to the alveolar air so the ethanol content of expired air bears a constant relationship to pulmonary arterial blood ethanol levels. The partition coefficient is 2100:1. This means that 2100 ml of expired air contains the same amount of ethanol as 1 ml of blood. If the blood contains 100 mg of ethanol, the expired air will contain 232 ppm. This is the basis for the breath tests of intoxication. Intoxication occurs at 150 mg/100 ml of blood, but most states prosecute drivers having blood levels exceeding 100 mg/dl.

Of the ethanol consumed, 90 to 98% is oxidized to carbon dioxide and water. The rest is excreted as ethanol in the breath or in the urine. The metabolism of ethanol is shown in Figure 22. This is in contrast to other metabolizable carbohydrates in that the rate of oxidation is fairly constant at about 10 to 20 mg/ml. This indicates that the first rate limiting reaction catalyzed by alcohol dehydrogenase is saturated at this level. This is a zero order reaction. The average rate at which alcohol can be metabolized is about 10 ml/hr (or 7 g/hr). The ethanol in 4 oz of whisky requires 5 to 6 hr to metabolize completely to CO_2 and water. One mole of ethanol requires 16 moles of ATP for its conversion to CO_2 and HOH.

While ethanol is distributed throughout the body, the liver is the chief site for its oxidation. As mentioned, the first rate limiting reaction is catalyzed by alcohol dehydrogenase and converts ethanol to acetaldehyde. Acetaldehyde is quite damaging to cellular proteins and part of the hepatic injury found in alcoholics is due to this metabolite. It binds covalently to protein, impairs the microtubular assembly and the mitochondrial respiratory chain, depletes pyridoxine supplies, stimulates inappropriate collagen synthesis, and inhibits DNA repair. Acetaldehyde is also produced when ethanol is metabolized by the microsomal ethanol oxidizing system (MEOS). This system uses peroxide (H_2O_2) and produces a molecule of water as well as the acetaldehyde. The acetaldehyde is converted to acetate which can either be joined with a CoA or released to the circulation. If too much acetate is released, acidosis develops. Acetyl CoA can either be used for fatty acid synthesis or be shuttled into the mitochondria via carnitine to be oxidized as through the citric acid cycle. A fatty liver typifies the alcoholic. The fatty liver may progress to alcoholic hepatitis, to cirrhosis, liver failure, and death. The fatty liver is due to accelerated hepatic fatty acid synthesis as well as due to an ethanol-induced impairment in hepatic lipid output. If the hepatocyte accumulates too much lipid, the cell will burst and die. Areas of dead tissue within the liver is known as cirrhosis. When too much tissue dies, the liver may cease to function and the alcoholic dies.

In addition to the direct effects of ethanol on cell function, there are a number of auxiliary health concerns related to ethanol consumption. In the person who consumes large quantities of ethanol, their needs for thiamin, niacin, pyridoxine, and pantothenic acid increase dramatically. The alcoholic frequently manifests symptoms of beriberi, pellagra, and other deficiency diseases. In part, this is due to the increased need for these vitamins when ethanol is metabolized and in part because alcoholics may choose to consume alcoholic beverages in preference to nourishing food. Those alcoholics who continue to eat nourishing food in addition to consuming ethanol do not develop overt deficiency diseases as frequently. Nonetheless, the nutritionist should be aware of ethanol-induced increases in the needs for the B vitamins.

Lastly, there is another concern with respect to ethanol consumption. That is the development of fetal malformations in women who drink ethanol during pregnancy. In 1973, eight cases of unrelated children were described having similar congenital defects. Particularly noticeable were the facial malformations involving eye placement and nose and mouth development. All of these children had mothers who were alcoholic. In a subsequent report, it was noted that alcoholism in mothers was associated with an increased incidence of spontaneous abortions, premature delivery of fetuses who were poorly developed for their gestational age, and infants born with respiratory distress syndrome. Many of these children failed to grow and develop normally with full intellectual capacity. Various learning disabilities (partial hearing or visual loss) also characterized these children. How the ethanol affects fetal development, particularly the development of the central nervous system, is not known. Yet, awareness of the potential damage of ethanol to the developing embryo and fetus would dictate abstinence prior to and during the gestational period.

IX. CARBOHYDRATE REQUIREMENTS

Carbohydrates are not considered to be essential nutrients aside from their use as providers of energy. As discussed in Section VI.E, the body can usually synthesize sufficient glucose to sustain its absolute need for this fuel. Those cells that require other of the monosaccharides likewise can synthesize them. The mammary gland, for example, can convert glucose to galactose (see Figure 12) and use it to make the milk sugar lactose. The seminal vesicles likewise can isomerize glucose to fructose (see Figure 11) to meet its need for this particular monosaccharide. Thus, the traditional definition of nutrient essentiality is not met. The normal human, as well as members of other animal species, does not need to consume glucose in any set amount if synthesis is sufficiently active to meet the need and if the diet provides sufficient gluconeogenic precursors. It has been estimated that the average human uses about 125 g of glucose/day to sustain neural activity. If this glucose is supplied by gluconeogenesis, 40% will come from lipid precursors and 60% will come from protein components (see Table 8). As mentioned, this synthesis is very expensive with respect to the energy needed and, more importantly, with respect to the amount of dietary protein that must be consumed in order to support glucose synthesis. If no dietary carbohydrate is consumed, more than 155 g of protein (2 to 3 times the usual protein need) must be consumed to provide the 75 g of the 125 g glucose per day that is needed.

Are there circumstances where this is not true? Are there times when glucose serves a vital function that is in addition to its role as an energy provider? The answer to these questions is yes. Just as the growing child needs dietary histidine and arginine while the adult does not, the traumatized or septic patient needs glucose when otherwise this need could be met by gluconeogenesis.

In trauma or sepsis, the energy requirement is greatly increased (see Unit 3) because trauma or sepsis elicit a stress response. This stress response means an increase in levels of the catabolic hormones which are anti-insulin hormones as well as anti-inflammatory hormones. The stress hormones mobilize the body protein and fat stores to provide the means for repair of the injured tissues. When this catabolic response is prolonged (days to weeks), it must be reversed or the patient could die if his/her protein and energy stores are insufficient to sustain the prolonged mobilization. If sufficient glucose is provided in a hypertonic solution via a central vein such as the subclavian, it can reverse this catabolic response. This treatment is called parenteral nutrition. This will minimize the loss in body muscle mass. The effect of this hypertonic solution of glucose is to overcome (through mass action) the anti-insulin effects of the catabolic hormones and thereby stimulate glycolysis and glycogenesis, and inhibit proteolysis and lipolysis.

The questions are how much carbohydrate (glucose) is needed to have the above effect and how long should glucose be provided at this high level? The estimates vary. If the liver is functioning normally, 50 to 80% of the energy intake should have the desired anticatabolic effect. This would mean a 5 to 30% increase over the usual carbohydrate intake of 45 to 55% of the total energy intake, presuming that the patient can and will eat. This is not always possible. The patient may be in a coma or have a broken jaw or the injury/sepsis may involve the gastrointestinal tract. In this instance, all of the needed nutrients including glucose must be supplied by the parenteral route. This creates other kinds of problems with respect to our knowledge about micronutrient needs in the absence of the protective role of the gastrointestinal system. Micromineral needs are especially difficult to manage under these circumstances. Humans need small amounts of most of these nutrients. If supplied in excess, a toxic state can develop.

With respect to the absolute amount of glucose that must be provided to the traumatized or septic patient, the estimates vary from 4 g/kg body weight (280 g/day/70 kg man) to 7 g/kg body weight (490 g/day/70 kg man). This would provide between 1120 to 1960 kcal from glucose per day. The period of administration of this high a level of glucose to achieve anticatabolism has been estimated to be from four days to two weeks. After this period, a more normal distribution of macronutrients may be more appropriate.

SUPPLEMENTAL READINGS

ARTICLES

Baily, D. L. and Horuk, R. (1988) The biology and biochemistry of the glucose transporter, *Biochem. Biophys. Acta,* 947:541–590.

Barnard, R. J. and Youngren, J. F. (1992) Regulation of glucose transport in skeletal muscle, *FASEB J.,* 6:3238–3244.

Beale, E. G., Clouthier, D. E., and Hammer, R. E. (1992) Cell-specific expression of cytosolic phosphoenolpyruvate carboxykinase in transgenic mice, *FASEB J.,* 6:3330–3337.

Bowman, B. A., Forbes, A. L., White, J. S., and Glinsman, W. H., Eds. (1993) Health effects of dietary fructose, *Am. J. Clin. Nutr.,* 58:721S–823S (Special issue).

Chiu, K. C., Tanizawa, Y., and Permutt, M. A. (1993) Glucokinase gene variants in the common form of NIDDM, *Diabetes,* 42:579–582.

Devor, E. J. and Cloninger, C. R. (1989) Genetics of alcoholism, *Ann. Rev. Genet.,* 23:19–39.

Elwyn, D. H. and Bureztein, S. (1993) Carbohydrate metabolism and requirements for nutritional support, *Nutrition,* 9:50–66; 164–175; 255–267.

Goering, H. K. and van Soest, J. P. (1970) Forage fiber analysis. Agriculture Handbook No. 379, Agriculture Research Service, U. S. Department of Agriculture, Washington, D.C.

Gould, G. W. and Bell, G. I. (1990) Facilitative glucose transporters: an expanding family, *TIBS,* 15:18–23.

Hoek, J. B., Thomas, A. P., Rooney, T. A., Higashi, K., and Rubin, E. (1992) Ethanol and signal transduction, *FASEB J.,* 6:2386–2396.

Jensen, B. A., Rosenberg, H. S., and Notkins, A. L. (1980) Postmortem tissue changes in children with fatal viral infections, *Lancet,* 2:354–358.

Joost, H. G. and Weber, T. M. (1989) The regulation of glucose transport in insulin sensitive cells, *Diabetologia,* 32:831–838.

Kahn, B. B. and Pedersen, O. (1992) Tissue specific regulation of glucose transporters in different forms of obesity, *Proc. Soc. Exp. Biol. Med.,* 200:214–217.

Lieber, C. S. (1993) Herman Award Lecture, 1993. A personal perspective on alcohol, nutrition and the liver, *Am. J. Clin. Nutr.,* 58:430–442.

Makino, H., Taire, M., Shimada, F., Hasimoto, N., Suzuki, Y., Nozaki, O., Hatanaka, Y., and Yoshida, S. (1992) Insulin receptor gene mutation: A molecular and functional analysis, *Cell. Signaling,* 4:351–363.

McCrane, R. A., Widdowson, E. M., and Shackelton, L. B. (1936) The nutritive value of fruits, vegetables, and nuts, Medical Research Council Special Report Series No. 213, London.

Nandan, S. D. and Beale, E. G. (1992) Regulation of phosphoenolpyruvate carboxykinase mRNA in mouse liver, kidney, and fat tissues by fasting, diabetes and insulin, *Lab. Anim. Sci.,* 42:473–477.

Nordlie, R. C., Bode, A. M., and Foster, J. D. (1993) Recent advances in hepatic glucose 6 phosphatase regulation and function, *Proc. Soc. Exp. Biol. Med.,* 203:274–285.

Olansky, L., Janssen, R., Welling, C., and Permutt, M. A. (1992) Variability of the insulin gene in American Blacks with NIDDM, *Diabetes,* 41:742–749.

Sharp, S. C. and Diamond, M. P. (1993) Sex steroids and diabetes, *Diabetes Rev.,* 1:318–342.

Short, M. K., Clouthier, D. E., Schaefer, I. M., Hammer, R. E., Magnuson, M. A., and Beale, E. G. (1992) Tissue specific, developmental, hormonal and dietary regulation of rat phosphoenolpyruvate carboxykinase-human growth hormone fusion genes in transgenic mice, *Mol. Cell. Biol.,* 12:1007–1020.

Smith, G. N., Patrick, J., and Sinervo, K. R. (1991) Effects of ethanol exposure on the embryo-fetus: experimental considerations, mechanisms, and the role of prostaglandins, *Can. J. Physiol. Pharmacol.,* 69:550–569.

Southgate, D. A. T. (1969) Determination of carbohydrates in food. II. Unavailable carbohydrates, *J. Sci. Food Agric.,* 20:331.

Steiner, D. F., Tager, H. S., Chan, S. J., Nanjo, K., Sanke, T., and Rubenstein, A. H. (1990) Lessons learned from molecular biology of insulin gene mutations, *Diabetes Care,* 13:600–609.

Stoffel, M., Froguel, P. H., Takeda, J., Zouali, H., Vionnet, N., Nishi, S., Weber, I. T., Harrison, R. W., Pilkis, S. J., Lesage, S., Vaxillaire, M., Velho, G., Sun, F., Iris, F., Passa, P. H., Cohen, D., and Bell, G. I. (1992) Human glucokinase gene: isolation, characterization, and identification of two missense mutations linked to early onset-non insulin-dependent (type 2) diabetes mellitus, *Proc. Natl. Acad. Sci. U.S.A.,* 89:7689–7702.

Thacker, S. B., Veech, R. L., Vernon, A. A., and Rutstein, D. D. (1984) Genetic and biochemical factors relevant to alcoholism, *Clin. Exp. Res.,* 8:375–383.

van Soest, P. J. and McQueen, R. W. (1973) The chemistry and estimation of fibre, *Proc. Nutr. Soc.,* 32(1936):123.

Yoon, J.-W., Austin, M., Onodera, T., and Notkins, A. L. (1979) Virus induced diabetes mellitus. Isolation of a virus from the pancreas of a child with diabetic ketoacidosis, *N. Engl. J. Med.,* 300:1173–1179.

BOOKS

Bjorntorp, P. and Brodoff, B. N. (Eds.) (1962) *Obesity,* J. B. Lippincott Co., Philadelphia, 805 pages.

Dickens, F., Randle, P. J., and Whelan, W. J. (Eds.) (1968) *Carbohydrate Metabolism and its Disorders,* Academic Press, New York, 105 pages.

Ellenberg, M. and Rifkin, H. (Eds.) (1985) *Diabetes Mellitus, Theory and Practice,* 3rd ed., Medical Examination Publishing Co., New Hyde Park, NY, 1105 pages.

Leiter, E. H. and Wilson, G. L. (1988) Viral interactions in pancreatic β cells. In: *Pathology of the Endocrine Pancreas* (Ripeleers, D. and Lefebore, P., Eds.), Springer-Verlag, New York, pp 8–105.

Magnuson, M. A. and Jetton, T. L. (1993) Tissue specific regulation of glucokinase. In: *Nutrition and Gene Expression* (Berdanier, C. D. and Hargrove, J. L., Eds.), CRC Press, Boca Raton, FL, pp. 143–167.

Marble, A., Krall, L. P., Bradley, R. F., Christlieb, A. R., and Soeldner, J. S. (1985) *Joslin's Diabetes Mellitus,* Lea & Febiger, Philadelphia, 1007 pages.

Notkins, A. L., Yoon, J. W., Onodera, T., Toniolo, A., and Jenson, A. B. (1981) Virus-induced diabetes mellitus. In: *Perspectives in Virology XI* (Pollard, M., Ed.), Alan R. Liss, Inc., New York, pp 141–162.

Shafrir, E. and Renold, A. E. (Eds.) (1988) *Frontiers in Diabetes. Lessons from Animal Diabetes II,* Vol. III, John Libby, London, 682 pages.

Shallenberger, R. S. and Birch, G. G. (1975) *Sugar Chemistry,* Avi Publishing Co., Westport, CT.

Sipple, H. L. and McNutt, K. W. (Eds.) (1974) *Sugars in Nutrition,* Academic Press, New York, 768 pages.

LIPIDS

TABLE OF CONTENTS

I. INTRODUCTION

The lipids comprise the third macronutrient group. The lipids are calorically more dense than carbohydrate, having 9 kcal/g. Americans consume approximately 32 to 42% of their total calories as fat. The lipids comprise a group of compounds which, in general, are insoluble in water and soluble in such solvents as diethyl ether, carbon tetrachloride, hot alcohol, chloroform, and benzene. They are present in various amounts in all living mammalian cells. Nerve cells and adipose cells are rich in lipid; muscle cells and epithelial cells have considerably less.

In addition to being a very important source of energy, lipids serve a variety of other needs. They perform a basic role in the structure and function of biological membranes. In the body, they are the precursors of several hormones and serve as important cellular signals. They help to regulate the uptake and excretion of nutrients by the cell. Each cell has a characteristic lipid content.

II. CLASSIFICATION

Lipids, as has been mentioned, have the property of being: (1) relatively insoluble in water; and (2) relatively soluble in such solvents as ether, chloroform, benzene, and some alcohols. Additionally, some lipids are saponifiable; others are not. Saponifiable lipids, when treated with alkali, undergo hydrolysis at the ester linkage resulting in the formation of an alcohol and a soap. Triacylglycerol (triglyceride), for example, when treated with sodium hydroxide is hydrolyzed, yielding a mixture of soaps and free glycerol. Traditionally, saponifiable lipids have been classified into three groups, each with subgroups.

Simple lipids: esters of fatty acids with various alcohols.

1. Fats: esters of fatty acids with glycerol (acylglycerols).
2. Waxes: esters of fatty acids with long chain alcohols.
3. Cholesterol esters.

Compound lipids: esters of fatty acid which contain chemical groups in addition to fatty acids and alcohol.

1. Phospholipids: esters of fatty acids, alcohol, a phosphoric acid residue, and usually an amino alcohol, sugar, or other substituent.
2. Glycolipids: esters of fatty acids which contain carbohydrates and nitrogen (but not phosphoric acid) in addition to fatty acids and alcohol.
3. Lipoproteins: loose combinations of lipids and proteins.

Derived lipids: substances derived from the above groups by hydrolysis. They are the results of saponification.

Two other terms that are frequently used in the classification of lipids (but are not a division of the system just described) are neutral and polar lipids. Neutral lipids are uncharged lipids and include triacylglycerols (also called triglycerides), cholesterol, and cholesterol esters. Polar lipids have positive and negative charges on certain atoms of the molecule. Examples of these are the phospholipids which comprise the cell membrane. Phosphatidyl inositol, phosphatidyl choline, and phosphatidyl ethanolamine are membrane phospholipids and are polar.

III. STRUCTURE AND NOMENCLATURE OF SAPONIFIABLE LIPIDS

A. SIMPLE LIPIDS

1. Fatty Acids

Fatty acids are carboxylic acids. They have a polar group (the carboxyl group) at one end, and a methyl group at the other end. A hydrocarbon chain is in the middle. Fatty acids can have as few as 4 carbon atoms or more than 20; however, chain lengths of 16 and 18 carbons are the most prevalent. There are usually an even number of carbon atoms (with no branching) in the chain. The chain may be saturated (containing no double bonds) or unsaturated (containing one or more double bonds). Monounsaturated acids have one double bond; polyunsaturated acids have two or more.

Nomenclature of fatty acids is frequently confusing because the same fatty acid can have more than one name: its common (or trivial) name and its systematic name. The common name is rarely, if ever, related to the structure of the molecule. It is sometimes derived from the plant or animal source from which the acid was first isolated. The student has no choice but to memorize these names. Common names for nutritionally important fatty acids are given in Table 1.

The systematic method of naming fatty acids is based on a modification of the name of the straight chain hydrocarbon having the same number of carbon atoms. The final -*e* from the hydrocarbon name is removed and -*oic* added, followed by the word *acid*. To name the salt of the acid, the -*e* from the hydrocarbon base is replaced with -*ate*. For example, the saturated, 18-carbon hydrocarbon, $C_{18}H_{38}$, has as its systematic name *n*-octadecane (the *n* means normal or no branching); its saturated fatty acid counterpart is *n*-octadecan*oic acid* (its common name is stearic acid); the salt is *n*-octadecan*ate*. The monounsaturated 18-carbon is 9-octadecen*e*; one form of the unsaturated acid is *cis*-9-octadecan*oic acid* (common name, oleic acid). The salt is *cis*-9-octadecan*ate*.

In the systematic name it is possible to address each carbon atom (as was done in the last example just cited). There are two ways of doing this: with lower-case Greek letters or with Arabic numerals. With Greek letters the carbon adjacent to the carboxyl group is α (alpha), the next one is β (beta), and the last in the molecule is ω (omega). The carboxyl carbon is not given a designation. With Arabic numerals the carboxyl carbon is 1, the next carbon, 2, the next, 3, and so on. The number 9 in the above example means that a double bond exists between carbons 9 and 10.

Other conventions are also used to indicate the position of the double bond. In one of them $\Delta 9$ indicates a double bond between carbons 9 and 10. In another, the number of carbon atoms, the number of double bonds, and the position of each double bond are all clearly shown. For example, oleic acid is 18:1 $\Delta 9$, or *18* carbons with one double bond between the ninth and tenth carbon. Similarly, the 18-carbon acid with two double bonds is linoleic acid; in this system it would be referred to as 18:2 $\Delta 9$, 12. In yet another convention, the position of the double bond from the terminal carbon is indicated. The number of carbon atoms and the number of double bonds are shown as in the previous convention. The position of the double bond from the terminal carbon is then shown. For instance, oleic acid is 18:1ω9; linoleic acid is 18:2ω6. This convention is particularly useful in discussions about the interconversion of fatty acids; since carbon atoms are added between this double bond and the carboxyl group, it remains the terminal carbon.

As mentioned, fatty acids are either saturated or unsaturated. These two forms of fatty acids differ significantly in their structural considerations. In the saturated fatty acid, the hydrocarbon tail can exist in an infinite number of conformations because each carbon atom can rotate freely.

Unsaturated fatty acids, on the other hand, have a rigid feature to their structure because the carbons in the double bonds are not free to rotate; they exist as the *cis* or *trans* geometrical

TABLE 1
Structure and Names of Fatty Acids Found in Food

Structure	No. of carbons:double bonds	Systematic name	Trivial name	Source
Saturated Fatty Acids				
CH$_3$(CH$_2$)$_2$COOH	4:0	n-Butanoic	Butyric	Butter
CH$_3$(CH$_2$)$_4$COOH	6:0	n-Hexanoic	Caproic	Butter
CH$_3$(CH$_2$)$_6$COOH	8:0	n-Octanoic	Caprylic	Coconut oil
CH$_3$(CH$_2$)$_8$COOH	10:0	n-Decanoic	Capric	Palm oil
CH$_3$(CH$_2$)$_{10}$COOH	12:0	n-Dodecanoic	Lauric	Coconut oil, nutmeg, butter
CH$_3$(CH$_2$)$_{12}$COOH	14:0	n-Tetradecanoic	Myristic	Coconut oil
CH$_3$(CH$_2$)$_{14}$COOH	16:0	n-Hexadecanoic	Palmitic	Most fats and oils
CH$_3$(CH$_2$)$_{16}$COOH	18:0	n-Octadecanoic	Stearic	Most fats and oils
CH$_3$(CH$_2$)$_{18}$COOH	20:0	n-Eicosanoic	Arachidic	Peanut oil, lard
Unsaturated Fatty Acids				
CH$_3$(CH$_2$)$_5$CH>CH(CH$_2$)$_7$COOH	16:1	9-Hexadecanoic	Palmitoleic	Butter and seed oils
CH$_3$(CH$_2$)$_7$CH>CH(CH$_2$)$_7$COOH	18:1	9-Octadecanoic	Oleic	Most fats and oils
CH$_3$(CH$_2$)$_5$CH>CH(CH$_2$)$_9$COOH	20:1	11-Octadecanoic	trans-Vaccenic	Hydrogenated vegetable oils
CH$_3$(CH$_2$)$_4$CH>CHCH$_2$CH>CH(CH$_2$)$_7$COOH	18:2	9,12-Octadecadienoic	Linoleic	Linseed oil, corn oil, cottonseed oil
CH$_3$(CH$_2$(CH>CHCH$_2$)$_3$(CH$_2$)$_7$COOH	18:3	9,12,15-Octadecatrienoic	Linolenic	Soybean oil, marine oils
CH$_3$(CH$_2$)$_4$(CH>CHCH$_2$)$_4$(CH$_2$)$_2$COOH	20:4	5,8,11,14-Eicosatetraenoic	Arachidonic	Cottonseed oil

isomers. The *cis* configuration produces a bond in the hydrocarbon chain so that it resembles the shape of the letter U. Each *cis* configuration in the tail will add another bend. The *trans* configuration has nearly the same shape as the extended conformation of the saturated fatty acid. These structural features of the unsaturated fatty acids have a biological significance, as will be discussed in later sections.

In polyunsaturated fatty acids, the double bonds are not conjugated; that is, the double bonds will be separated by more than one covalent bond as in: $-CH_2-CH=CH-CH_2-CH=CH-CH_2-$. The unsaturated fatty acids of higher plants and animals are usually palmitoleic, oleic, linoleic, and linolenic acids, and the first double bond will be between atoms 9 and 10; others, if present, will be at carbon 12 or greater. Most of these unsaturated fatty acids will exist in the *cis* configuration. When vegetable oils are made into solids to make margarine, some of the double bonds will be converted to single bonds through the addition of hydrogen. The process is called hydrogenation and the oils must be heated before hydrogenation will take place. When this occurs, some of the residual unsaturated fatty acids will change from the *cis* to the *trans* residual form. Margarine and vegetable shortening are thus sources of the *trans* fatty acids in the human diet. Some fatty acids exist naturally in the *trans* configuration; 8% of the total fat in cows' milk is in the *trans* form. In this instance, the presence of *trans* fatty acids is due to their production by the rumen flora.

Fatty acids with odd numbers of carbon atoms are found in limited amounts in natural products. Less than 0.4% of the total fatty acids in olive oil and 0.8% of those in lard contain an odd number of carbon atoms. In contrast, 60% of olive oil and 40% of lard consists of the even-numbered fatty acid, oleic acid. Few oils or waxes contain significant amounts of odd-numbered fatty acids.

Of the polyunsaturated fatty acids, linoleic and linolenic are designated as the *essential fatty acids* (EFA). Most mammals require these fatty acids and cannot synthesize them. Felines, in addition, cannot convert linoleic acid to arachidonic acid. Hence, for these animals, arachidonic acid is an esential fatty acid. Shown in Figure 12 are the structures of linoleic, γ-linolenic, and linolenic. The latter two differ only in the positions of the double bonds.

2. Fats

Fats are formed when one or more fatty acids react with the hydroxyl group(s) of glycerol to make an ester. They are called neutral fats, glycerides, or acylglycerols. The fat most frequently found in nature has all three hydroxyl positions esterified; it is known as triacylglycerol. Triacylglycerols which contain the same fatty acid residue on all three carbons are simple triacylglycerols. An example would be tripalmitin. In nature, the triacylglycerols usually contain more than one fatty acid and thus are called mixed triacylglycerols or triglycerides.

Most fats in nature are complex mixtures of simple and mixed triacylglycerols. As yet, no general rule has been devised to determine the manner in which the fatty acids attach to glycerol. Many oils and fats contain between six and ten different saturated and unsaturated fatty acids. The number of possible combinations with this many fatty acid residues is very large.

The ratio of unsaturated to saturated fatty acids is defined as the P/S ratio. A high value for the ratio means that few saturated fats are present. Animal fats and the foods rich in these fats usually have a low P/S ratio. Most vegetable oils have a high P/S ratio. There are some exceptions to the notion that lipids of plant origin have high P/S ratios. The tropical plants (palm and coconut) provide a solid fat with a low P/S ratio. These fats, although called "oils", are rich in medium-chain (chain lengths of 8–14 carbons) saturated fatty acids. By convention, these lipids are called oils because they are fluid at much lower temperatures than are the fats of animal origin. Thus, we have coconut oil, palm oil, and palm kernel oil as solids at room temperature. The P/S ratio of the fat in the adipose tissue of humans reflects the P/S ratio of the food these humans consumed. If one wished to assess the usual fat intake of populations, one need only obtain a small sample of adipose tissue and analyze it for its fatty acid content.

IV. SOURCES OF LIPIDS

When discussing food sources of lipids, one means primarily food sources of triacylglycerols, for they are the lipids that occur in foods in large quantities. Lipids are found in almost every natural food. Fruits and vegetables have small amounts of lipids while meat, milk, and table spreads have large amounts. A few plant foods, olives and avocados, contain as much as 20% (by weight) fat. Nuts are rich sources of fat: pecans are 71% fat and walnuts are 60% fat. Table 2 shows the total fat content of several foods and also gives some values for the saturated fatty acid content and the amount of two common unsaturated fatty acids, oleic and linoleic.

More than one half of dietary fat is contributed from invisible sources: from the homogenized fat in milk and eggs, whole grain cereals, baked products, and convenience foods. The other fraction of dietary fat is visible. The marbling in meat, butter on bread or vegetables, and salad oil on lettuce are examples of the latter.

The fatty acid composition of several fats and oils is given in Table 2. Of the saturated fatty acids, palmitic (16:0) and stearic (18:0) are the most prevalent in nature. Of the unsaturated fatty acids, oleic (18:1) and linoleic (18:2) are the most abundant. Together, these two fatty acids make up 90% of the unsaturated fatty acids in the American diet.

As mentioned earlier, fats of plant origin tend to be less saturated than animal fats. Beef contains a lot of stearic acid. Mutton fat (tallow) and cocoa butter contain a similar array of fatty acids but not in the same amounts. Mutton fat has as much as 27% saturated fatty acids by weight whereas cocoa butter has 2.5%. This accounts for the marked difference in the physical properties of these two fats. Milk fat is similar to lard (pig fat) because it contains large amounts of palmitic and oleic acid. Fish, on the other hand, tends to have much more polyunsaturated fatty acids in its glycerides. Freshwater fish contain more unsaturated C_{18} and less unsaturated C_{20} and C_{22} than do marine fish. Fatty marine fish such as mackerel contain long-chain polyunsaturated fatty acids of the omega ω-3 or n-3 type.

Cholesterol, cholesterol esters, free fatty acids, and phospholipids are also present in the foods humans consume. These compounds represent only a small fraction of the total fat consumed. Because of the population studies linking heart disease to cholesterol levels in the blood, nutritionists are frequently interested in the levels of this lipid in the food. Listed in Table 3 are some human foods and their cholesterol content. Greater detail on the composition of the tremendous variety of foods that humans consume may be found in the USDA Handbook of Food Composition (U.S. Government Printing Office, Washington, D.C.). Other handbooks are also available. The figures shown in these tables are averages of several different figures and are not absolute. Variation in the source of the food, how it is prepared, and how much fat is removed prior to preparation and consumption contributes to the uncertainty associated with these values.

V. DIGESTION AND ABSORPTION

The digestion and absorption of the various food lipids involves the mouth, stomach, and intestine (Figure 1). The digestion of lipid is begun in the mouth with the mastication of food and the mixing with the acid-stable lingual lipase. Digestion can proceed only when the large particles of the food are made smaller through chewing. The action of the tongue, and later the churning action of the stomach, mix the food particles with the various digestive juices and with hydrochloric acid. These actions separate the lipid particles, exposing more surface area for enzyme action and providing the opportunity for emulsion formation. The changes in physical state, illustrated in Figure 2, are essential steps that precede absorption. In the

TABLE 2
Percent Fat in 100 g Portions of Common Foods

Item	Total fat % by weight	% of the total fatty acids in the fat		
		Total sat'd fatty acids	Unsaturated: oleic	Fatty acids: linoleic
Animal				
Bacon	53	20	27	7
Butter	81	45	27	3
Chicken, broiled	3.5	1	1	1
Egg, whole	12	4	5	Trace
Hamburger	12	6	4.7	Trace
Ice cream, 10% fat	10	6	4	Trace
Lamb, leg, roasted	19	10	7	Trace
Milk, whole	3.5	2	1.2	Trace
Milk, 2%	2	1.2	0.8	Trace
Milk, skim	Trace	Trace	Trace	Trace
Pork chops	21	8	9	2
Salmon, pink	6	1	1	Trace
Vegetable				
Avocados	13	2.3	6	1.8
Bread, whole wheat	2.6	0.4	1.3	0.4
Bread, white enriched	3.3	0.7	1.8	0.4
Broccoli	0.6	Trace	Trace	Trace
Cereal, 40% bran	2.8	Trace	Trace	Trace
Cereal, oatmeal	0.8	Trace	Trace	Trace
Orange juice, fresh	0.4	Trace	Trace	Trace
Peanut butter	50	12.5	25	12.5
Pecans	71	4.6	44	14
Potato, baked	Trace	Trace	Trace	Trace
Strawberries, raw	0.7	Trace	Trace	Trace
Walnuts	60	3	24	33

Source: Nutritive Values of the Edible Part of Foods, Home and Garden Bulletin No. 72, U.S. Department of Agriculture, Washington, D.C., 1970.

stomach, lipid-protein complexes are cleaved releasing lipid when the proteins of these complexes are denatured by gastric hydrochloric acid and attacked by the proteases (pepsin, parapepsin I, and parapepsin II) of the gastric juice. The remaining lipid components of the diet are mixed with other diet ingredients by the churning action of the stomach.

Little degradation of fat occurs in this organ except that catalyzed by lingual lipase. Lingual lipase is thought to originate from glands in the back of the mouth and under the tongue. This lipase is active in the acid environment of the stomach. However, because of the tendency of lipid to coalesce and form a separate phase, this lipase has limited opportunity to attack triacylglycerols. Those that are attacked release a single fatty acid, usually a short- or medium-chain one. The remaining diacylglycerol is subsequently hydrolyzed in the duodenum. In adults consuming a mixed diet, lingual lipase is relatively unimportant. However, in infants having an immature duodenal lipase, lingual lipase is quite important. In addition, this lipase has its greatest activity on the triacylglycerols commonly present in whole milk. Milk fat has more short- and medium-chain fatty acids than fats from other food sources.

Although the action of lingual lipase is slow relative to lipases found in the duodenum, its action to release diacylglycerol and short- and medium-chain fatty acids serves another function: these fatty acids serve as surfactants. Surfactants spontaneously adsorb to the water-lipid interface conferring a hydrophilic surface to lipid droplets and thereby provide a stable interface with the aqueous environment. The dietary surfactants are the free fatty acids, lecithin, and phospholipids. The action of acid-stable lingual lipase provides more fatty acids

TABLE 3
Total Lipid and Cholesterol Content in 100 g
Portions of Several Common Foods[a]

Food	% Fat	% Cholesterol
Codfish	0.67	0.043
Halibut	2.94	0.041
Mackerel	6.30	0.076
Salmon	3.45	0.052
Beef steak, cooked	31.8	0.36
Hamburger, cooked	12.8	0.10
Stew meat	18.8	1
Lamb chops, cooked	36.0	1.11
Pork chops, cooked	21.1	1.03
Pork sausage	46.2	1.35
Bologna	28.6	1.04
Chicken, white meat	3.5	0.64
Eggs, whole	12	4.2
Egg white	<3	—
Whole milk	3.3	0.32
Skim milk	Trace	Trace
Cheddar cheese	32	1.0
Cottage cheese (4%)	4.29	0.21
Mozzarella cheese, skim milk	17.9	4.5
Butter	81.4	2.4
Margarine	81.4	—
Fruits, all kinds	<1	—
Avocado	13	—
Leafy vegetables	<1	—
Legumes (except peanuts)	1	—
Root vegetables	<1	—
Cereals and grains	1-2	0
Crackers	1	0
Bread, white, enriched	4	<0.1

[a]   Foods are selected from the vast array of foods presented in
     Handbooks 8 to 15, United States Department of Agricul-
     ture, Human Nutrition Information Service, U.S. Govern-
     ment Printing Office, Superintendent of Documents, Wash-
     ington, D.C.

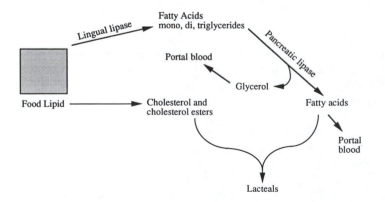

FIGURE 1.   Overview of digestion and absorption of food lipid.

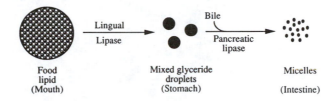

FIGURE 2. Changes in the physical state of food lipid as it is prepared for absorption.

to supplement the dietary supply. All together, these surfactants plus the churning action of the stomach produce an emulsion which is then expelled into the duodenum as chyme.

Once the chyme enters the duodenum, its entry stimulates the release into the bloodstream of the gut hormone, cholecystokinin. Cholecystokinin stimulates the gall bladder to contract and release bile. Bile salts serve as emulsifying agents and serve to further disperse the lipid droplets at the lipid-aqueous interface, thus facilitating the hydrolysis of the glycerides by the pancreatic lipases. The bile salts impart a negative charge to the lipids, which in turn attracts the pancreatic enzyme, colipase.

Cholecystokinin stimulates the exocrine pancreas to release pancreatic juice which contains three lipases (lipase, lipid esterase, colipase) which act at the water-lipid interface of the emulsion particles. One lipase acts on the fatty acids esterified at positions 1 and 3 of the glycerol backbone leaving a fatty acid esterified at carbon 2. This 2-monoacylglyceride can isomerize and the remaining fatty acid can move to carbon 1 or 3, or be freed of the glycerol entirely. The pancreatic juice contains another less specific lipase (called lipid esterase) which cleaves the fatty acid from cholesterol esters, monoglycerides, or esters such as vitamin A ester. Its action requires the presence of the bile salts. The lipase that is specific for the ester linkage at carbons 1 and 3 does not have a requirement for the bile salts and, in fact, is inhibited by them. The inhibition of pancreatic lipase by the bile salts is relieved by the third pancreatic enzyme, colipase. Colipase is a small protein (12,000 Da) which binds both the lipid at the water-lipid interface and to lipase, thereby anchoring and activating the lipase. The products of the lipase-catalyzed reaction, a reaction that favors the release of fatty acids having 10 or more carbons, are these fatty acids and monoacylglyceride. The products of the lipid esterase-catalyzed reaction are cholesterol, vitamins, fatty acids, and glycerol. Phospholipids present in food are attacked by phospholipases specific to each of the phospholipids. The pancreatic juice contains these lipases as prephospholipases which are activated by the enzyme trypsin.

As mentioned, the release of bile from the gall bladder is essential to the digestion of dietary fat. Bile contains the bile acids, cholic acid and chenodeoxycholic acid, which are biological detergents or emulsifying agents. At physiological pH, these acids are present as anions so they are frequently referred to as bile salts. At pH values above the physiological range, they form aggregates with the fats at concentrations above 2 to 5 mM. These aggregates are called micelles (Figure 3). These micelles are much smaller in size than the emulsified lipid droplets. Micelle sizes vary depending on the ratio of lipids to bile acids, but typically range from 40 to 600 Å.

Micelles are structured such that the hydrophobic portions (triacylglycerols, cholesterol esters, etc.) are toward the center of the structure while the hydrophilic portions (phospholipids, short-chain fatty acids, bile salts) surround this center. The micelles contain many different lipids. Mixed micelles have a disc-like shape whereby the lipids form a bilayer and the bile acids occupy edge positions, rendering the edge of the disc hydrophilic. During the process of lipase and esterase digestion of the lipids in the chyme, the water-insoluble lipids are rendered soluble and transferred from the lipid emulsion of the chyme to the micelle. In turn, these micelles transfer the products of digestion (free fatty acids, glycerol, cholesterol, etc.) from the intestinal lumen to the surface of the epithelial cells where absorption takes place. The micellar fluid layer next to this cell surface is homogenous, yet the products of lipid digestion are presented to the cell surface and, by passive diffusion, these products are

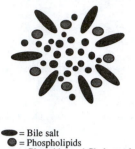

= Bile salt
= Phospholipids
= Glycerides and Cholesterol

FIGURE 3.   Cartoon of a micelle.

transported into the absorptive cell. Thus, the degree to which dietary lipid is absorbed once digested, depends largely on the amount of lipid to be absorbed relative to the amount of bile acid available to make the micelle. This, in turn, is dependent on the rate of bile acid synthesis by the liver and bile release by the gall bladder. People who have had their gall bladders removed still have their bile acids. Instead of stockpiling them in the gall bladder to be released upon the cholecystokinin signal, surgeons simply remove the gall bladder and make a direct connection between the liver and the duodenum. Once the fat has been absorbed, the bile acids pass on through the intestine where they are either reabsorbed or conjugated and excreted in the feces.

The primarily bile acids, cholic and chenodeoxycholic acids, are produced from cholesterol by the liver. They are secreted into the intestine and the intestinal flora convert these acids to their conjugated forms by dehydroxylating carbon 7 (see Figure 4). Further metabolism occurs at the far end of the intestinal tract where lithocholate is sulfated. While the dehydroxylated acids can be reabsorbed and sent back to the liver via the portal blood, the sulfated lithocholate can not. It appears in the feces. All four of the bile acids, the primary and dehydroxylated forms, are recirculated via the enterohepatic system such that very little of the bile acid is lost. It has been estimated that the bile acid lost in the feces (~0.8 g/day) equals that newly synthesized by the liver, such that the total pool remains between 3 to 5 g. The amount secreted per day is on the order of 16 to 70 g. Since the pool size is only 3 to 5 g, this means that these acids are recirculated as much as 14 times a day.

The function of the bile acids is thus quite similar to that of enzymes. Neither are "used up" by the processes they participate in and facilitate. In the instance of fat absorption, the bile acids facilitate the formation of micelles which, in turn, facilitate the uptake of the dietary fatty acids, monoglycerides, sterols, phospholipids, and other fat-soluble nutrients by the enterocyte of the small intestine. Not only do these bile acids recirculate, so too does cholesterol. Gall stones develop when the resecreted material is supersaturated with cholesterol and this cholesterol-laden bile is stored in the gall bladder. With time, the cholesterol precipitates out providing a crystalline structure for the stone. Since the bile also contains a variety of minerals, these minerals form salts with the bile acids and are deposited within and around the cholesterol matrix. Eventually these stones irritate the lining of the gall bladder or may lodge themselves in the duct connecting the bladder to the duodenum. When this happens, the bladder becomes inflamed, the duct may be blocked, and the patient becomes unable to tolerate food. In some cases, treatment consists of reducing the irritation and inflammation through drugs, but often the patient has the gall bladder and its offending stones removed. This surgery is called a cholecystectomy.

Virtually all of the fatty acids, monoacylglyceride, and glycerol are absorbed into the enterocyte. The structure of the intestinal absorbing cell is shown in Figure 5. Only 30 to 40% of the dietary cholesterol is absorbed. The percent cholesterol absorbed depends on a number of factors including the fiber content of the diet, the gut passage time, and the total amount of cholesterol present for absorption. At higher intake levels less is absorbed, and vice versa

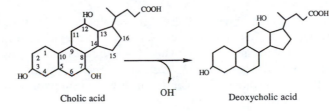

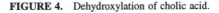

FIGURE 4. Dehydroxylation of cholic acid.

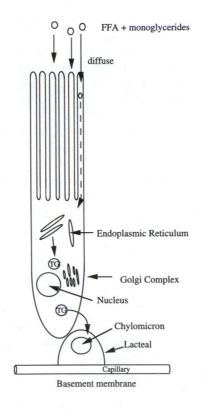

FIGURE 5. Structure of the enterocyte.

at lower intake levels. Compared to fatty acids and the acylglycerides, the rate of cholesterol absorption is very slow. It is estimated that the half-life of cholesterol in the enterocyte is 12 hours. With high fiber intakes, less cholesterol is absorbed because the fiber acts as an adsorbent, reducing cholesterol availability. Unit 5 discusses the different fibers and their biological activity. Cellulose and lignins are good adsorbents of cholesterol while transit time can be decreased by hemicellulose. Pectins and gums increase transit time yet they lower serum cholesterol levels by creating a gel-like consistency of the chyme, rendering the cholesterol in the chyme less available. High-fiber diets also reduce gut passage time, which, in turn, results in less time for cholesterol absorption.

The fate of the absorbed fatty acids depends on chain length. Those fatty acids having 10 or fewer carbons are quickly passed into the portal bloodstream without further modification. They are carried to the liver bound to albumin. Those fatty acids remaining are bound to a fatty acid binding protein and transported through the cytosol to the endoplasmic reticulum, whereupon they are converted to their CoA derivatives and reesterified to glycerol or the residual monoacylglycerides to reform the triacylglyceride. These reformed triacylglycerides adhere to phospholipids and a fat-transporting protein called apolipoprotein b. This relatively large lipid-protein complex migrates to the Golgi complex in the basolateral basement membrane of the enterocyte. The lipid-rich vesicles fuse with the Golgi surface membrane, whereupon the lipid-protein complex is exocytosed or secreted into the intercellular space which, in turn, drains into the lymphatic system. The lymphatic system contributes these lipids to the circulation as the thoracic duct enters the jugular vein prior to its entry into the heart.

VI. TRANSPORT

Blood lipid values vary depending on the age, sex, lifestyle, genetics, and the diet of the population. Typical values for the different lipids are shown in Table 4. After a meal the blood lipids rise. The time it takes for the peak value to appear depends on a variety of factors, but most notably it depends on the proximate composition of the meal. A high-fat meal leaves the stomach at a slower rate than does a low-fat meal. A high-fat meal will result in more total lipid entering the blood than a low-fat meal but this lipid will enter the blood at a slower rate.

The majority of the lipids leaving the enterocyte leaves as a chylomicron. A small percentage (~10%) leaves as a very low-density lipoprotein (VLDL). The apolipoprotein that is part of the chylomicron is unique to the intestinal cell. While it has the same function (that of carrying lipid in the bloodstream) as the gut VLDL or the lipoprotein of the liver (hepatic VLDL), it does not have the same amino acid structure. The characteristics of the various lipoprotein classes in the blood are given in Table 5. The hepatic and intestinal apolipoproteins can be distinguished using electrophoresis, a technique of separating proteins based on their electrophoretic mobility. A typical electrophoretic separation of a human serum sample is shown in Figure 6.

The intestinal cell has two apolipoproteins called A-1 and β. Apolipoprotein β is essential for chylomicron release by the intestinal cell. A-1 is the lipoprotein of the gut VLDL. Should apolipoprotein β be aberrant in function, as happens in the genetic disorder called A-β-lipoproteinemia, there will be a total or partial (depending on the genetic mutation) absence of lipoproteins in the blood. This terminology is confusing. The prefix A used for the disorder name refers to a lack of this protein, whereas lipoprotein A-1 is the lipid-carrying protein of the gut VLDL. It is quite similar to the lipoprotein of the liver VLDL. Patients with A-β-lipoproteinemia are characterized by very low blood lipids and lipid malabsorption (steatorrhea). The feces contain an abnormally large amount of fat and have a characteristic peculiar odor. In this disorder, not only is the triacylglyceride absorption affected, but so too are the fat-soluble vitamins. Without the ability to absorb these energy-rich food components and the vital fat-soluble vitamins, the patient does not thrive and survive. Fortunately this genetic mutation is not very common. It is inherited as an autosomal recessive trait.

The chylomicron is a relatively stable way of ensuring the movement, in an aqueous medium (blood), of hydrophobic molecules such as cholesterol and triacylglycerols from their point of origin, the intestine, to their point of use or storage. As mentioned, there are several unique proteins that facilitate this movement. These lipid transporting proteins determine which cells of the body receive which lipids. At the target cell, the chylomicron and VLDL lose their lipid through hydrolysis facilitated by an interstitial lipoprotein lipase which is found in the capillary beds of muscle, fat cells, and other tissues using lipid as a fuel. Lipoprotein lipase is synthesized by these target cells but is anchored on the outside of the cells by a polysaccharide chain on the endothelial wall of the surrounding capillaries. Should this lipoprotein lipase be missing or genetically aberrant (Type I lipemia or chylomicronemia) so that the chylomicrons cannot be hydrolyzed, these chylomicrons accumulate, and the individual would have a lipemia characterized by elevated levels of triacylglyceride- and cholesterol-containing chylomicrons. Also

TABLE 4
Blood Lipid Levels for Normal
Fasting Humans

Fraction	Range of values
Total	450 to 1000 mg/dl
Triacylglycerides	40 to 150 mg/dl
Phospholipids	9 to 16 mg/dl as lipid P
Cholesterol	120 to 220 mg/dl
Free fatty acids	6 to 16 mg/dl

TABLE 5
Characteristics of the Various Lipoproteins

Fraction	% Protein	Density	% Lipid as: Triacylglycerol	Phospholipid	Cholesterol
Chylomicrons	1.5 to 2.5	<0.95	84 to 89	7 to 9	1 to 5
VLDL	5 to 10	0.95 to 1.006	50 to 65	15 to 20	5 to 15
LDL[a]	20 to 25	1.006 to 1.019	7 to 10	15 to 20	35 to 401
LDL[b]	20 to 25	1.019 to 1.063	7 to 10	15 to 20	7 to 102
HDL	40 to 55	1.068 to 1.210	5	20 to 35	4 to 12

[a] Primarily esterified cholesterol.
[b] Primarily unesterified cholesterol.

characteristic of this condition is the presence of an enlarged liver and spleen, considerable abdominal discomfort, and the presence of subcutaneous xanthomas (clusters of hard, saturated fatty acid and cholesterol-rich nodules). Like A-β-lipoproteinemia, this condition is rare. Of interest is the observation that despite the very high blood lipid levels of these people, few die of coronary vessel disease. Their shortened life span is due to an inappropriate lipid deposition in all of the vital organs which, in turn, has a negative effect on organ function.

Other genetic errors in lipoprotein metabolism have been described. One is a mutation in the codes for the low-density lipoprotein receptor found on the surface of the target cells. This disorder is called Type II lipemia. The receptor may be "missing" or "partly missing". What is meant by this is that the amino acid sequence of the receptor structure is so abnormal that it either cannot function as a receptor at all (i.e., is missing) or functions only partly (partly missing). This set of genetic errors is fairly common and occurs in 1 person in 500. Goldstein and Brown described this error in the receptors for the low-density lipoprotein in the early 1970s. The work was recognized by the Nobel committee in the late 1980s.

The low-density lipoproteins originate in both the intestine and liver and have a fairly high cholesterol content (see Table 5). The level of cholesterol in the blood depends on the diet consumed and how much cholesterol is being synthesized. The cholesterol content of the gut LDL of a person on a low-cholesterol diet might run as low as 7 to 10% of the total lipid in the lipoprotein while the hepatic LDL of this same individual might be as high as 58% of total lipid. People consuming a low-cholesterol, low-saturated-fat diet may reduce the contribution of the diet to the blood cholesterol while increasing the hepatic *de novo* cholesterol synthesis. Persons having an LPL receptor deficiency are characterized by high serum cholesterol levels, and in some cases by high serum triacylglycerides. The reason these blood lipids are elevated is because the individuals cannot utilize the lipids carried by the LDL due to the error(s) in the receptor molecule. Further, because these circulating lipids do not enter into the adipose and hepatic cell in normal amounts, the synthesis of triacylglycerides and cholesterol is not

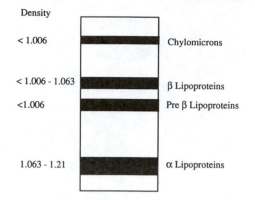

FIGURE 6. Electrophoretic separation characteristics of human plasma lipoproteins.

appropriately down regulated. Hence, this individual has elevated serum lipids not only because the LDL lipid is not appropriately cleared from the blood but also because of high rates of lipid synthesis. Individuals with this disorder have lipid deposits in unusual places such as immediately under the skin, around the eyes, on the tendons, and in the vascular tree. It is this last feature that probably accounts for the shortened life span of these people, with the cause of death being cardiovascular disease.

As can be seen from the metabolic characteristics of this disorder, low-fat diets are probably useless in reducing serum cholesterol levels since *de novo* synthesis of triacylglycerides and cholesterol from nonlipid precursors can and does occur. Treatment with lipid adsorbents (high-fiber diets and the drug, cholestyramine) will help reduce the cholesterol (but not triacylglycerides) coming from the intestine, and there are drugs that can safely lower *de novo* cholesterol synthesis as well as increase intracellular lipid oxidation. All of these therapies may help reduce the serum lipid levels, but even doing this only treats the symptoms and not the genetic disorder. For that, gene therapy is needed to correct the genetic disorder that is the basic underlying cause of the symptoms.

Heart disease in its various forms is also associated with elevated levels of the very low-density lipoproteins (VLDL). A specific genetic error has not been identified; however, the disorders have been subdivided into three general categories. In one, Type III lipemia, the patients are characterized by elevated serum cholesterol, phospholipid, and triacylglyceride levels, elevated VLDL levels (and sometimes LDL levels), fatty deposits on the tendons and in areas on the arms just under the skin, vascular atheromas, and ischemic heart disease. This type of lipemia is inherited as an autosomal dominant trait in 1 person in 5000. Another lipemia (type IV) having a normal cholesterol level but an elevated triacylglyceride level and elevated VLDL levels is also associated with ischemic heart disease and premature atherosclerosis. It is frequently seen in obese patients with noninsulin-dependent diabetes mellitus (NIDDM). People with diabetes mellitus have five times the risk of normal people of developing premature atherosclerosis and its associated coronary events. Cardiovascular disease, followed by renal disease, are the leading causes of death for people with diabetes mellitus.

Those people with insulin-dependent diabetes mellitus are more likely to develop a lipemia (Type V lipemia) that is slightly different from the aforementioned NIDDM-related lipemia. While the incidence of both is 2 in 1000, those with the latter problem inherited their trait in an autosomal recessive manner while those with the NIDDM-related lipemia inherited their trait as an autosomal dominant trait. Elevated chylomicron and VLDL levels and reduced dietary fat tolerance characterize this type of lipemia. Patients with this disorder are usually of normal body weight.

VII. METABOLISM

Once the dietary lipids are transferred to the target tissues, one of several processes occur. The fatty acids of the triacylglycerols either are oxidized for energy, or are stored as resynthesized triacylglycerols, or are incorporated into the membranes within and around the cells. An overview of these processes is shown in Figure 7. Certain of the fatty acids, the essential fatty acids linoleic and linolenic, have a special role as precursors for the 20-carbon compounds called eicosanoids. Diet can affect all of these processes and, as well, stimulate lipid synthesis.

A. FATTY ACID SYNTHESIS

In humans consuming a typical American diet containing 35 to 45% of its energy as fat, very little fatty acid synthesis occurs. However, in certain circumstances, such as humans consuming a very low fat diet that is high in refined sugar, for example, synthesis can and does occur. The magnitude of this synthesis is dependent on a variety of factors of which diet is one. In laboratory rats accustomed to a very low fat diet comprised mainly of cereal grains, lipid synthesis occurs at a significant rate. Furthermore, in people that are obese, it is suspected that significant fatty synthesis also occurs despite their high fat intake. In humans, primates, and birds, the liver is the primary site for fat synthesis. In rats and mice, lipogenesis occurs in the adipose tissue as well as in the liver. In pigs, lipogenesis occurs primarily in the fat depots. In those humans having a very high synthetic rate, a fatty liver may be observed. Humans sustained by parenteral nutrition (nutrients provided through a catheter placed in the subclavian vein) or those who derive a significant (more than 60%) amount of their energy from carbohydrate may have high lipogenic rates and a fatty liver if the export of these newly synthesized lipids via VLDL synthesis and hepatic release is impeded. If VLDL synthesis keeps pace with the high lipogenic rate, a fatty liver does not develop. In rats fed high (65% by weight) sugar diets, lipogenesis is quite high. However, normal rats will adapt to this diet such that the initial fatty liver will disappear as the hepatic lipid output increases to match the increased synthesis.

Fatty acid synthesis (Figure 8) begins with acetyl CoA. Acetyl CoA arises from the oxidation of glucose or the carbon skeletons of deaminated amino acids. Acetyl CoA is converted to malonyl CoA with the addition of one carbon (from bicarbonate) in the presence of the enzyme acetyl CoA carboxylase. The reaction uses the energy from one molecule of ATP and biotin as a coenzyme. This reaction is the first committed step in the reaction sequence that results in the synthesis of a fatty acid. In many respects, it resembles the carboxylation of pyruvate, the first committed step in gluconeogenesis. In both reactions activated carbon dioxide attached to the biotin-enzyme complex is transferred to the methyl end of the substrate. Although most fatty acids synthesized in mammalian cells have an even number of carbons, this first committed step yields a three-carbon product. Figure 9 illustrates these initial reactions. This results in an asymmetric molecule which becomes vulnerable to attack (addition) at the center of the molecule with the subsequent loss of the terminal carbon. The vulnerability is conferred by the fact that both the carboxyl group at one end and the $\overset{\displaystyle O}{\underset{\displaystyle -C \sim S - CoA}{\|}}$ group at the other end are both powerful attractants of electrons from the

hydrogen of the middle carbon. This leaves the carbon in a very reactive state and a second acetyl group carried by a carrier protein with the help of phosphopantethine, which has a sulfur group connection, can be joined to it through the action of the enzyme, malonyl transferase. Subsequently, the "extra" carbon is released via the enzyme β-ketoacyl enzyme synthase, leaving a four-carbon chain still connected to an SH group at the carboxyl end. This SH group is the docking end for all the enzymes that comprise the fatty acid synthase complex. These

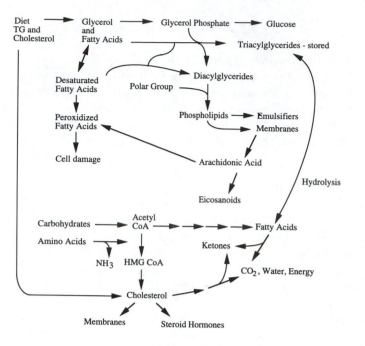

FIGURE 7.   Overview of fatty acid metabolism.

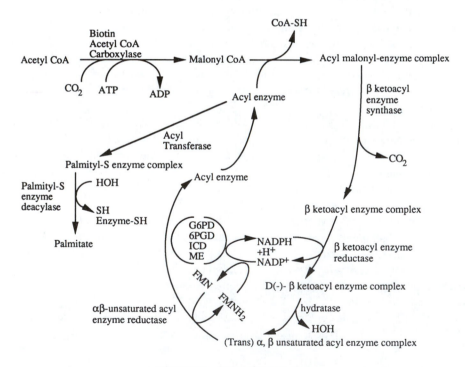

FIGURE 8.   Fatty acid synthesis.

enzymes catalyze the addition of two carbon acetyl groups in sequence to the methyl end of the carbon chain until the final product, palmityl CoA, and then palmitic acid, is produced. Members of this fatty acid synthase complex include the aforementioned malonyl transferase and β-ketoacyl synthase, β-ketoacyl reductase, which catalyzes the addition of reducing equivalents carried by FMN, and an acyl transferase. Upon completion of these six steps, the

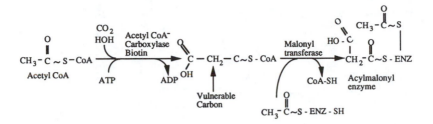

FIGURE 9. Details of initial steps in fatty acid synthesis.

process is repeated until the chain length is 16 carbons long. At this point, the SH-acyl carrier protein is removed through the action of the enzyme palmityl-S-enzyme deacylase and the palmitic acid is available for esterification to glycerol to form a mono-, di-, or triacylglyceride.

Fatty acid synthesis does not occur as an uncontrolled sequence of reactions. It has a number of direct and indirect controllers. As mentioned above, the synthesis of malonyl CoA is the first committed step in the pathway. It also is the first rate limiting reaction. Acetyl CoA carboxylase as a rate limiting enzyme has been studied in detail. It is synthesized as an inactive protomer which, when citrate levels increase, aggregate to form the active enzyme. Other tricarboxylates can stimulate aggregation but citrate is the preferred anion. Citrate, a citric acid cycle intermediate in the mitochondria, is exchanged for malate or pyruvate. Figure 10 illustrates the relationship of the citric acid cycle to fatty acid synthesis. The malate-citrate shuttle is very active in cells also having a very active lipogenic process. It, too, is regarded as a rate limiting step. Pyruvate, from the oxidation of glucose via the glycolytic sequence (see Unit 5), is also actively exchanged for citrate in the lipogenic cell. These exchanges are described and discussed in Unit 3. Citrate is cleaved through the action of the ATP-citrate lyase (citrate cleavage enzyme) producing oxalacetate and acetyl CoA. This acetyl CoA is the beginning substrate for fatty acid synthesis. Feedback inhibition of acetyl CoA carboxylase is exerted when palmitoyl CoA accumulates.

Acetyl CoA carboxylase is sensitive to the phosphorylation state of the cytosol. High levels of ATP are needed to provide the initial energy for the formation of acetyl CoA from citrate and for the carboxylation of this acetyl CoA to form malonyl CoA. Thus, high phosphorylation states (high concentrations of ATP relative to ADP and inorganic phosphate) are a characteristic requirement for lipogenesis. Acetyl CoA carboxylase is also controlled by a cAMP-mediated phosphorylation-dephosphorylation mechanism in which the phosphorylated enzyme is less active than the dephosphorylated enzyme. Insulin promotes dephosphorylation while glucagon promotes phosphorylation. Thus, when insulin levels are high, one would anticipate high rates of lipogenesis, and the reverse when insulin levels are low and glucagon levels are high. One might also anticipate an increase in lipogenesis in hyperinsulinemic individuals and, indeed, obese people as well as genetically obese experimental animals are characterized by both. As a corollary, one might also anticipate that the consumption of a high-glucose, low-fat diet which stimulates insulin release and also provides ample glucose for conversion to fatty acids would be characterized by high rates of lipogenesis, particularly in the liver. In rodents, this anticipation is justified. However, in humans, there is some discussion as to whether the human diet is sufficiently high in simple sugar and sufficiently low in fat to have the same sort of lipogenic response. Species differences in habitual diet composition as well as species differences in biological time frame complicate the discussion. A 24-hour day in a rat is roughly equivalent to a 30-day time span in the human with respect to total life span. The peaks and nadirs in the lipogenic rates in the rat will thus be further apart within a 24-hour period than will lipogenic rates in the human. Thus, one can elicit an increase in acetyl CoA carboxylase activity and in lipogenesis in the rodent with a short interval (1 to 2 days) of high-glucose diet feeding where that same interval for the human will show little, if any, change.

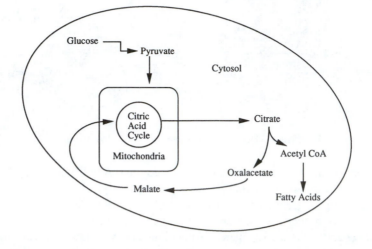

FIGURE 10.   Citric acid cycle activity is important to active lipogenesis.

Genetic factors also influence acetyl CoA carboxylase activity. In the human, the gene for acetyl CoA carboxylase is located on chromosome 17. Should this gene mutate, a nonfunctional enzyme will be produced and *de novo* fatty acid synthesis will not occur. Such an inborn error has been reported in humans. However, since humans consuming a high-fat diet such as that consumed in the U.S. synthesize very little lipid *de novo*, the absence of a functioning acetyl CoA carboxylase is not as devastating as the absence of an important rate limiting step in some other pathway. In contrast, such a deficiency in rats, animals that usually consume a low-fat, high-carbohydrate diet, would seriously impair survival unless the rat was fed a human-like diet.

The molecular biology of acetyl CoA carboxylase has recently been reviewed by Allred and Bowers (1993). Detailed studies of transcription, translation, and posttranslational processing of the enzyme support and explain how the enzyme is activated and suppressed by various hormones and dietary ingredients. Suffice it to say that this enzyme and the reaction it catalyzes is a critical step in the regulation of the *de novo* synthesis of fatty acids.

Another control of fatty acid synthesis is exerted by the complex of enzymes known as the fatty acid synthase. All of the dietary and hormonal factors described above for activating or inhibiting acetyl CoA carboxylase have the same effects on the fatty acid synthase complex. Further, phosphorylated sugars have allosteric effects on this enzyme complex. An allosteric effect is one which promotes (or inhibits) the activity of an enzyme or enzyme complex by binding to a site other than the active catalytic site which promotes (or inhibits) the activity of the active catalytic site. An allosteric effector may not be involved in the reaction itself, but through its binding causes a change in the conformation of the enzyme. In the case of inhibition, such a conformational change may "hide" the active catalytic portion of the molecule. In promotion, the reverse occurs; the "business end" of the molecule is readily accessible to substrate, cofactors, and coenzymes.

While dietary ingredients affect the activity of fatty acid synthase through effects on the supplies of acetyl CoA, they have other effects as well. These effects occur at the level of the genes for fatty acid synthase. Diets high in simple sugars increase the synthesis of fatty acid synthase. Diets rich in polyunsaturated fatty acids decrease this synthesis. Clarke and Jump (1993) have reviewed the literature on this aspect of fatty acid synthesis and have concluded that polyunsaturated fatty acids suppress the rapid transcription of genes coding for fatty acid synthesis. They speculate that in liver cells there is a nuclear fatty acid binding protein which selectively binds 18:2(ω6 or N6) polyenoic fatty acids and their metabolites. Upon binding, the putative *trans*-acting protein would bind to a *cis*-acting element linked to the fatty acid synthase (or S14) gene which, in turn, would result in a suppression of gene transcription.

In the conditions described by Clarke and Jump, suppression of gene transcription is not complete. While less enzyme is being synthesized, some of this decrease in enzyme amount may be countered by an increase in the activity of the enzyme present. One of the ways nutrition scientists have of measuring enzyme activity is to isolate the fraction of the cell known to contain the enzyme and to measure the amount of substrate used or product produced where all components of the reaction are in optimal amounts.

Numerous publications exist reporting in detail how the various enzymes in metabolism work *in vitro*. However, one must appreciate the fact that most *in vitro* studies of enzyme activity are conducted with idealized amounts of substrate and cofactors and with little subsequent product removal. Usually, the enzyme is studied at saturation, a condition that seldom occurs in the living organism. *In vivo*, enzymes are rarely saturated; they usually are working so rapidly that 10 to 20% saturation is more likely. This allows for greater control of the flux of metabolites through the system by factors other than the amount and activity of the enzyme per se. Thus, in cells having 50% less of a given enzyme as measured *in vitro* compared with normal cells, the flux of substrate through the pathway *in vivo* would not necessarily be slower. In fact, the inheritance of a number of the genetic diseases characterized by an absence of activity of a certain enzyme can be tracked within a given family by the activity of that enzyme in unaffected homozygotes and heterozygotes. Heterozygotes will have reduced enzyme activity yet be normal with respect to their metabolism. This may also be true for the fatty acid synthase complex in animals fed polyunsaturated fatty acids. That is, they may have less enzyme but the flux of acetyl CoA through the fatty acid synthesis pathway, as reflected in the total amount of accumulated lipid in the tissue, may differ from animals fed a low polyunsaturated fatty acid diet. There are many reasons why this occurs. Suffice it to say that the amount of rate limiting enzyme does not always predict the activity of the pathway of which it is a part and the amount of product the pathway produces that accumulates.

Despite the gaps in our knowledge about the details of acetyl CoA carboxylase and fatty acid synthase, the reaction sequence shown in Figure 8 is well established as is the effects of certain dietary ingredients and hormones on fatty acid synthesis in living creatures. We know that the fatty acid chain is continually bound to the fatty acid synthase complex and is sequentially transferred between the 4'-phosphopantetheine (pantothenic acid) group of the acyl carrier protein and the sulfhydryl group of a cystein residue on β-ketoacyl-ACP synthase during the condensation step.

There are other aspects of fatty acid synthesis that should be mentioned. Although the hexose monophosphate shunt NADP-linked enzymes are not rate controlling, it is recognized that the reactions catalyzed by these enzymes provide about 50% of the reducing equivalents needed in the reaction sequence catalyzed by the fatty acid synthase complex. The remaining reducing equivalents are provided by the NADP-linked isocitrate dehydrogenase (~10%) and the malic enzyme (~40%). Fatty acid synthesis is one of the few synthetic pathways that incorporate reducing equivalents into the product. Most pathways for synthesis release reducing equivalents as part of their condensation reactions. Because fatty acid synthesis incorporates these reducing equivalents, one can measure the rate of incorporation of ^{3}H (from radiolabeled water) into palmitate. This technique was devised by Lowenstein and refined by Fain and Jungas.

The pathway for the synthesis of fatty acids shown in Figure 8 has been well studied. It produces the 16-carbon saturated fatty acid, palmitate. This fatty acid is then the substrate for a variety of other reactions to produce the full array of endogenously produced fatty acids found in the body. Palmitate can be elongated, desaturated, hydroxylated, oxidized, and esterified. Descriptions of all of these processes follows.

1. Elongation

Elongation occurs in either the endoplasmic reticulum or the mitochondria. The reaction differs depending on where it occurs. In the endoplasmic reticulum, the reaction sequence is similar to that just described for the cytosolic fatty acid synthase complex. The source of the two-carbon unit is malonyl CoA, and NADPH provides the reducing power. The intermediates are CoA esters, not the acyl carrier protein 4'-phosphopantetheine. The reaction sequence (Figure 11) produces stearic acid in all tissues that make fatty acids except the brain. In the brain, elongation can proceed further, producing fatty acids containing up to 24 carbons. In the mitochondria, elongation uses acetyl CoA rather than malonyl CoA as the source of the two-carbon unit. It uses either $NADH^+H^+$ or $NADPH^+H^+$ as the source of reducing equivalents and as substrate uses carbon chains of less than 16 carbons. Mitochondrial elongation is the reversal of fatty acid oxidation which also occurs in this organelle.

2. Desaturation

Desaturation occurs in the endoplasmic reticulum and microsomes. The enzymes that catalyze this desaturation are the $\Delta 9$, or $\Delta 6$, or $\Delta 3$ desaturases. They are sometimes called mixed function oxidases because two substrates (fatty acid and NADPH) are oxidized simultaneously. Desaturation of stearic acid to form oleic acid results in the formation of a double bond at the $\Delta 9$ position. This is the first committed step of the desaturation pathway. Fatty acid desaturation can be followed by elongation and repeated such that a variety of mono- and polyunsaturated fatty acids can be formed. These fatty acids contribute fluidity to membranes because of their lower melting point. An increase in the activity of the desaturation pathway is a characteristic response of rats fed a diet high in saturated fatty acids. The body can convert the dietary saturated fatty acids to unsaturated fatty acids, thus maintaining an optimal P/S ratio in the tissues. There are two unsaturated fatty acids the body cannot make. These are the so-called essential fatty acids, linoleic (18:2, ω6) and linolenic (18:2, ω3) acids (Figure 12). The consequences of inadequate essential fatty intake are both subtle and various. In the absence of linoleic acid in the diet, microsomal desaturation and elongation activity increases and $\Delta^{5,8,11}$ eicosatrienoic acid (20:3, ω9) accumulates in the blood. The essential fatty acids can be synthesized in the plant kingdom and, when consumed by animals, find their way into the food chain. Linoleic acid is used to make arachidonic acid (20:4, ω6) while linolenic acid is used to make eicosapentanoic acid (20:5, ω3) through elongation and desaturation. Figure 11 shows the overall pathway for the synthesis of these unsaturated fatty acids, including the conversion of linoleic to arachidonic acid.

The activity of the desaturases can be increased through feeding saturated fat and/or high-sugar diets. Both dietary maneuvers increase the need to synthesize unsaturated fatty acids. Desaturase activity is stimulated by insulin, triiodothyronine, and glucocorticoid. Desaturase activity is decreased when highly polyunsaturated fats are fed.

3. Autooxidation

Unsaturated fatty acids, particularly the polyunsaturated fatty acids, are more reactive than saturated fatty acids. The double bonds can be attacked by oxygen radicals in a process called autooxidation. Autooxidation occurs in food and is responsible for the deterioration of food quality. The discoloration of red meat upon exposure to air at room temperature is an indication of the autooxidation process. The off odor that accompanies this discoloration is the result of the autooxidation of the fatty acids in the meat fat. In living systems, the process of autooxidation is suppressed to a large extent because the products of this oxidation, fatty acid peroxides, can be very damaging. Peroxides denature proteins, rendering them inactive, and attack the DNA in the nucleus and mitochondria resulting in base pair deletions or breaks in the DNA which, in turn, result in mutations or errors in this DNA. In the nucleus, these breaks or deletions can be repaired. In the aging animal, the repair mechanism loses its efficiency and

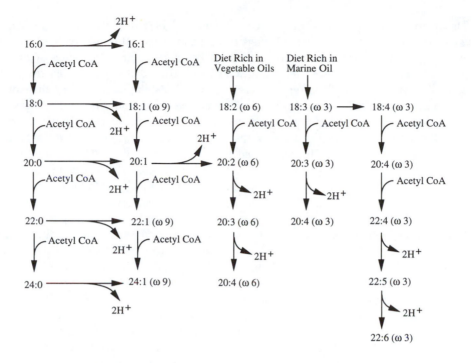

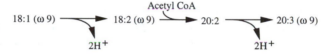

In the absence of dietary 18:2 (ω 6) the following sequence occurs:

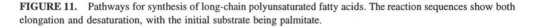

FIGURE 11. Pathways for synthesis of long-chain polyunsaturated fatty acids. The reaction sequences show both elongation and desaturation, with the initial substrate being palmitate.

$$CH_3CH_2CH_2CH_2C=C-CH_2-C=CCH_2CH_2CH_2CH_2CH_2CH_2CH_2COOH \quad \text{linoleic acid } [18:2, (9, 12)]$$

$$CH_3CH_2CH_2CH_2CH_2C=C-CH_2-C=C-CH_2-C=CCH_2CH_2CH_2CH_2COOH \quad \gamma \text{ linolenic acid } [18:3, (6, 9, 12)]$$

$$CH_3CH_2C=C-CH_2-C=C-CH_2-C=C-(CH_2)_7COOH \quad \text{linolenic acid } [18:3 (9, 12, 15)]$$

FIGURE 12. Essential fatty acids.

one of the characteristics of aged cells is the loss of its DNA repair ability. Mitochondria have no DNA repair mechanism so base pair deletions occurring as a result of free radical attack cannot be reversed. Fortunately, there are many mitochondria (~50,000) in each cell so that if a few are damaged in this way the effect is not as devastating as happens with unrepaired DNA damage in the nucleus. To prevent widespread damage to cellular proteins and DNA by these radicals, there is a potent antioxidation system in all cells. This antioxidation system includes the selenium-containing enzyme, glutathione peroxidase, catalase, and superoxide dismutase. These enzymes are found in the peroxisomes. Superoxide dismutase is also found in the mitochondria. All of these components serve to suppress free radical formation.

The free radical chain reaction is shown in Figure 13. Free radicals can form when the oxygen atom is excited by a variety of drugs and contaminants and by ultraviolet light. The excited oxygen atom is called singlet oxygen ($O_2 \cdot^-$). Pollutants such as the oxides of nitrogen or carbon tetrachloride can provoke this reaction. *In vivo*, the detoxification reactions catalyzed by the cytochrome P450 enzymes generate free radicals. In the respiratory chain of the mitochondria the possibility of oxygen radical production exists, and it is for this reason the mitochondria possess a particularly potent peroxide suppressor, superoxide dismutase or SOD. SOD in the mitochondria requires the manganese ion as a cofactor. The cytosol also has SOD but this enzyme requires the copper and zinc ions. Both forms of the enzyme catalyze the reaction $O_2 \cdot^- + O_2 \cdot^- + 2H^+ \rightarrow H_2O_2 + O_2$. Two superoxides and two hydrogen ions are joined to form one molecule of hydrogen peroxide and a molecule of oxygen. In turn, the peroxide can be converted to water through the action of the enzyme catalase. Peroxides can also be "neutralized" through the action of glutathione-S-transferase. This reaction requires two moles of reduced glutathione and produces two molecules of oxidized glutathione and two molecules of water. Fatty acid radicals can also be neutralized by glutathione peroxidase, producing a molecule of an alcohol with the same chain length as the fatty acid. Glutathione-S-transferase can duplicate the action of glutathione peroxidase. These enzymes and the reactions they catalyze are listed in Table 6.

In addition to the reactions that counteract the *in vivo* formation of oxygen radicals or fatty acid peroxides, certain of the vitamins have this role as well. Ascorbic acid has an antioxidant function as it can donate reducing equivalents to a peroxide, converting it to an alcohol. β-Carotene can quench singlet oxygen and thus convert it into O_2. Vitamin E is perhaps the best known antioxidant vitamin and its action is similar to that of ascorbic acid. It donates reducing equivalents to a peroxide converting it to an alcohol.

Although the foregoing has emphasized the negative aspects of the partial reduction products of oxygen, there is some evidence that peroxide formation has some benefit. For example, leukocytes produce peroxides as a means of killing invading bacteria. Other examples no doubt will emerge as scientists struggle to understand the role of peroxidation (and the peroxisomes) in mammalian metabolism.

4. Esterification

Most fats in food as well as those stored in the adipose tissue depots and those present in small amounts in other tissues exist as triacylglycerides. Triacylglycerides are hydrolyzed to their component fatty acids and glycerol and reesterified at each of several points in their metabolism. Already described is the process of fat absorption that involves hydrolysis and reesterification prior to entry into the bloodstream as either chylomicrons or VLDL. This hydrolysis and reesterification also occurs when lipids arrive at the hepatocyte or the myocyte or the adipocyte. The triacylglyceride is hydrolyzed by interstitial lipoprotein lipase, the fatty acids are transported into the target cell and reesterified to glycerol-3-phosphate. In the fat cell, this glycerol-3-phosphate usually is a product of glycolysis rather than the glycerol liberated when the triacylglycerol is hydrolyzed. The liberated glycerol usually passes back to the liver which has a very active glycerokinase to phosphorylate it. In the liver, the phosphorylated glycerol is either used as a substrate for glucose synthesis, recycled into hepatic phospholipids or triacylglycerides, or oxidized to CO_2 and water.

The formation of triacylglycerides regardless of the source for the glycerol-3-phosphate follows the same pattern in all tissues. With some modification as will be described, it is the pathway used for the synthesis of phospholipids. These pathways are shown in Figure 14.

Triacylglycerides are formed in a stepwise fashion. First, a fatty acid (usually a saturated fatty acid) is attached at carbon 1 of the glycerophosphate. The phosphate group at carbon 3 is electronegative and because it pulls electrons toward it, it leaves carbon 1 more reactive than carbon 2. The fatty acid (as an acyl CoA) is transferred to carbon 1 through the action of a

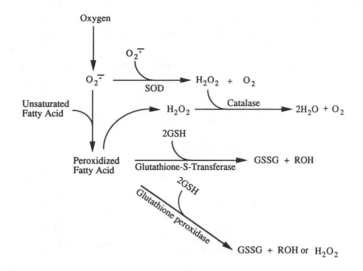

FIGURE 13. Free radical formation and suppression *in vivo*. GSH — reduced glutathione; GSSH — oxidized glutathione; ROH — organic alcohol; H_2O_2 — hydrogen peroxide; and SOD — superoxide dismutase.

TABLE 6
Antioxidant Enzymes Found in Mammalian Cells

Enzyme	Required mineral cofactor	Reaction catalyzed
Superoxide dismutase	CuZn or Mn	$2O_2 + 2H^+ \rightarrow H_2O_2 + O_2$
Glutathione peroxidase	Se	$H_2O_2 + 2GSH \rightarrow GSSG + 2H_2O$
		$ROOH + 2GSH \rightarrow GSSG + ROH + H_2O$
Catalase	Fe	$2H_2O_2 \rightarrow 2H_2O + O_2$
Glutathione-S-transferases	—	$ROOH + 2GSH \rightarrow GSSG + ROH + H_2O$

transferase. The attachment uses the carboxy end of the fatty acid chain and makes an ester linkage releasing the CoA. Now the molecule has electronegative forces at each end: the phosphate group on carbon 3 and the oxygen plus carbon chain at carbon 1. Now carbon 2 is vulnerable and reactive and another carbon chain can be attached. In this instance the fatty acid is usually an unsaturated fatty acid. At this point, the 1,2-diacylglyceride phosphate loses its phosphate group so that carbon 3 is now reactive. The 1,2-diacylglyceride can either be esterified with another fatty acid to make triacylglyceride or can be used to make the membrane lipids; phosphatidylcholine, phosphatidylethanolamine, phosphatidylinositol, cardiolipin, and phosphatidylserine. These membrane lipids have very special functions as will be discussed later.

In the stored triacylglycerides, most unsaturated fatty acids are found at carbon 2. In the membrane phospholipids the unsaturated fatty acid at carbon 2 is usually arachidonic acid. This arachidonic acid, produced by elongation and desaturation of dietary linoleic acid, is preferentially used in the membrane phospholipid. It can either be attached to the glycerol backbone when the phospholipid is made, or exchanged for another fatty acid as the lipids in and around the cells remodel themselves. There is constant hydrolysis and reesterification in the cell. Thus, there is a rapid exchange of fatty acids between those in the membranes and those inside the cell. In fact, if one were to change the fatty acid composition of the diet it would take less than a week to observe corresponding changes in the fatty acid composition of the stored lipids *and* even less time to observe changes in membrane phospholipid fatty acids. Scientists wanting to confirm food intake data with respect to the kinds of fats consumed

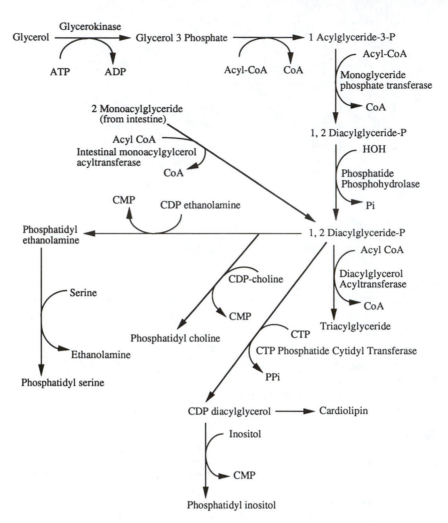

FIGURE 14.   Pathways for the synthesis of triacylglycerides.

need only examine the fatty acid composition of the membrane and stored lipids to learn how accurate their food intake reports are.

Shown in Table 7 are some data giving the phospholipid fatty acid composition of livers from rats fed either a 6% corn oil or hydrogenated coconut oil diet. Recall that corn oil is a good source of polyunsaturated fatty acids having 16 and 18 carbons. Note that the corn-oil-fed rats had a phospholipid fatty acid profile that reflected their corn oil intake. Note too that rats fed the hydrogenated coconut oil, which has *no* linoleic or arachidonic acid, likewise had less of these fatty acids in their profile. These rats tried to compensate for their essential fatty acid-deficient diet by increasing their desaturase and elongase activity. Thus, the increases in unsaturated fatty acids (16:1, 18:1, 20:2, 20:3, 22:2, 22:6) can be seen. Hydrogenated coconut oil is rich in medium-chain saturated fatty acid. These medium-chain saturated fatty acids account for the fact that hydrogenated coconut oil is a solid at room temperature. One might like to assume that animals consuming this fat would have more rigid (less fluid) membranes but Mother Nature has designed a fairly competent compensatory system that can partially overcome the diet fat effect on the membrane.

TABLE 7
Effect of Corn or Coconut Oil Diets on the Phospholipid Fatty Acid Composition of the Livers of Rats

Fatty acids[a]	Diet	
	Corn oil	Coconut oil
	(% of the total)	
14:0	0.09 ± 0.03	0.30 ± 0.03
14:1	0.10 ± 0.02	0.05 ± 0.01
15:0	0.17 ± 0.03	0.20 ± 0.03
16:0	15.2 ± 0.03	15.4 ± 0.03
16:1	0.70 ± 0.08	2.26 ± 0.07
17:0	0.38 ± 0.04	0.13 ± 0.02
17:1	0.09 ± 0.02	0.11 ± 0.02
18:0	20.8 ± 0.8	22.0 ± 0.4
18:1	7.17 ± 0.6	12.0 ± 0.5
18:2	14.4 ± 0.4	7.98 ± 0.27
20:0	0.01 ± 0.01	0.16 ± 0.04
18:3	0.41 ± 0.06	0.35 ± 0.04
20:1	—	0.18 ± 0.04
20:2	0.89 ± 0.17	6.44 ± 0.50
20:3	0.82 ± 0.16	2.20 ± 0.13
20:4	29.4 ± 0.5	18.0 ± 0.7
22:1	0.34 ± 0.02	0.35 ± 0.03
22:2	0.14 ± 0.02	0.48 ± 0.03
24:0	0.96 ± 0.01	0.95 ± 0.03
22:4	1.37 ± 0.09	0.54 ± 0.02
22:5	2.14 ± 0.25	2.24 ± 0.12
22:6	3.53 ± 0.31	6.64 ± 0.30
20:5	—	0.41 ± 0.04

[a] Designations used: number of carbons in chain followed by number of double bonds.

Note: Hydrogenated coconut oil is deficient in essential fatty acid but is a good source for 8-, 10-, 12-, and 14-carbon fatty acids.

Adapted from Berdanier, *Nutr. Rep. Internat.* 37:269, 1988.

Note in Table 7 that the unsaturation to saturation [fatty acid] ratios in the hepatic membranes of the rats fed these two different fats were nearly the same. Despite this compensation, however, the consumption of a diet lacking the essential fatty acids results in some profound effects on metabolism and bodily function. Shown in Table 8 are some of the features of essential fatty acid deficiency. Detailed studies of cells from deficient rats have revealed diet-induced changes in energetic efficiency which includes a partial loss of the ability of mitochondria to trap energy in the high-energy bond of ATP, an impairment in the glucose transporter activity in selected cells, and an alteration in insulin receptor number. While none of these effects are especially dramatic, collectively they help explain why animals fed such a deficient diet are growth impaired and have poor food efficiency. Some of the effects shown in Table 8 can be due to an effect on membranes per se, while other effects are attributable to a lack of arachidonic acid to serve as precursor for eicosanoid synthesis.

TABLE 8
Major Effects of EFA Deficiency in the Rat

1. Skin symptoms   Scaly, dry skin
2. Weight   Decrease
3. Circulation   Heart enlargement; decreased capillary resistance (lower blood pressure at periphery);
                       increased permeability
4. Kidney   Enlargement; intertubular hemorrhage
5. Lung   Cholesterol accumulation
6. Endocrine glands   (a) Adrenals. Weight decreased in females and increased in males
                       (b) Thyroid. Reduced weight.
7. Reproduction   (a) Females. Irregular estrus and impaired reproduction and lactation
                       (b) Males. Degeneration of seminiferrous tubules
8. Metabolism   (a) Changes in fatty acid composition of most organs
                       (b) Increase in cholesterol levels in liver, adrenals, and skin
                       (c) Decrease in plasma cholesterol
                       (d) Changes in swelling of heart and liver mitochondria and uncoupling of oxidative
                            phosphorylation
                       (e) Increased triglyceride synthesis and release by the liver

From M. I. Gurr and A. T. James, *Lipid Biochemistry: An Introduction*, Cornell University Press, Ithaca, New York, 1971, 56. With permission.

5. Eicosanoids

Eicosanoids are 20-carbon molecules having hormone-like activity. In their various forms they are produced and released by many different mammalian cells rather than being produced by highly specialized cells as is the instance of insulin and the β cell in the islets of Langerhans. When each of these compounds is produced, their site of action is local. That is, whereas insulin may be transported from the pancreas to peripheral target cells, the eicosanoids are produced, released, and have as their targets the surrounding cells. For this reason, the eicosanoids are called local hormones. They have a variety of actions. Table 9 lists the eicosanoids and their functions.

The eicosanoids fall into three general groups of compounds: the prostaglandins (compounds of the PG series), the thromboxanes (compounds of the TBX series), and the leukotrienes (compounds of the LKT series). All of these compounds arise from a 20-carbon polyunsaturated fatty acid. This fatty acid is usually arachidonic acid (20 carbons, 4 double bonds at 5, 8, 11, 14). However, in instances where the diet is rich in omega-3 (n-3) fatty acids the precursor may be a 20-carbon 5-double-bond fatty acid, eicosapentaenoic acid (double bonds at 5, 8, 11, 14, 17). Other eicosanoids can be synthesized from a 20-carbon fatty acid, dihomo-γ-linoleic acid which has only 3 double bonds at carbons 8, 11, and 14. Each of these precursors yields a particular set of eicosanoids. They are called eicosanoids because they have 20 carbons; during their synthesis they take up oxygen and are cyclized. Dihomo-γ-linoleic acid is the precursor of prostaglandin E_1 (PGE$_1$) and prostaglandin $E_{1\alpha}$ (PGE$_{1\alpha}$) and subsequent prostaglandins. Arachidonic acid is the precursor of prostaglandins of the 2 series (PGE$_2$, PGF$_{2\alpha}$, etc.) and eicosapentaenoic acid is the precursor of prostaglandins of the 3 series (PGE$_3$, PGF$_{3\alpha}$, etc.).

The cyclization of these 20-carbon fatty acids is accomplished by a complex of enzymes called the prostaglandin synthesis complex. The first step is the cyclooxygenase step which involves the cyclization of C-9 to C-12 of the precursor to form the cyclic 9,11-endoperoxide-15-hydroperoxide (PGG$_2$) shown in Figure 15. PGG$_2$ is then used to form prostaglandin H_2 (PGH$_2$) through the removal of one oxygen from the carbonyl group at carbon 15. Glutathione peroxidase and prostaglandin H synthase catalyze the reaction shown in Figure 16. Prostaglandin H synthase is a very unstable short-lived enzyme with a messenger RNA that is one of the shortest-lived species so far found in mammalian cells. The expression of genes for this

TABLE 9
Functions of Eicosanoids

Eicosanoids	Function
PGG$_2$	Precursor of PGH$_2$
PGH$_2$	Precursor of PGD$_2$, PGE$_2$, PGI$_2$, PGF$_{2\alpha}$
PGD$_2$	Promotes sleeping behavior
	Precursor of PGF$_2$
PGE$_2$	Enhances perception of pain when histamine or bradykinin is given. Induces signs of inflammation. Promotes wakefulness. Precursor of PGF$_{2\alpha}$. Reduces gastric acid secretion, induces partuition. Vasoconstrictor in some tissues. Vasodilator in other tissues. Maintains the patency of the ductus arteriosis prior to birth
PGF$_{2\alpha}$	Bronchial constrictor. Vasoconstrictor especially in coronary vasculature. Increases sperm motility. Induces partuition; stimulates steroidogenesis corpus luteum; induces luteolysis
PGI$_2$	Inhibits platelet aggregation
PGE$_1$	Inhibits motility of nonpregnant uterus increases motility of pregnant uterus
	Bronchial dilator
TXA$_2$	Stimulates platelet aggregation. Potent vasoconstrictor
TXB$_2$	Metabolite of TXA$_2$
LTA$_4$	Precursor of LTB$_4$
LTB$_4$	Potent chemotaxic agent

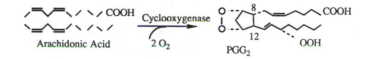

FIGURE 15. Cyclization of C-9 to C-12 to form PGG$_2$.

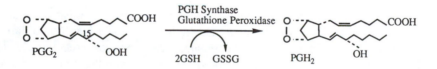

FIGURE 16. Oxygen removal to form PGH$_2$.

enzyme is under the control of polypeptide growth factors such as interleukin 1α and colony stimulating factor 1.

Interferon α and β inhibit expression and prostanoid production by the macrophages. Glutathione peroxidase is a selenium-containing enzyme and in animals fed a highly polyunsaturated fat diet one might expect to see a higher than normal requirement for selenium in the diet to accommodate the need for this enzyme. However, such an expectation is without merit. Studies of rats fed a highly polyunsaturated fat diet such as a marine oil-rich diet require more vitamin E to accommodate the increased need to support the antioxidation system (see Section VII.3 this unit) but not an increased need for selenium. The need to make the eicosanoids is quite low compared to the need to suppress the formation of fatty acid radicals. This probably explains why the selenium requirement is not increased under these dietary conditions.

PGH$_2$ is then converted through the action of a variety of isomerases to PGD$_2$ or PGE$_2$ or prostacyclin I$_2$ (PGI$_2$) or prostaglandin F$_{2\alpha}$ (PGF$_{2\alpha}$). These are the primary precursors of the prostaglandins of the D, E, and F series and PGI or thromboxane. The conversion to subsequent prostaglandins is mediated by enzymes that are specific to a certain cell type and tissue. Not all of these subsequent compounds are formed in all tissues. Thus, PGE$_2$ and PGF$_{2\alpha}$ are produced in the kidney and spleen. $PGF_{2\alpha}$ and PGE are also produced in the uterus only when signals from the pituitary induce their production, and so stimulate parturition. PGI_2 is primarily produced by endothelial cells lining the blood vessels. This prostaglandin inhibits platelet aggregation and thus is important to maintaining a blood flow free of clots. It is counteracted by thromboxane A_2 which is produced by the platelets when these cells contact a foreign surface. PGE_2, $PGF_{2\alpha}$, and PGI_2 are formed by the heart in about equal amounts. All of these prostaglandins have a very short half-life. No sooner are they released than they are inactivated. The thromboxanes are highly active metabolites of the prostaglandins. As mentioned above, they are formed when PGH_2 has its cyclopentane ring replaced by a six-membered oxane ring shown in Figure 17. Imidazole is a potent inhibitor of thromboxane A synthase and is used to block TXA_2 production and platelet aggregation.

Thromboxane A_2 has a role in clot formation and the name thromboxane comes from this function (thrombus means clot). The half-life of TXA_2 is less than one minute. TXB_2 is its metabolic end product and has little biological activity. Measuring TXB_2 levels in blood and tissue can give an indication of how much TXA_2 had been produced. PGD_2 and PGE_2 are involved in the regulation of sleep-wake cycles in a variety of species.

The cyclooxygenase reaction illustrated in Figure 15 can be inhibited by certain antiinflammatory drugs such as aspirin, indomethacin, and phenylbutazone. These are the nonsteroidal antiinflammatory drugs that are commonly available in drug stores. These drugs block the action of cyclooxygenase by acetylating the enzyme. While occasional use of these drugs for the occasional injury or headache is harmless, long-term chronic use can result in untoward effects. Long-term chronic use of aspirin, for example, can affect vascular competence and blood clotting. People consuming large amounts of aspirin over long periods of time may find an increase in bruises (subcutaneous hemorrhages). Small contact injuries that normally would not result in a bruise will do so in these people. Gastric bleeding is another possible complication with long-term chronic aspirin ingestion. Aplastic anemia can result from long-term phenylbutazone therapy. Again, the occasional use of these drugs is not likely to have these effects.

A second group of antiinflammatory agents are the steroids: hydrocortisone, prednisone, and other similar compounds. These drugs are prescription drugs which act by inhibiting the enzyme, phospholipase A_2. Phospholipase A_2 stimulates the release of arachidonic acid from the membrane phospholipids. Hence, inhibition of this reaction will result in a decreased supply of arachidonic acid for prostaglandin synthesis. When the conversion of arachidonic acid to prostaglandins is inhibited as above, or when either of the other 20-carbon fatty acids are abundantly available, a different series of prostaglandins and leukotrienes are produced. Eicosapentaenoic acid is not as good a substrate for cyclooxygenation as is arachidonic acid. As a result, less of the arachidonic acid related prostaglandins (even-numbered PGs and TBXs) are produced and more of the odd-numbered prostaglandins and leukotrienes are produced. Figure 18 shows the overall metabolic pathway for eicosanoid synthesis and degradation.

Although the cyclooxygenase pathway is quite important in the production of prostaglandins, equally important is the lipoxygenase pathway. This pathway is catalyzed by a family of enzymes called the lipoxygenase enzymes. These enzymes differ from the cyclooxygenase enzymes in the catalytic site for oxygen addition to the unsaturated fatty acid. One lipoxygenase is active at the double bond at carbon 5, while a second is active at carbon 11, and a third is active at carbon 15. The products of these reactions are monohydroperoxy-eicosatetraenoic acids (HPETEs) and are numbered according to the location of the double bond to which the oxygen is added. 5HPETE is the major lipoxygenase product in basophils, polymorphonuclear leukocytes, macrophages, mast cells, and any organ undergoing an inflammatory response. 12HPETE is the major product in platelets, pancreatic endocrine cells, vascular smooth muscle, and glomerular cells. 15HPETE predominates in reticulocytes, eosinophils, T-lymphocytes, and tracheal epithelial cells. The HPETEs are not in themselves active hormones;

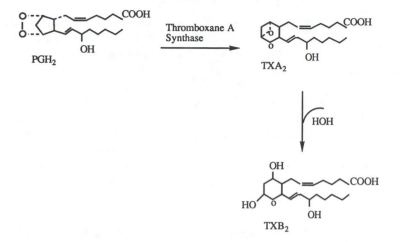

FIGURE 17. Reaction sequence that produces TXA₂ and TXB₂.

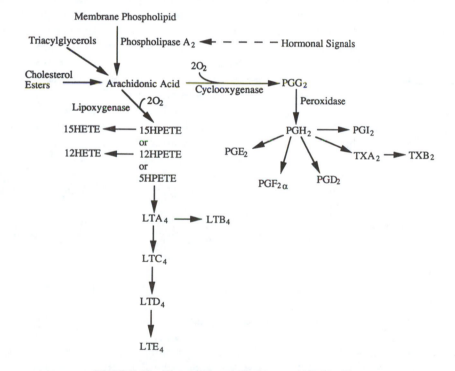

FIGURE 18. Eicosanoid synthesis from arachidonic acid.

rather, they serve as precursors for the leukotrienes. The leukotrienes are the metabolic end products of the lipoxygenase reaction. These compounds contain at least three conjugated double bonds. The unstable 5HPETE is converted to either an analogous alcohol (hydroxy fatty acid) or is reduced by a peroxide or converted to leukotriene. The peroxidative reduction of 5'HPETE to the stable 5HETE (5-hydroxyeicosatetraenoic acid) is similar to that of 12HPETE to 12HETE and of 15HPETE to 15HETE. In each instance the carbon-carbon double bonds are unconjugated and the geometry of the double bonds is *trans, cis, cis,* respectively.

In contrast to the active thromboxanes which have very short half-lives, the leukotrienes can persist as long as four hours. These compounds comprise a group of substances known as the slow acting anaphylaxis substances. They cause slowly evolving but protracted contractions of smooth muscles in the airways and gastrointestinal tract. Leukotriene C_4 is rapidly converted to LTD_4 which, in turn, is slowly converted to LTE_4. Enzymes in the plasma are responsible for these conversions.

The products of the lipoxygenase pathway are potent mediators of the response to allergens, tissue damage (inflammation), hormone secretion, cell movement, cell growth, and calcium flux. Within minutes of stimulation, lipoxygenase products are produced. In an allergy attack, for example, an allergen can instigate the release of leukotrienes which are the immediate mediators of response. The leukotrienes are more potent than histamine in stimulating the contraction of the bronchial nonvascular smooth muscles. In addition, LTD_4 increases the permeability of the microvasculature. The mono HETEs and LTB_4 stimulate the movement of eosinophils and neutrophils, making them the first line of defense in injury resulting in inflammation.

As mentioned, when dihomo-γ-linoleic acid or eicosapentaenoic acid serve as substrates for eicosanoid production, the products are either of the 1 series or 3 series. The products they form may be less active than those formed from arachidonic acid and this decrease in activity can be of therapeutic value. Hence, ingestion of omega-3 fatty acids leads to the decreased production of prostaglandin E_2 and its metabolites; a decrease in the production of thromboxane A_2, a potent platelet aggregator and vasoconstrictor; and a decrease in leukotriene B_4, a potent inflammatory hormone and a powerful inducer of leukocyte hemotaxis and adherence. Counteracting these decreases are an increase in thromboxane A_3 (TXA_3) a weak platelet aggregator and vasoconstrictor, an increase in the production of PGI_3 without an increase in PGI_2 which stimulates vasodilation and inhibits platelet aggregation, and an increase in leukotriene B_5 which is a weak inducer of inflammation and a weak chemotoxic agent. Marine oils, rich in omega-3 unsaturated fatty acids, affect (decrease) platelet aggregation because they stimulate the synthesis of thromboxane A_3. Thromboxane A_3 does not have the platelet aggregating property of the other eicosanoids. In addition, eicosapentaenoic acid is used to make the anti-aggregating prostaglandin, PGI_3. Animals fed omega-3-rich oils produce significantly more of the eicosanoids of the LTB_5 series. LTB_4 is an important inflammatory mediator whereas LTB_5 is not.

Fish oil consumption results in an increased neutrophil LTB_5 production with a concomitant decrease in LTB_4 production. This diet-influenced change in LTB_4 and LTB_5 production seems to be related to a reduced incidence of autoimmune-inflammatory disorders such as asthma, psoriasis, and rheumatoid arthritis in populations consuming omega-3 fatty acids routinely. Thus, eicosanoid synthesis can be used as an explanation of the beneficial effects of fish oil ingestion on rheumatoid arthritis. In arthritics, the joints are inflamed and painful. The prostaglandins PGE_2 and leukotriene are both produced from arachidonate. PGE_2 induces the signs of inflammation which include redness and heat due to arteriolar vasodilation, and swelling and localized edema resulting from increased capillary permeability. Leukotriene prevents platelet aggregation. If there is less arachidonate available for the synthesis of these prostaglandins, then the inflammation is inhibited.

Tumorigenesis likewise can be influenced by the relative amounts of the various eicosanoids. Prostaglandin G of the 2-series acts as a tumor promoter. It down regulates macrophage tumoricidal activities and inhibits interleukin-2 production. Increased PGE_2 levels (from omega-6 fatty acids) have been associated with aggressive growth patterns of both basal and squamous cell skin carcinomas in humans. Vegetable oils are rich in these fatty acids. Products of the lipooxygenase pathway (stimulated by the omega-3 fatty acids) have the reverse effect.

While the various eicosanoids have different (and sometimes conflicting) effects on inflammatory processes and on tumor promotion, one might anticipate that susceptibility to pathogenic organisms would be similarly affected. Studies with mice exposed to a variety of pathogens and fed either a fish oil or a control diet did not show any diet fat-related differences in susceptibility to these organisms. Other research has suggested that a dietary fat effect on immunological competence might be related to the age of the animal and whether the diet contained sufficient vitamin E to suppress the formation of peroxides which can facilitate the entry of pathogens into target cells. Both age and vitamin E status apparently affect the disease resistance of animals fed different fats.

All of these observations have prompted nutrition scientists to investigate the possible benefits of consuming foods rich in omega-3 fatty acids. A number of years ago, a group of Danish scientists compared the food intake and health status of Danes and Greenland Eskimos. Both populations consume high-protein high-fat diets; however, where the Danish diet includes a variety of milk and meat products, the Eskimo diet includes primarily fish and marine creatures such as whale, walrus, seal, and so forth. These marine foods contain fat which is rich in the omega-3 fatty acids such as linolenic acid, eicosapentanoic acid, and docosahexanoic acid. The P/S ratio of the Greenland Eskimo diet was 0.84 compared to 0.24 for Danes. The Eskimo diet contained more fatty acids with a single double bond than did the Danish diet. The Eskimo diet also contained significant amounts of long-chain fatty acids having 5 or 6 double bonds. While omega-3 fatty acids (or N-3 fatty acids) are usually found in marine foods (ocean fish and sea mammals), some vegetable oils such as primrose oil, canola oil, wheat germ oil, linseed oil, and walnut oil also contain significant amounts. Small amounts are also found in a number of other foods such as spinach, certain margarines, broccoli, and lettuce. Hens fed omega-3 fatty acid-rich fats will lay eggs containing these fatty acids in the yolk.

The Danish investigators observed these diet differences between Danes and Eskimos and also noticed the differences in blood lipid profiles as well as differences in the incidence of cardiovascular disease (CVD). While CVD was one of the leading causes of death in the Danes, the leading cause of death in Eskimos was cerebral hemorrhage (stroke). The Eskimos had prolonged bleeding times and a nosebleed was a serious problem. The prolonged clotting time was probably due to the omega-3 fatty acid effect on those eicosanoids involved in clot formation. These death statistics considered age-matched groups, but were not age adjusted. That is, the investigators compared the two populations using age-matched groups without correcting for total population longevity or for early death due to communicable diseases, malnutrition (in infants particularly), or the hazards of daily life. For the Eskimo, these factors could have been quite important. Furthermore, one must realize that all causes must add up to 100%. Thus, if fewer die of CVD more may have died from communicable disease or something else. Nonetheless, the findings of the Danes regarding omega-3 fatty acid intake and cardiovascular disease set off a whole flurry of animal and human studies directed toward understanding how the omega-3 fatty acids affected metabolism.

Consistent with the Danish report of lower levels of blood lipids in the Eskimos, others found that the consumption of marine oils was associated with a significant decline in blood lipid levels. The decrease in serum lipids in humans and experimental animals with fish oil consumption has been demonstrated many times. The reasons for this serum lipid lowering effect have been explored. Fish oil in the diet easily oxidizes and forms peroxides. These peroxides are what gives these oils their peculiar and oftimes objectionable odor. Diets containing large amounts of these oils are not as well liked by experimental animals and appetite is suppressed. Food intake may be decreased by as much as 20%. Even when the scientist takes stringent care of the diet by preventing autooxidation, the food intake of fat-rich diets is reduced. Despite a reduction in food intake, animals utilize their diet very well and a marine oil diet usually is characterized by an increase in feed efficiency. That is, the animal will gain more weight per unit of food consumed than an animal consuming a diet containing some other fat source. This is not always true however. Genetically obese rats and mice gain less weight when fed a marine oil diet than fed a corn oil or tallow or safflower oil diet.

At any rate, a decrease in food consumption despite an increase in feed efficiency means that there is less food for the liver to metabolize and convert to VLDL for transport to the peripheral fat depots for storage and, in part, this explains the effect of the marine oils on serum lipid levels. Dietary marine oils have two other equally important effects that can also explain their serum lipid lowering action. The first of these is an inhibition of hepatic fatty acid, phospholipid, and cholesterol synthesis. In part, this attenuation of lipid synthesis by marine oils occurs at the level of specific genes that encode for the lipogenic enzymes. The transcription of genes encoded for enzymes necessary for lipogenesis is suppressed in hepatic tissue from rats fed the marine oils. While we realize that enzymes are never fully active *in vivo* and that the amount of enzyme may not fully predict the amount of product (in this case, lipid) produced, these findings do contribute to our understanding of how dietary marine oils can lower serum lipid levels.

Added to the decrease in lipogenic enzyme activity and decreased rates of lipid synthesis observed in animals fed marine oils is the observation that marine oil-fed animals also have a reduced hepatic lipid output. This means that lipids formed in the liver are not as readily exported and the liver of the animal fed the marine oils contains more fat than the liver of the rat fed a control diet. Reduced hepatic lipid output by humans consuming fish oil supplements has been reported. This too results in a lowering of serum triglycerides and serum cholesterol. Accumulated lipids in the liver may be an additional reason why lipid synthesis is down regulated. Product inhibition, in this case newly synthesized lipid, is a well-recognized metabolic control mechanism.

Consumption of omega-3 fatty acids nonetheless does result in lower blood lipid levels, and this effect is presumed to explain the lower incidence of cardiovascular disease in the Eskimos. Whether this presumption is correct or not cannot be taken for granted. Cardiovascular disease has a complicated pathophysiology that is not well understood. Genetic factors as well as life style choices can influence its development and can determine whether it is a life-threatening condition.

B. FATTY ACIDS AND MEMBRANE FUNCTION

Biological membranes contain a large number of lipids, proteins, lipid-protein complexes, glycolipids, and glycoproteins. The arrangement of these many compounds within the membrane structure has been studied extensively.

The membranes exist as a lipid bilayer because the phospholipids have amphipathic characteristics. They have both polar (the phosphorylated substituent at carbon 3) and nonpolar (the fatty acids) regions. The polar region is hydrophilic and is positioned such that it is in contact with the aqueous media around and within the cells. The nonpolar or fatty acid region is oriented towards the center of the bilayer so that it is protected from contact with the contents of the cell and the fluids that surround it.

The ability of these amphipathic compounds to self-assemble into a bilayer can be demonstrated *in vitro*. Lipid vesicles can be made by the addition of these phospholipids to water. A lipid bilayer will form just as described above. This feature of the phospholipids is consistent with one of the many roles a membrane serves. It is a permeability barrier for the cells and cell compartments. The lipid bilayer forms the matrix into which specific proteins are placed. Each of the individual phospholipids and the cholesterol provide specific regional characteristics that satisfy the insertion requirements of each of the many membrane proteins. The lipid bilayer serves as a seal around these membrane proteins and thus prevents nonspecific leakage. These lipids also serve to maintain the proteins in their most appropriate functional conformations. The polar position of the phospholipids satisfies the requirements for the electrostatic charge that is needed for the surface associations of specific cell surface proteins. All of these characteristics are needed and are critical to normal cell function. For example, an intact permeability barrier to sodium, potassium, calcium, and hydrogen ions is needed so that electrochemical gradients, which, in turn, drive other membrane transport process, are maintained.

Cell membranes usually work best when their lipids are in the liquid crystal state. This means that there are regional differences in the physical state of the lipid. Some portions may be fairly fluid whereas other regions may be fairly solid. The localized difference in physical state or fluidity has to do with the chain length and saturation of the fatty acids attached at carbons 1 and 2 of the phospholipid; it is this portion of the molecule that extends into the center of the bilayer. Membranes whose phospholipid fatty acids are saturated are less fluid than those membranes containing polyunsaturated fatty acids in their phospholipids. Even within a membrane there can be regional differences in fluidity due to the nature of the fatty acids in the phospholipids of that region. Differences in fluidity are due not only to the ratio of saturated fatty acids to unsaturated fatty acids, but also to the ratio of cholesterol to fatty acids. This ratio varies according to the location of the membrane. Plasma membranes, for example, contain more cholesterol than do mitochondrial membranes.

1. Membrane Phospholipid Composition

There are three major classes of lipids in membranes: glycolipids, cholesterol, and phospholipids. The glycolipids have a role in the cell surface-associated antigens whereas the cholesterol serves to regulate fluidity. The phospholipids have fatty acids attached at carbons 1 and 2. It is usual to find a saturated fatty acid attached at carbon 1 and an unsaturated fatty acid at carbon 2. In addition, phosphatidylethanolamine and phosphatidylserine usually have fatty acids that are more unsaturated than phosphatidylinositol and phosphatidylcholine. Less than 10% of the membrane phospholipid is phosphatidylinositol. Plasma membranes have no cardiolipin and the mitochondrial membranes have very little phosphatidylserine. Several of these phospholipids have important roles in the signal transduction processes that mediate the action of a variety of hormones. Phosphatidylinositol and its role in the phosphatidylinositol cycle is one of the most important. Phosphatidylcholine and phosphatidylethanolamine also play a role in these systems. Shown in Figure 19 is the PIP cycle. Its importance relates to the action of inositol-1,4,5-phosphate in moving the calcium ion from its intracellular store to where it can stimulate protein kinase C. Phosphatidylinositol also serves to anchor glycoproteins to the membrane. Glycoproteins are tethered to the external aspect of the plasma membrane and play a role in the cell recognition process. Antigens, pathogens, and foreign proteins are recognized by these structures.

2. Disease Effects on Membrane Lipids

There are numerous reviews on the effects of essential fatty acids and disease on the fatty acid content of membranes. While the primary focus has been on the abnormalities of the proteins in the membrane lipid bilayer, there is a role for the lipid in some of these disorders. Muscular dystrophy and multiple sclerosis are characterized by changes in the lipid structure of the membrane. In the former, the change consists of an increase in the amount of lysophosphatidylcholine and cardiolipin. In multiple sclerosis there is a degeneration of the myelin of both central and peripheral nerves. The myelin is 75% lipid and 25% protein. Although the disease could be attributed to a specific abnormality in either component, there are reports that the protein contains about 27% fatty acid (palmitate and oleate) in a covalent linkage and that multiple sclerosis is associated with a derangement in this association and a reduction in the amount of phosphatidylserine. There have been many reports of these lipid changes or a lack of change in myelin; however, it is generally agreed that the disease is not primary to the lipid portion of the membrane. Rather, it is the specific myelin protein that somehow becomes abnormal. Such other diseases as renal disease, hepatic disease, ethanol intoxication, spur cell anemia, and diabetes, likewise result in secondary effects on the membrane lipids. These changes can, however, make the disease state worse by compromising the functionality of the membrane and its role in metabolic regulation. In humans with cirrhotic liver disease, the erythrocyte membrane fatty acids change. In cirrhotic subjects, the membranes contain less phosphatidylethanolamine and more phosphatidylcholine than membranes from normal subjects. In these subjects, the membrane cholesterol and fatty acid content remains unchanged, but the ratio of cholesterol to phospholipid increases.

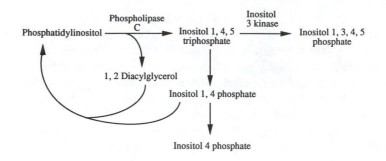

FIGURE 19. Phosphatidylinositol (PIP) cycle.

3. Hormonal Effects on Membrane Lipids

The hormone insulin can affect the fatty acid profile of the membrane phospholipids through its effect on glucose conversion to fatty acids and through its effect on the desaturases. Other hormones have an influence on this profile as well. Examples of this influence are shown in Table 10. Daily injections of the synthetic glucocorticoid, dexamethasone, resulted in an increase in the mole percent of linoleic (18:2) acid and a decrease in arachidonic acid (20:4). Thyroidectomy resulted in a small increase in rat liver mitochondrial levels of 18:2 and 20:4. This is probably due to the reduction in fatty acid turnover that occurs in the absence of the thyroid gland. Hypophysectomy, which causes a decrease in growth hormone levels, resulted in an increase in 18:2 and a decrease in 20:4 in hepatic mitochondria. Studies on the influence of all the many hormones that affect fatty acid synthesis, phospholipid synthesis, and membrane phospholipid fatty acid levels are not as readily available as are reports on the dietary fat effects on these parameters. However, they are of interest because these hormones may also have a large influence on the function of the protein components that are embedded in the various membranes. These hormones may act directly on the synthesis and activation of these proteins, which in turn may affect their conformation and hence their activity. Thyroxine, for example, negatively affects the activity of the Δ9 desaturase which, because it is less active, results in less unsaturated fatty acids in the membrane. In turn, microsomal cytochrome b_5 activity is less dependent on the lipid environment. That is, it must be surrounded by a very fluid lipid, and this lipid must have a number of unsaturated fatty acids in it. Just as thyroidectomy results in a decrease in membrane phospholipid fatty acid unsaturation, hyperthyroidism has the reverse effect. The thyroid hormones also affect fatty acid elongation by inducing an increase in the activity of the microsomal fatty acid elongation system while having little effect on mitochondrial elongation. It has been reported that the incorporation of labeled choline into brain and liver phosphatidylcholine was less in thyrotoxic rats than in normal rats.

4. Age Effects on Membrane Lipids

As animals age, their hormonal status changes, as does the lipid component of their membranes. With age, there is a decrease in growth hormone production, an increase followed by a decrease in the hormones for reproduction and, as the animal ages, larger fat stores. Larger fat cells are resistant to insulin, and insulin levels may rise as a result of increased fat cell size (insulin resistance). As mentioned in the preceding section, these hormones can affect the lipid portion of the membranes within and around the cells and hence affect how these cells regulate their metabolism. With age, the degree of unsaturation of the membrane fatty acids decreases and the cholesterol level rises.

There is also an increase in the number of superoxide radicals. This increase may be responsible for the degradation of the membrane lipids which, in turn, might explain the age-related changes in membrane function. Membranes from aging animals are less fluid and have reduced transport capacities. As animals age there is a decline in heptic mitochondrial

TABLE 10

**Effects of Glucocorticoid or Thyroid Deficiency or Diabetes on
Fatty Acid Profiles of Liver or Isolated Liver Mitochondria[a]**

Treatment	Fatty acids (mole %)						Tissue
	16:0	18:0	18:1	18:2	20:4	22:6	
1 mg GC/day	14.6	22.7	6.6	28.5	19.0	3.5	Liver
Control	17.0	20.3	7.6	15.1	27.4	1.5	Liver
Thyroidectomy	12.5	21	8.6	19.5	19.0	8.1	RLM
Control	13.0	20	9.0	17.4	15.7	7.0	RLM
Hypophysectomy	27.1	21.5	13.5	17.0	14.5	2.0	RLM
Control	27.4	22	12.2	12.1	17.4	2.8	RLM
Diabetes[b]	24.5	23.3	7.0	22.4	15.2	4.2	RLM
Control	16.9	23.2	9.3	22.7	22.2	3.1	RLM

[a]   GC, synthetic glucocorticoid, dexamethasone; RLM, rat liver mitochondria.
[b]   Streptozotocin-induced diabetes.

respiratory rate and a decrease in the respiratory ratio and the ADP/O ratio. In addition, there are reports of an age-related decrease in membrane fatty acid unsaturation coupled with a decrease in membrane fluidity and a decrease in the exchange of ATP for ADP across the mitochondrial membrane, a decrease in ATP synthesis, and an amelioration of these age-related decreases in mitochondrial function by restricted feeding (caloric intake reduced by 50% over the lifetime of the animals).

5. Membrane Function

In the previous section, the importance of diet, age, and hormonal status was described in terms of their influence on the composition of the membrane lipids. Although not emphasized, these compositional differences have important effects on metabolic regulation. This regulation consists of the control of the flux of nutrients, substrates, and/or products into, out of, and between the various compartments of the cell.

The cellular membranes serve as geographical boundaries of the cell, and they are the "gatekeepers" of the cells and their compartments. They regulate the influx and efflux of nutrients, substrates, hormones, and metabolic products produced or used by the cell or compartment in the course of its metabolic activity. For example, the mitochondrial membrane, through its transport of two- and four-carbon intermediates and through its exchange of ADP for ATP, regulates the activity of the respiratory chain and ATP synthesis. If too little ADP enters the mitochondria because of decreased ADP transport across the mitochondrial membrane, respiratory chain activity will decrease, less ATP will be synthesized, and there may be a decrease in other mitochondrial reactions that are either driven by ADP influx or dependent on ATP availability. Through its export of citrate from the matrix of the mitochondria it regulates the availability of citrate to the cytosol for cleavage into oxaloacetate and acetyl CoA, the beginning of fatty acid synthesis. If more citrate is exported from the mitochondria than can be split to oxaloacetate and acetyl CoA, this citrate will feed back onto the phosphofructokinase reaction, and glycolysis will be inhibited. Thus, the activity of the mitochondrial membrane tricarboxylate transporter has a role in the control of cytosolic metabolism. Other transporters such as the dicarboxylate transporter or the adenine nucleotide translocase have similar responsibilities vis-á-vis the control of cytosolic and mitochondrial metabolic activity. In the plasma membrane, receptors embedded in the membrane have a similar function. That is, they control the entry of nutrients or hormones into the cell. Further, the plasma membrane hormone receptor may bind a given hormone and, with binding, elicit a cascade of reactions characteristic of the hormone effect without permitting the entry of the hormone itself into the cystosolic compartment. An example here is the hormone insulin.

Insulin binds to its receptor and, in so doing, elicits the cascade of events that include the transport and metabolism of glucose by the cell. The insulin, bound to the receptor site, is inactivated and is brought into the cell by pinocytosis for further degradation. Other hormones, notably the nonprotein steroids and the low molecular weight hormones such as epinephrine and thyroxine, pass through the plasma membrane and attach to receptors in the cytosol and/ or nuclear membrane or on the endoplasmic reticulum. Once attached to their respective binding sites, they also elicit a metabolic response.

In the membranes are a variety of closely packed proteins and lipids. The membrane-bound proteins have extensive hydrophobic regions and usually require lipids for the maintenance of their activity. Adenylate cyclase, cytochrome b_5, and cytochrome c oxidase have all been shown to have phospholipid affinities. Cytochrome c oxidase from mitochondria has a tightly bound aldehyde lipid that cannot be removed without destroying its activity as the enzyme that transfers electrons to molecular oxygen in the final step of respiration. A number of other membrane proteins have tightly bound fatty acids as part of their structures. These fatty acids are covalently bound to their proteins as a posttranslational event and act to direct, insert, and anchor the proteins in the cell membranes. Other lipids are bound differently to membrane proteins. Some are acylated with fatty acids during their passage from their site of synthesis on the rough endoplasmic reticulum to the membrane, whereas others acquire their lipid component during their placement in the membrane. β-Hydroxybutyrate dehydrogenase, for example, requires the choline head of phosphatidylcholine for its activity. If hepatocytes are caused to increase their synthesis of phosphatidylmethylethanolamine, which substitutes for phosphatidylcholine in the membrane, β-hydroxybutyrate dehydrogenase activity is reduced.

All of these examples illustrate the importance of the cellular and intracellular membranes in the regulation of metabolism. They illustrate the fact that the gatekeeping property of the membrane is vested in the structure and function of the various transporters and receptors or binding proteins embedded in the membrane. Whereas the genetic heritage of an individual determines the amino acid sequence of the proteins, and hence their function, this function can be modified by the lipid milieu in which they exist. Diet, hormonal state, and genetics, in turn, control the lipid milieu in terms of the kinds and amounts of the different lipids that are synthesized within the cell and incorporated into the membrane.

C. FATTY ACID OXIDATION

While fatty acids are important components of membranes, and while certain ones are important precursors of the eicosanoids, the main function of these molecules in the body is to provide energy to sustain life. This provision is accomplished through oxidation. Regardless of whether the fatty acids come from the diet or are mobilized from the tissue triacylglyceride store, the pathway for oxidation is the same once the triacylglyceride has been hydrolyzed.

The hydrolysis of stored lipid is catalyzed in a three-step process by one of the lipases specific to mono, di, or triacylglycerol. Intracellular hormone-sensitive lipase hydrolyze fatty acids one at a time from all three carbon positions of the glycerol moiety and these fatty acids are then available for oxidation. Interstitial hormone-insensitive lipase has a similar mode of action. The lipases that act on the phospholipids to release arachidonic acid for eicosanoid synthesis or to release inositol-1,3,4-phosphate and diacylglyceride or other components of the phospholipids also provide fatty acids for oxidation, but that is not their primary role.

The lipases in the adipose tissue are the key to the regulated release of fatty acids from the stored triacylglycerides. These fatty acids can be oxidized *in situ* by the adipocyte, but usually they are released for transport to other tissues as energy sources. The fatty acids are carried by albumin or by lipoproteins to where they are needed. At the target cell, the fatty acids are liberated from the triacylglycerides carried by the lipoproteins through the action of lipoprotein lipase or liberated from albumin by an (as yet) undefined mechanism. The liberated fatty acids diffuse through the plasma membrane, bind to the cytosolic fatty acid binding protein, and migrate through the cytoplasm to the outer mitochondrial membrane or to the peroxisomes, microsomes, or the endoplasmic reticulum. At each of these destinations, they are activated by conversion to their CoA thioesters.

This activation requires ATP and the enzyme acyl CoA synthase or thiokinase. There are several thiokinases which differ with respect to their specificity for the different fatty acids. The activation step is dependent on the release of energy from two high-energy phosphate bonds. ATP is hydrolyzed to AMP and two molecules of inorganic phosphate.

Figure 20 shows the initial steps in the oxidation of fatty acids. Once the fatty acid is activated it is bound to carnitine with the release of CoA. The acyl carnitine is then translocated through the mitochondrial membranes into the mitochondrial matrix via the carnitine acylcarnitine translocase. As one molecule of acylcarnitine is passed into the matrix, one molecule of carnitine is translocated back to the cytosol and the acylcarnitine is converted back to acyl CoA. The acyl CoA can then enter the β oxidation pathway shown in Figure 21. Without carnitine, the oxidation of fatty acids, especially the long-chain fatty acids, cannot proceed. Acyl CoA can not traverse the membrane into the mitochondria and thus requires a translocase for its entry. The translocase requires carnitine. Carnitine is synthesized from methionine and lysine as shown in Figure 22.

While most of the fatty acids that enter the β oxidation pathway are completely oxidized via the Krebs cycle and respiratory chain to CO_2 and HOH, some of the acetyl CoA is instead converted to the ketone, acetoacetate, and β-hydroxybutyrate. The condensation of two molecules of acetyl CoA to acetoacetyl CoA occurs in the mitochondria via the enzyme β-ketothiolase. Acetoacetyl CoA then condenses with another acetyl CoA to form HMG CoA. Finally, the HMG CoA is cleaved into acetoacetic acid and acetyl CoA. The acetoacetic acid is reduced to β-hydroxybutyrate and this reduction is dependent on the ratio of NAD^+ to $NADH^+H^+$. The enzyme for this reduction, β-hydroxybutyrate dehydrogenase is tightly bound to the inner aspect of the mitochondrial membrane. Because of its high activity, the product (β-hydroxybutyrate) and substrate (acetoacetate) are in equilibrium. Measurements of these two compounds can thus be used to determine the redox state (ratio of oxidized to reduced NAD) of the mitochondrial compartment.

HMG CoA is also synthesized in the cytosol, however, because this compartment lacks the HMG CoA lyase, the ketones are formed only in the mitochondria. In the cytosol, HMG CoA is the beginning substrate for cholesterol synthesis. The ketones can ultimately be used as fuel but may appear in the blood, liver, and other tissues at a level of less than 0.2 mM. In the starving individuals, or in people consuming a high-fat diet, blood and tissue ketone levels may rise above normal (3 to 5 mM). However, unless these levels greatly exceed the body's capacity to use them as fuel (as is the case in uncontrolled diabetes mellitus with levels up to 20 mM) a rise in ketone levels is not a cause for concern. Ketones are choice metabolic fuels for muscle and brain. Although both tissues may prefer to use glucose, the ketones can be used when glucose is in short supply. Ketones are used to spare glucose wherever possible under these conditions.

The oxidation of unsaturated fatty acids follows the same pathway as the saturated fatty acids until the double bonded carbons are reached. At this point, a few side steps must be taken that involve a few additional enzymes. An example of this pathway is shown in Figure 23 using linoleate as the fatty acid being oxidized.

Linoleate has two double bonds in the *cis* configuration. β Oxidation removes three acetyl units leaving a CoA attached to the terminal carbon just before the first *cis* double bond. At this point an isomerase enzyme, Δ^3 *cis* Δ^6 *trans* enoyl CoA isomerase, acts to convert the first *cis* bond to a *trans* bond. Now this part of the molecule can once again enter the β oxidation sequence and two more acetyl CoA units are released. The second double bond is then opened and a hydroxyl group is inserted. In turn, this hydroxyl group is rotated to the L position and the remaining product can then reenter the β oxidation pathway. Other unsaturated fatty acids

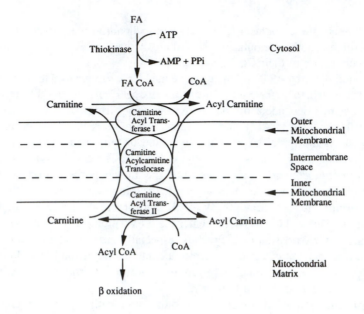

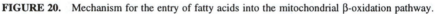

FIGURE 20.　Mechanism for the entry of fatty acids into the mitochondrial β-oxidation pathway.

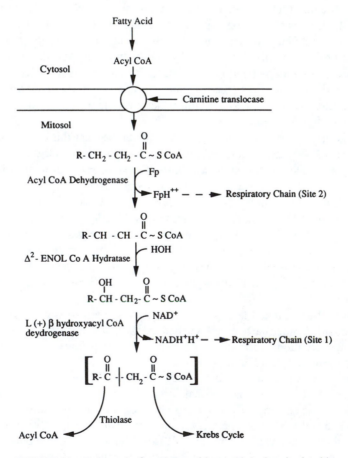

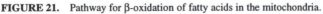

FIGURE 21.　Pathway for β-oxidation of fatty acids in the mitochondria.

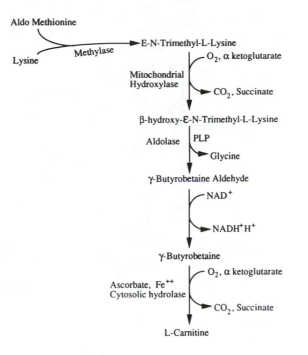

FIGURE 22. Synthesis of carnitine from lysine and methionine.

can be similarly oxidized. Each time the double bond is approached the isomerization and hydroxyl group addition takes place until all of the fatty acid is oxidized.

While β oxidation is the main pathway for the oxidation of fatty acids, some fatty acids undergo α oxidation so as to provide the substrates for the synthesis of sphingolipids. These reactions occur in the endoplasmic reticulum and mitochondria and involve the mixed function oxidases because they require molecular oxygen, reduced NAD, and specific cytochromes. The fatty acid oxidation that occurs in organelles other than the mitochondria are energy wasteful reactions because these other organelles do not have the Krebs cycle nor do they have the respiratory chain which takes the reducing equivalents released by the oxidative steps and combine them with oxygen to make water, releasing energy that is then trapped in the high-energy bonds of the ATP.

Peroxisomal oxidation in the kidney and liver is an important aspect of drug metabolism. The peroxisomes are a class of subcellular organelles that are important in the protection against oxygen toxicity. They have a high level of catalase activity which suggests their importance in the antioxidant system. The peroxisomal fatty acid oxidation pathway differs in three important ways from the mitochondrial pathway. First, the initial dehydrogenation is accomplished by a cyanide-insensitive oxidase which produces H_2O_2. This H_2O_2 is rapidly extinguished by catalase. Second, the enzymes of the pathway prefer long-chain fatty acids and are slightly different in structure from those (with the same function) of the mitochondrial pathway. Third, β oxidation in the peroxisomes stops at eight carbons rather than proceeding all the way to acetyl CoA. It may be that peroxisomal oxidation helps the body get rid of fatty acids that are in excess of 20 carbons in length. The peroxisomes also serve in the conversion of cholesterol to bile acids and in the formation of ether lipids (plasmalogens). Of interest are the reports of a rare fatal genetic disorder which is characterized by the absence of the peroxisomes. This is called the Zellweger syndrome. Victims of this disorder do not make bile acids or plasmalogens nor are they able to shorten the very long fatty acids. These biochemical deficiencies are seemingly unrelated to the structural abnormalities observed in liver, kidney, muscle, and brain. Efforts to circumvent the genetic mutation have been unsuccessful. It is possible to detect its presence by the absence of peroxisomal enzymes in amniotic fluid.

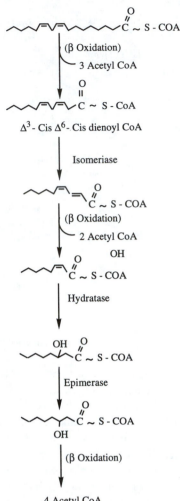

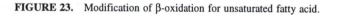

FIGURE 23.   Modification of β-oxidation for unsaturated fatty acid.

D. DYNAMIC CONSIDERATIONS IN FATTY ACID SYNTHESIS AND USE

The body consists of many different organs and cell types whose fuel needs differ appreciably. Most of the foregoing discussion has focused on the individual reactions that comprise fatty acid synthesis and use. However, one must appreciate the complexity of the system that dictates the ebb and flow of these energy-rich molecules. In this we acknowledge the role of the many hormones that regulate or influence lipogenesis and lipolysis. Fatty acid synthesis in the liver and fat cell is stimulated by insulin and high-carbohydrate diets. Fatty acid release is stimulated by thyroid hormone, growth hormone, epinephrine and norepinephrine, glucocorticoid, glucagon, ACTH, and starvation. Fatty acid oxidation is increased by many of the same hormones that stimulate lipolysis as well as by high-fat feeding. Communication and transport of fatty acids and glycerides via the blood to tissues which use these lipids from tissues which make them involves the synthesis and degradation of lipoproteins. All of these components are shown in Figure 24.

E. CHOLESTEROL SYNTHESIS, DEGRADATION, AND USE

Cholesterol is widely distributed in all cells and is an important lipid constituent of membranes. Membranes differ in the amount of cholesterol they contain; mitochondrial

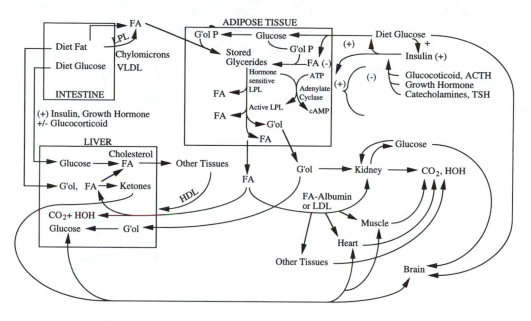

FIGURE 24. Integration of diet and hormone effects on fatty acid metabolism. Inactive LPL = hormone sensitive lipoprotein lipase.

membranes contain very little while plasma membranes contain somewhat more. Cholesterol is not very soluble in water but is carried in the blood by the low density and very low density lipoproteins (LDL and VLDL). About 70% of the cholesterol carried by these proteins is esterified to a fatty acid while the remaining 30% is unesterified. Cholesterol, either from dietary sources or synthesized *de novo*, is the precursor for the synthesis of the bile acids, the adrenal steroids, active vitamin D, and the sex hormones, as shown in Figure 25.

Cholesterol is abundant in the bile where the normal concentration is about 380 to 400 mg/dl. In the bile 96% of the cholesterol exists in the unesterified form. The bile is the chief route for cholesterol excretion. Any cholesterol that is not reabsorbed by the jejunum and ileum is excreted in the feces. Humans consuming a low (~200 mg/day) cholesterol diet have approximately 1300 mg/day returned to the liver. Some of this is the reabsorbed cholesterol via the enterohepatic circulation. Some is carried by the HDL from the periphery as lipids are mobilized and used. The bile does not contain any lipid- or cholesterol-carrying protein, but does contain some phospholipid whose detergent properties keep the cholesterol in solution. If there is a reduction in the amount of phospholipid in the bile, the cholesterol will fall out of solution and form cholesterol aggregates or gall stones. Bile acids also assist in keeping the cholesterol in solution and, again, if there is a reduction in bile acid production cholesterol will precipitate out and collect in the gall bladder.

1. Synthesis

As mentioned, the synthesis of cholesterol begins with acetyl CoA. This synthesis occurs in all cells to varying degrees. The liver, adrenals, gonads, and intestine have the greatest cholesterol synthesizing capacity for obvious reasons. The pathway for cholesterol synthesis is shown in Figure 26.

The total cholesterol pool in the body is carefully regulated. It comes from two sources: the diet and *de novo* synthesis. It is excreted as free cholesterol and as bile acids in the bile. When the amount of cholesterol in the diet is reduced, there is a compensatory increase in *de novo* synthesis by both the liver and the intestine. Once synthesized, it is carried in the blood by lipoprotein B. The liver and intestine are the only tissues that can synthesize apolipoprotein B, hence the cholesterol synthesized in these tissues will be transported primarily by this protein and will be found in the LDL or VLDL lipoprotein class. The LDL is formed when

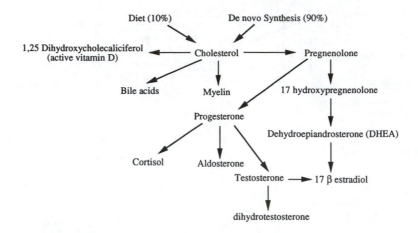

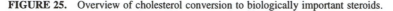

FIGURE 25.   Overview of cholesterol conversion to biologically important steroids.

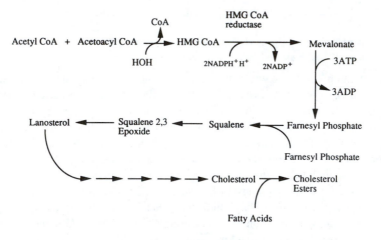

FIGURE 26.   Cholesterol biosynthesis.

the apolipoprotein C components and triacylglycerides are removed from the VLDL. When the diet contains a lot of cholesterol, *de novo* synthesis is almost totally suppressed. Thus, there is an inverse relationship between intake and synthesis. The cholesterol present in the diet is carried in the chylomicrons, not by the VLDL. The high-density lipoproteins (HDL) and the enzyme, lecithin:cholesterol acyl transferase (LCAT), are important in the regulation of cholesterol turnover. LCAT catalyzes the transfer of fatty acid in the carbon 2 position of phosphatidylcholine to the 3-hydroxyl group of cholesterol. LCAT is a plasma enzyme and its substrate is the cholesterol carried by HDL. The cholesterol ester generated by the LCAT reaction is carried in the core of the HDL particle, where it is transported to the liver and prepared for excretion as free cholesterol or bile acid in the bile. HDL is thus the vehicle for transporting cholesterol generated in the periphery to the liver for excretion.

Synthesis is controlled primarily at the level of the HMG CoA reductase step. There is feedback inhibition of the enzyme by mevalonate and cholesterol. Mevalonate inactivates the existing enzyme as well as inhibits the activation of the preexisting enzyme. Blood cholesterol levels rise when the cholesterol biosynthesis is not suppressed. This can occur when the LDL-bound cholesterol fails to enter the cell to suppress the synthesis and activation of HMG CoA reductase. This failure occurs when the LDL receptor fails to bind the LDL and extract the carried cholesterol. The receptor recognizes only the apolipoprotein B (the lipid-carrying protein synthesized in the intestine and liver). It does not recognize any other lipoprotein or any other protein which carries lipid material. All of these have their own receptors. People with a mutation in the gene which encodes the receptors are therefore characterized by high blood levels of cholesterol as well as high rates of endogenous cholesterol synthesis.

VIII. HEALTH CONCERNS IN LIPID NUTRITION

A. CARDIOVASCULAR DISEASE

There are a number of human diseases that are of interest to the lipid nutritionist. In the 1950s and 1960s, epidemiologists attracted much attention to the association between the incidence of coronary vessel disease (CVD) and the customary fat intakes of a number of countries throughout the world. Countries with food intakes that were low in saturated fat had low incidences of heart disease and vice versa. These associations neglected all other considerations, such as death from communicable disease or malnutrition.

Epidemiologists have not only pointed out an association between saturated fat intake and CVD, they have also identified an association between CVD and blood cholesterol levels. People with high (greater than 240 mg/dl) serum cholesterol values are at greater risk of having CVD than are people with serum cholesterol levels of less than 200 mg/dl. Regression analysis of the many studies on the effects of dietary fatty acids and cholesterol on serum cholesterol and lipoprotein cholesterol showed that diet can affect the blood lipid levels. However, regression analysis is simply a mathematical array of relating intake to blood lipid levels. It cannot show the next step; that is, that increasing blood lipids are *causal* with respect to CVD. It is not possible for ethical reasons to conduct experiments that show causality in humans. As pointed out in the earlier sections on lipid transport and metabolism, the genetics of the consumer is as potent (or perhaps more so) a determinant of blood lipid levels as is the habitual fat intake. Thus, the jury is still out on the question of whether dietary fat is responsible for the high death rate in developed nations from CVD. More than likely we will find that CVD results from an interaction of genetic factors with lifestyle choices of which the dietary fat intake is but a part.

The observations on marine oils and CVD have stimulated considerable research on the responses of humans and animals to the inclusion of marine oils in the diet. Rats, mice, swine, monkeys, and rabbits have been studied in addition to normal humans and humans having a variety of diseases thought to benefit from the consumption of these oils. Whether the inclusion of omega-3 fatty acids in the diets of hyperlipidemic subjects was of benefit was tested by Phillipson et al. (1985). Twenty hyperlipemic subjects were studied. Ten of these subjects had Type IIb lipemia (cholesterol range: 238 to 411 mg/dl, triglyceride range: 198 to 720 mg/dl) and ten had Type V lipemia (cholesterol range: 274 to 840 mg/dl, triglyceride range: 896 to 5775 mg/dl). The subjects consumed either a corn-oil-based diet or a fish-oil-based diet or a control diet for four weeks each. In the Type IIb group, fish oil consumption resulted in a 27% decrease in plasma cholesterol and a 64% decrease in triglyceride. In the Type V group, the reductions were 45 and 79%, respectively. In the Type V group, the consumption of the corn oil diet resulted in a significant rise in plasma triglyceride levels. These and other investigators reported that fish oil consumption resulted in a decrease in VLDL levels in the blood.

B. MARINE OILS AND DIABETES

Not only has there been interest in the relationship of dietary omega-3 fatty acids to cardiovascular disease, there has also been interest in its relationship to diabetes. People with diabetes mellitus have five times the risk of nondiabetics of having cardiovascular disease. Diabetes and heart disease are closely related. With respect to diabetes, Feldman et al. studied two groups of Alaskan Eskimos. One group consumed a typical Western diet while the other consumed the traditional Alaskan Eskimo diet which, like the Greenland Eskimo diet, is high in marine foods and low in total carbohydrates as well as sugar. As found in the Greenland Eskimos, serum lipids were very low and glucose tolerance normal when the traditional diet was consumed. When the Eskimos consumed Western diets which are higher in carbohydrate, particularly sugar, they had significantly higher free fatty acid and triglyceride levels as well as minor abnormalities in their glucose tolerance. Although Alaskan Eskimos, in general, have a very low prevalence of diabetes, these findings suggest that as these Eskimos begin to include significant amounts of carbohydrate, particularly sweets, in their diet, the prevalence of diabetes may change. In addition, since the Eskimos studied by Feldman consumed significant quantities of marine foods, one might also infer that the development of glucose intolerance was genetically controlled and unaffected by the presence of omega-3 fatty acids in the diet.

C. CANCER AND DIETARY FAT

The many different forms of cancer account for the second largest number of deaths due to disease in developed nations. It, too, is probably influenced by the fat intake, but in these disorders it is not the saturated fat that is culpable. Studies on the development of mammary tumors in rats and mice have shown that high intakes of polyunsaturated fat containing the omega-6 fatty acids promote the development of the cancer. Carcinogenesis is thought to occur in two steps. The first is the initiation step. This step concerns the conversion of normal DNA to the DNA typical of a cancer cell. Large segments of the gene code are deleted or so changed that the translation products are either not present or are not normal in function. This conversion can be instigated by chemicals such as 7,12-dimethylbenz-(α)-anthracene (DMBA), by viruses, radiation, and perhaps oxidized (free radical) food components. By itself, this step, the initiation step, will not progress to the metastatic cell unless the next step, the promotion step, also occurs. Cells whose DNA has been injured will and can repair this DNA. However, if the "right" environment is provided this does not occur and a metastatic cell is produced *and reproduced*. Dietary corn oil has been shown to be a very good promoter of DMBA-induced breast cancer in rats and mice while dietary beef tallow is not. How corn oil has this effect is not known and, of course, cause and effect studies cannot be conducted in humans. Just as epidemiological studies cannot provide definitive proof of the role of diet in CVD development, the same is true for cancer. Both the level of intake and the type of fat have been implicated, but strong proof is lacking. As with CVD, the genetic influence is quite strong. Glauert (1993) has recently reviewed the literature on the role of dietary fat in the expression of genes related to cancer development.

D. OTHER DISEASES

No discussion of the role of dietary fat in human disease would be complete without the mention of obesity. As discussed in Unit 3, this disorder has a multiplicity of causes of which the total energy intake is but a part. The excess energy consumed could easily be provided by the dietary fat since it has twice the energy value per gram as does dietary carbohydrate and protein. However, intake alone does not fully explain the obese state. Genetic factors which control energy intake, storage, and use are also important.

Gall bladder disease is frequently associated with excess body fatness (or its loss) and, as explained in Section V of this unit, may be attributable to the precipitation of cholesterol from the bile whilst in the gall bladder. Other genetic diseases involving lipid metabolism are shown in Table 11. These diseases are due to mutations in genes for specific enzymes important to the synthesis and degradation of neuronal lipids. Many are associated with mental retardation and early death. None seem to be related to nutrition or dietary fat intake.

TABLE 11
Genetic Diseases in Lipid Metabolism

Disease	Mutation	Characteristics
Tay-Sachs Disease	Hexosaminidase A deficiency	Early death, CNS degeneration, ganglioside GM$_2$ accumulates
Gaucher's Disease	Glucocerebrosidase deficiency	Enlarged liver and spleen; erosion of long bones and pelvis; mental retardation; glucocerebroside accumulates
Fabry's Disease	α-Galactosidase A deficiency	Skin rash, kidney failure, pain in legs and feet, ceramide trihexoside accumulates
Neimann-Pick disease	Sphingomyelinase deficiency	Enlarged liver and spleen, mental retardation, sphingomyelin accumulates
Krabbe's Disease (Globoid Leukodystrophy)	Galactocerebroside deficiency	Mental retardation, absence of myelin
Metachromatic Leukodystrophy	Arylsulfatase A deficiency	Mental retardation, sulfatides accumulate
Generalized gangliosidosis	Gmi, Gandioside: β-galactosidase deficiency	Mental retardation, enlarged liver
Sandhoff-Jatzkewitz Disease	Hexosaminidase A and B deficiency	Same as Tay-Sachs but develops quicker
Fucosidosis	α-L-fucoisidase	Cerebral degeneration, spastic muscles, thick skin
Acetyl CoA carboxylase deficiency	Acetyl CoA carboxylase deficiency	No *de novo* fatty acid synthesis
Hypercholesterolemia	LDL receptor deficiency	Premature atherosclerosis and death from CVD
Refsum's Disease	α-Hydroxylating enzyme	Neurological problems: deafness, blindness, cerebellar ataxia, phytanic acid accumulates

Lastly, although already described above in Section VII, mention should be made of the impact on health of essential fatty acid deficiency and of carnitine deficiency. In today's world these deficiencies are uncommon except under the special circumstance of long-term sustained intravenous nutritional support of the patient who cannot or will not eat, or when using the special formulas needed to sustain the premature infant. In both instances, care must be given to provide useful linoleic and linolenic acids in the intravenous nutrient support solution and to provide these nutrients and carnitine in the formula that supports the premature infant. In both instances, failure to provide these important nutrients can compromise the ability of the individual to survive and thrive. It is generally accepted that 1 to 2% of the total energy intake from fat be provided by the essential fatty acids. The usual mixed diet of Americans provides far more than this amount so the chances of an essential fatty acid deficiency in the normal individual are very slim indeed.

With respect to carnitine, intake recommendations for normal humans have not been made because carnitine usually can be synthesized in adequate amounts in the body. There are circumstances where this is not the case and in these situations sufficient carnitine must be supplied. The premature infant, the individual consuming a lysine-poor diet, the elderly, and persons being sustained by parenteral nutrition are all suspected to need more carnitine than their bodies can synthesize. While we know that these people probably would benefit from carnitine supplementation, we do not have a sufficiently large data base to use in order to develop an intake recommendation.

SUPPLEMENTAL READINGS

ARTICLES

Allred, J. B. and Bowers, D. F. (1993) Regulation of acetyl CoA carboxylase and gene expression, chap. 12, p. 269–295. In: *Nutrition and Gene Expression,* Berdanier C. D. and Hargrove, J. L., Eds., CRC Press, Boca Raton, FL.

Arner, P. (1992) Adrenergic receptor function in fat cells, *Am. J. Clin. Nutr.,* 55:228S–236S.

Bartolini, G., Orlandi, M., Chricolo, M., Licastro, F., Zambonelli, P., Minghetti, L., and Tomasi, V. (1990) Interleukins, interferons: Yen-yang modulators of PGH synthase in human macrophages, *Bio Factors,* 2:267–270.

Blom, W., DeMunck-Keizer, S. M. P. F., and Scholte, H. R. (1981) Acetyl CoA carboxylase deficiency: an inborn error of de novo fatty acid synthesis, *N. Engl. J. Med.,* 305:465.

Buettner, G. R. (1993) The pecking order of free radicals and antioxidants: lipid peroxidation, α tocopherol and ascorbate, *Arch. Biochem. Biophys.,* 300:535–543.

Clarke, S. D. and Jump, D. B. (1993) Regulation of hepatic gene expression by dietary fats: A unique role for polyunsaturated fatty acids, chap. 10, pp. 227–246. In: *Nutrition and Gene Expression,* Berdanier, C. D. and Hargrove, J. L., Eds., CRC Press, Boca Raton, FL.

Coates, P. M. and Tanaka, K. (1992) Molecular basis of mitochondrial fatty acid oxidation defects, *J. Lipid Res.,* 33:1099–1110.

Cockcroft, S. and Thoms, G. M. H. (1992) Inositol-lipid-specific phospholipase C isoenzymes and their differential regulation by receptors, *Biochem. J.,* 288:1–14.

Duval, D. and Freyss-Beguin, M. (1992) Glucocorticoids and prostaglandin synthesis: we cannot see the wood for the trees, *Prostaglandins, Leukotrienes, Essential Fatty Acids,* 45:85–112.

Esterbauer, H. (1993) Cytotoxicity and genotoxicity of lipid oxidation products, *Am. J. Clin. Nutr.,* 57:779S–786S.

Field, C. J., Ryan, E. A., Thomson, A. B. R., and Clandinin, M. T. (1990) Diet fat composition alters membrane phospholipid composition, insulin binding and glucose metabolism from control and diabetic animals, *J. Biol. Chem.,* 265:11143–11150.

Fisher, M., Levine, P. H., and Leaf, A. (1989) n-3 Fatty acids and cellular aspects of atherosclerosis, *Arch. Int. Med.,* 149:1726–1728.

Glauert, H. P. (1993) Dietary fat, gene expression and carcinogenesis, chap. 11. In: *Nutrition and Gene Expression,* Berdanier, C. D. and Hargrove, J. L., Eds., CRC Press, Boca Raton, FL.

Harman, D. (1993) Free radical involvement in aging, *Drugs Aging,* 3:60–80.

Hayaishi, O. (1991) Molecular mechanisms of sleep-wake regulation: roles of prostaglandins D_2 and E_2, *FASEB J.,* 5:2575–2581.

Hegsted, D. M., Ausman, L. M., Johnson, J. A., and Dallal, G. E. (1993) Dietary fat and serum lipids: an evaluation of the experimental data, Am. J. Clin. Nutr., 57:875–883.

Horrobin, D. F. (1991) Interactions between n-3 and n-6 essential fatty acids in the regulation of cardiovascular disorders and inflammation, *Prostaglandins, Leukotrienes, Essential Fatty Acids,* 44:127–131.

Howard, B. V., Welty, T. K., Fabsitz, R. R., Cowan, L. D., Oopik, A. J., Lee, N.-A., Yeh, J., Savage, P. J., and Lee, L. T. (1992) Risk factors for coronary heart disease in diabetic and nondiabetic native Americans, *Diabetes,* 41:4–11.

Just, W. W. and Soto, U. (1992) Biogenesis of peroxisomes in mammals, *Cell. Biochem. Function,* 10:159–165.

MacDonald, J. I. S. and Sprecher, H. (1991) Phospholipid remodeling in mammalian cells, *B.B.A.,* 1084:105–121.

Mannaerts, G. P. and Van Veldhoven, P. P. (1993) Metabolic pathways in mammalian peroxisomes, *Biochimie,* 75(3–4):147–158.

Mayer, R. J. and Marshall, L. A. (1993) New insights on mammalian phospholipase A_2(s); comparison of arachidonyl-selective and non selective enzymes, *FASEB J.,* 7:339–348.

Meldolesi, J. and Magni, M. (1991) Lipid metabolites and growth factor action, *TIBS,* 12:362–364.

Milatovich, A., Plattner, R., Heeroma, N. A., Palmer, C. G., Lopez-Casselas, F., and Kim, K.-H. (1988) Localization of the gene for acetyl CoA carboxylase to human chromosome 17, *Cytogenet. Cell. Genet.,* 48:190.

Nishina, P. M., Johnson, J. P., Naggert, J. K., and Krauss, R. M. (1992) Linkage of atherogenic lipoprotein phenotype to the low-density lipoprotein receptor locus on the short arm of chromosome 19, *Proc. Natl. Acad. Sci. U.S.A.,* 89:708–712.

Parke, D. V., Ioannides, C., and Lewis, D. F. V. (1991) Role of cytochromes P450 in the detoxification and activation of drugs and other chemicals, *Can. J. Physiol. Pharmacol.,* 69:537–549.

Rebouche, C. J. (1992) Carnitine function and requirements during the life cycle, *FASEB J.,* 6:3379–3386.

Rossouw, J. E. and Rifkind, B. M. (1990) Does lowering serum cholesterol lower coronary heart disease risk? *Endocrinol. Metab. Clinic N.A.,* 19:279–297.

Rustan, A. C., Christiansen, E. N., and Drevon, C. A. (1992) Serum lipids, hepatic glycerolipid metabolism and peroxisomal fatty acid oxidation in rats fed ω3 and ω6 fatty acids, *Biochem. J.,* 283:333–339.

Smith, W. L. (1992) Prostanoid synthesis and mechanisms of action, *Am. J. Physiol.,* 263:F181–191.

Song, J. and Wander, R. C. (1991) Effects of dietary selenium and fish oil (Max EPA) on arachidonic acid metabolism and hemostatic function in rats, *J. Nutr.,* 121:284–292.

Suckling, K. E. and Jackson, B. (1993) Animal models of human lipid metabolism, *Prog. Lipid Res.,* 32:1–24.

Zeisel, S. H. (1993) Choline phospholipids: signal transduction and carcinogenesis, *FASEB J.,* 7:551–557.

BOOKS

Vance, D.E. and Vance, J.E. Eds. (1985) *Biochemistry of Lipids and Membranes.* Benjamin/Cummings Publishing Co., Menlo Park, CA, 593 pages.

C.K. Chow, Ed. (1992) *Fatty Acids in foods and Their Health Implications.* Marcel Dekker, New York, 890 pages.

GLOSSARY

ACAT — acyl coenzyme A:cholesterol acyl transferase. An enzyme that catalyzes the formation of an ester linkage between a fatty acid and cholesterol

ACP — acyl carrier protein. A pantothenic acid-protein-thio-ethanolamine structure upon which fatty acid biosynthesis occurs

Actuarial data — information used to create mortality tables and life expectancy numbers

ADH — antidiuretic hormone also called vasopressin. Acts to conserve body water by increasing water resorption by the renal distal tubule

ADP — adenosine diphosphate. Metabolite of ATP. Energy is released when ATP is split to ADP and Pi

Age adjusted death rate — the number of deaths in a specific age group for a given calendar year divided by the population of that same age group and multiplied by 1000

Albumin — small molecular weight protein found in blood and sometimes in urine

Allele — any one of a series of different genes that may occupy the same location (locus) on a specific chromosome

AMP — adenosine monophosphate — metabolite of ADP. Energy is released when ADP is split to AMP and Pi

Anabolism — the totality of reactions that account for the synthesis of the body's macromolecules

Android obesity — a form of obesity where fat distribution is mainly in the shoulders and abdominal area

Anemia — below-normal levels of red blood cells and/or hemoglobin

Angina pectoris — chest pain due to lack of oxygen supplied to the heart

Antecedents — events that precede or are causally linked to an event

Anthropometry — measurement of body features, i.e., weight, height, etc.

Antigen — a compound that elicits or stimulates the production and release of antibodies

Apoproteins — blood proteins that can carry lipid (or some other compound)

Archimedes principle — an object's volume when submerged in water equals the volume of the water it displaces. If the mass and volume are known, the density can be calculated

Arteriography — a method of examining the arteries using X-rays and an infusion of a radiopaque dye solution

Atherogenic — atherosclerosis producing

Atherosclerosis — a progressive degenerative condition occurring within the vascular tree and resulting in occlusions and loss of elasticity

ATP — the energy-rich compound that serves as the energy coinage in the cell

Attenuated — weakened, lessened

Autosomal trait — a genetic characteristic carried on any pair of chromosomes except the XX or XY chromosome pair which determines the sex of the individual

Balance method — intake, use, and excretion of a given nutrient is quantitated. When balance is positive, intake exceeds excretion; when negative, excretion exceeds intake

BCAA — branched chain amino acids

BEE — basal energy expenditure

BMI — body mass index = body weight $\div$ height^2

BMR — basal metabolic rate; the minimal amount of energy need to sustain the body's metabolism. Frequently expressed in terms of the amount of oxygen used to sustain this metabolism because of the constancy between energy flux and oxygen use

Beriberi — thiamin deficiency disease

Bias — a measure of inaccuracy or departure from accuracy

Bioelectrical impedance — the measure of resistance to an alternating current in a body. Used to estimate percent body fat and body water

Biopsy — the removal of a very small amount of tissue from a selected site

Body cell mass — the metabolically active energy requiring mass of the body

Body density — weight (mass) per unit volume

cAMP — cyclic 3′,5′-adenosine monophosphate. An activator of protein kinase; serves as a second messenger for certain hormones

Cancer — a group of diseases characterized by abnormal growth of cells which, because it is uncontrolled, subsume the normal functions of vital organs and tissues

Cardiovascular disease — a group of diseases characterized by a diminution of heart action. The oxygen and nutrient supply to the heart may be impeded and/or the heart muscle degenerated

Catabolism — the totality of those reactions that reduce macromolecules to usable metabolites, carbon dioxide, and water

Cerebrovascular disease — similar to cardiovascular disease in that the vascular tree of the brain has developed atherosclerotic lesions which restrict or occlude the blood supply to this organ

Cholecystokinin — CCK — a hormone released from duodenal cells and which stimulates the gall bladder to contract, releasing bile into the duodenum

Cholesterol — a four-ringed structure in the lipid class that is an important substrate for steroid hormone synthesis

Chromosomes — when DNA is extracted from the cell nucleus, it is not one continuous strand. Rather, it breaks up into fairly predictable arrangements called chromosomes. The chromosomes exist in pairs and have been numbered. Those determining the sex of the individual are labeled as X or Y. If the individual has one X and one Y, he is a male. If the individual has two X chromosomes, she is a female. Many characteristics have been localized to particular chromosomes. There are species differences in the number of chromosomes. There are 23 sets of chromosomes (46 total) in the human

Chronic disease — a disease which takes years to develop

Chylomicrons — fat-protein complex formed to carry absorbed dietary fats from the intestine to other tissues. Not normally found in the blood of a fasting individual

CoA — coenzyme A — pantothenic acid-containing activator of acyl compounds

CoQ — coenzyme Q — also called ubiquinone, a carrier of hydrogens and electrons in the mitochondrial electron transport chain

Concordance — the chance that an identical mutation will occur in related family members

Coronary heart disease — a disease of the heart resulting from an inadequate circulation of blood to the heart muscle

Creatine — a nitrogen-containing substance which, when phosphorylated to creatine phosphate, provides the energy needed for muscle contraction

Creatinine — the urinary excretion product of creatine breakdown

Cytotoxic agents — chemicals that destroy specific cells

Densitometry — measurement of body density

Deuterium — a hydrogen isotope having twice the mass of the common hydrogen atom

Deuterium oxide — heavy water which contains two molecules of deuterium and one of oxygen

DHHS — Department of Health and Human Services

Diabetes mellitus — a group of diseases characterized by an inappropriate glucose-insulin relationship. These diseases are divided into two major subgroups; insulin dependent and noninsulin dependent diabetes, IDDM and NIDDM. Insulin dependent mellitus, which includes juvenile onset diabetes, refers primarily to the treatment of the disease by insulin injections. Used to be called Type I diabetes. Noninsulin dependent diabetes mellitus used to be called adult onset or Type II diabetes mellitus. The term refers to the management of the disorder through diet and exercise

DNA — deoxyribonucleic acid — dictates all of our genetically determined biochemical characteristics. Each of these characteristics is coded by the sequence of purine and pyrimidine bases that are connected together in an enormous double stranded helix found in the nucleus of the cell. Some DNA is also found in the mitochondria

DE — digestive energy — the energy of food after the costs (and losses) of digestion are subtracted

Distal — away from the center of the body

Diurnal variation — cyclical changes in one or more features of the body over a 24-hour day

Dual energy radiographic absorptiometry (DRA) — a procedure based on X-rays that measures bone mineralization. Also known as dual X-ray absorptiometry (DXA) and dual energy absorptiometry (DEXA)

Dual photon absorptiometry — similar to DEXA but uses photons at two different energy levels to determine bone mineral content

Electrolyte — an electrically charged particle (anion or cation)

Enteral nutrition — the provision of nutrients as a solution infused via a nasogastric tube

ER — endoplasmic reticulum

Erythrocyte — red blood cell

ESADDI — estimated safe and adequate daily dietary intakes

Etiology — the study of the causes of a disease

FAD — flavin adenine nucleotide — a riboflavin-containing coenzyme serving as a hydrogen and electron carrier in certain dehydrogenase reactions. $FADH_2$ is its reduced form

FDA — Food and Drug Administration

Fibrous plaque — lipids that collect within the arterial walls during the atherogenic process, creating a projection into the lumen of the vessel and impeding flow

FMN — flavin mononucleotide. A nucleotide coenzyme containing riboflavin, functioning as a component of the mitochondrial respiratory chain

GABA — gamma amino butyric acid. A neurotransmitter formed from the decarboxylation of glutamic acid

GDP — guanosine diphosphate. A diphosphorylated form of GTP important in the activation of substances participating in the biosynthesis of proteins

Gene — carrier of the genetic codes for all of the characteristics of the organism

Genotype — the inherited character of the individual

GIP — gastric inhibitory peptide. A peptide hormone inhibiting gastric motility and acid secretion

GI tract — gastrointestinal tract

GRP — gastrin releasing peptide. A neuroactive peptide originating in nerves of the gut and stimulating the release of gastrin from gastrin cells

GSSG — glutathionine, oxidized. A tripeptide containing glutamic acid, cysteine, and glycine. Its sulfhydryl group can undergo reversible oxidation and reduction allowing the peptide to serve as a buffer. Its chief function is to serve as a reductant of toxic peroxides. It is designated GSH in its reduced form

Goiter — thyroid gland enlargement due to deficient iodine intake

GTP — guanosine triphosphate — a high-energy phosphate-containing compound needed for protein synthesis

Gynoid obesity — excess body fat deposited mainly on hips and thighs

HANES (NHANES I, II, III or HHANES) — Health and Nutrition Examination Survey height-weight indices — various ratios or indices used to express weight in terms of height. Body mass index is one such expression

Hemoglobin — the iron-containing protein pigment in the red blood cell responsible for carrying oxygen to the cells and returning carbon dioxide to the lungs

HDL — high density lipoprotein. A plasma lipid-protein complex found in the blood. Elevated HDL is associated with a decreased risk of cardiovascular disease

HMG CoA — 3-hydroxy-3-methylglutaryl coenzyme A. A metabolic intermediate in cholesterol synthesis

HNIS — Human Nutrition Information Service of the USDA

Homozygote — an individual who has two identical genes coding for a given characteristic

Hyperlipidemia — above normal levels of lipid in the blood of a fasted individual

Hypermetabolism — above normal metabolic rate

Hypertension — blood pressure that exceeds 120/80 by 20%

IBW — ideal body weight

Iliac crest — the crest or top of the ilium or the longest of the three bones comprising the pelvis. Sometimes called the top of the hip bone.

Impedance — the opposition to an alternating current composed of two elements: resistance and reactance

Incidence — the number of new events or cases of a disease in a population within a specified time period

Indirect calorimetry — determination of energy expenditure using the measurement of oxygen consumption

Infarct — death of local tissue fed by an obstructed artery or occluded vein

Infectious disease — any disease caused by the invasion and multiplication of an invading microorganism

IU — international unit. An amount defined by the International Conference for Unification of Formulae

Ischemia — impaired blood flow causing oxygen and nutrient deprivation resulting in pain and, if severe, death of some or all parts of the tissue

Islets of Langerhans — the particular segments of the pancreas having an endocrine function. These islets consist of several cell types, one of which is the β cell that produces the hormone insulin

ISF — interstitial fluid, fluid surrounding the extravascular cells providing a medium for passage of nutrients to and from cells

Joule — a unit of work or energy in the metric system. The amount of work done by a force of 1 newton acting over the distance of 1 meter

Kilocalorie — kcal. The amount of energy required to raise the temperature of 1 kg water 1°C. 1 kJ = 4.189 kcal

Kwashiorkor — protein-deficiency disorder

Locus — the position on a chromosome occupied by a gene or its allele

LDL — low density lipoprotein

LDL receptor — molecules on the surface of the cell which have a particular affinity for LDL

Lipoprotein — lipid-protein complex

LHA — lateral hypothalamus

LNAA — large neutral amino acids; branched chain and aromatic amino acids

μ — Greek letter prefix which indicates 10^{-6} fraction of a liter or gram

Magnetic resonance imaging — a technology allowing the imaging of a body without radiation hazard

Malnutrition — inadequate or unbalanced intake of essential nutrients

MAO — monoamine oxidase; an enzyme which reduces neural transmission by inactivating amine neurotransmitters such as serotonin

Marasmus — condition of deficient energy and protein intake

MCV — mean corpuscular volume

Mean — average value for a group of values

Median — value where half the values fall below and half fall above this value

Menopause — cessation of estrus cycles

mRNA — messenger RNA; short-lived species of RNA which carries the code for the synthesis of specific compounds (peptides or proteins)

Morbidity — illness

Mutation — when the sequence of base pairs in the DNA is disturbed by either a deletion or substitution of one or more of the nucleotide bases, the protein coded by this sequence will not be synthesized in its normal amino acid sequence. The amino acid sequence determines the shape and function of the protein. Many mutations occur that have an effect on this sequence but have *no effect* on function because the substitution or deletion does not occur in the active or working part of the protein molecule

Myocardial infarction — heart attack

Myocardium — heart muscle

NAD, NADH, NADP, NADPH — niacin-containing coenzymes which function as carriers for hydrogen ions in dehydrogenase-catalyzed reactions

NCHS — National Center for Health Statistics

NFCS — Nationwide Food Consumption Survey

NHES — National Health Examination Survey

NPU — net protein use

NDp Cal% — net protein calories percent. The percent of the total energy value of the diet provided by the protein

Nutrient density — the nutrient composition of food expressed in terms of nutrient quantity per 1000 kcal

Nutritional assessment — measurement of indicators of dietary status and the nutrition-related health status of individuals or populations

Obesity — excess accumulation of body fat (more than 20% of the body is fat)

Osteoporosis — disease where the bone loses its mineral content

Overweight — a body weight in excess of that thought to be normal for height

Parenteral nutrition — nutritional support furnished through the vascular system

Pellagra — niacin deficiency disorder

Peripheral vascular disease — atherosclerotic changes in the vessels of the limbs

PEP — phosphoenopyruvic acid, a key intermediate in glucose synthesis

PGI, PGE — prostaglandins of the I or E series

Phenotype — a category or group to which an individual is assigned based on one or more inherited characteristics; the overt expression of the genotype

PKU — phenyketonuria — a mutation in the gene for phenylalanine hydroxylase that results in mental retardation unless diagnosed early and managed with a low phenylalanine diet

PLP — pyridoxal phosphate; a coenzyme required in amino acid metabolism

PTH — parathyroid hormone — essential to the regulation of blood calcium levels

PUFA — polyunsaturated fatty acids

Postprandial — after a meal

Prevalence — the number of existing cases of X in a given population at a given time

Proximal — towards the center of the body

PVN — paraventricular nucleus in the hypothalamus — releases hormones that affect food intake

Quantitative computed tomography — an imaging technique consisting of an array of X-ray sources and radiation detectors aligned opposite each other. As X-ray beams pass through the subject they are weakened or attenuated by the tissues and picked up by the detectors. The signals are then compared using a computer which can construct a cross section of the body using sophisticated modeling techniques

RBC — red blood cell; erythrocyte

Receptor — this is a general term applied to any protein in any part of the cell that binds to a specific compound and allows that compound to do its job in the cell. Most hormones and many nutrients have specific receptors without which these hormones or nutrients would be ineffective

Recumbent — lying down

Regression equation — a statistical method for calculating the relationships between an independent variable such as age with a dependent variable

RDA — recommended daily allowance; not to be confused with requirement

RER — rough endoplasmic reticulum. That portion of the cell which appears granular due to the profusion of ribosomes

RIA — radioimmunoassay; technique useful for determining small quantities of biologically important substances such as hormones

Rickets — bone malformation usually due to inadequate intake of vitamins and minerals

RNA — ribonucleic acid. A polynucleotide; synthesis of RNA is directed by DNA

RQ — respiratory quotient. Ratio of CO_2 to O_2

SAM — S-adenosylmethionine, a principle methyl donor

Scurvy — ascorbic acid deficiency disease

SER — smooth endoplasmic reticulum. That portion of the endoplasmic reticulum where certain lipids are synthesized and drugs are detoxified

Sex-linked trait — a genetic characteristic carried on either the X or the Y chromosome of the XY pair of chromosomes

Skinfold thickness — a double fold of skin and underlying tissue which can be used as a measure of the subcutaneous fat store

SOD — superoxide dismutase

Stroke — blockage or rupture of blood vessel(s) supplying the brain with resulting loss of consciousness, paralysis and other symptoms

Supine — lying on one's back

Symptoms — signs or indications of disease

T_3 — triiodothyronine, the most active of the thyroid hormones

T_4 — thyroxine, the form of thyroid hormone released by the thyroid gland to the blood

T-cells — cells of the immune system that originated from the thymus gland. These cells recognize antigens and produce antibodies to them

TBF — total body fat

TBW — total body water

TBG — thyroxine binding globulin — the protein which carries the thyroxine from the thyroid gland to its target tissue

TDP, TPP — thiamin-containing coenzyme required for decarboxylation reactions

Thermic effect — heat-producing response of the body to such processes as exercise or digestion and absorption on the response to disease or injury (fever)

TPN — total parenteral nutrition. A method of providing all nutrient needs through a solution infused into a large blood vessel

TSH — thyroid stimulating hormone — a pituitary hormone which stimulates the thyroid gland to produce thyroid hormone

tRNA — transfer ribonucleic acid; form of nucleic acid responsible for transferring specific amino acids to specific sites on the mRNA in the process of protein synthesis

Tritium — radioactive hydrogen

TXA_2 — thromboxane A_2 — an eicosanoid involved in stimulating platelet aggregation

UDP, UTP — uridine di- or triphosphate. A high-energy compound essential to glycogen synthesis

VIP — vasoactive peptide. A neuropeptide originating in the neurons of the gastrointestinal system

VLDL — very low density lipoprotein. A lipid-protein complex involved in the transport of lipids from the liver and gut to storage sites

Xerophthalmia — vitamin A deficiency. One of the leading causes of blindness in the world

APPENDIX

SMALL-ANIMAL ANALOGS FOR HUMAN DEGENERATIVE DISEASES

INSULIN-DEPENDENT DIABETES MELLITUS (IDDM)
Streptozotocin treated animals of most species
Alloxan can be substituted for streptozotocin
Pancreatectomy will also produce IDDM
BB rat (autoimmune disease)
db/db mouse
NOD mouse (autoimmune disease)
FAT mouse
NZO mouse
TUBBY mouse
Adipose mouse
Chinese hamster (*cricetulus griseus*)
South African hamster (*mystromys alb*)
Tuco-Tuco (*clenomys tabarum*)

NONINSULIN-DEPENDENT DIABETES MELLITUS
ob/ob mouse
KK, yellow KK mouse
A^{vy}, Ay yellow mouse
P, PB 13/Ld mouse
db PAS mouse
BHE/cdb rat
Zucker diabetic rat
SHR/N-cp rat
Spiny mouse
HUS rat
LA/N-cp rat
Wistar Kyoto rat

OBESITY
Zucker rat
SHR/N-cp rat
LA/N-cp rat
ob/ob mouse
Ventral hypothalamus lesioned animals
Osborne-Mendel rats fed high-fat diets

HYPERTENSION
SHR rats   WKY rats
JCR:LA rats   Transgenic rats

GALLSTONES
(The rat does not have a gall bladder nor does it have stones)
Gerbil fed a cholesterol-rich, cholic acid-rich diet
Hamster, prairie dog, squirrel monkey, or tree shrew fed a cholesterol-rich diet

LIPEMIA
    Zucker fatty rat
    BHE/cdb rat
    NZW mouse
    Transgenic mice given gene for atherosclerosis

ATHEROSCLEROSIS
    Transgenic mice given gene for atherosclerosis
    NZW mouse
    JCR:LA cp/cp rat

There are several compilations of animal models for human disease. See the series of books edited by Shafrir having the general title, *Lessons from Animal Diabetes*, published by Smith Gordon, London. See also the NIH Guide for Animal Resources, updated annually, and the Jackson Laboratory Catalog, Bar Harbor, Maine. A number of review articles may also be helpful:

1. **Suckling, K. E. and Jackson, B.** (1993) Animal models of human lipid metabolism, *Prog. Lipid Res.,* 32:1–24.
2. **Kirkwood, T. B. L.** (1992) Comparative life spans of species: why do species have the life spans they do?, *Am. J. Clin. Nutr.,* 55:11915–1195S.

INDEX

X

Y

Z